The Fibromyalgia Advocate

Getting the Support You Need to Cope with Fibromyalgia and Myofascial Pain Syndrome

DEVIN J. STARLANYL, M.D.

New Harbinger Publications, Inc.

Distributed in the U.S.A. by Publishers Group West; in Canada by Raincoast Books; in Great Britain by Airlift Book Company, Ltd.; in South Africa by Real Books, Ltd.; in Australia by Boobook; and in New Zealand by Tandem Press.

The illustration on the top left-hand corner of the cover was prepared by Tracy Marie Powell.

The remaining seven cover illustrations were previously published in *Myofascial Pain and Dysfunction: The Trigger Point Manual, Volume I* and *II* by Janet G. Travell and David G. Simons, 1983 (Vol. I), 1992 (Vol. II), Williams and Wilkins, Baltimore, MD, and are reproduced here with permission of the copyright holder.

Copyright © 1998 by Devin J. Starlanyl, M.D.
        New Harbinger Publications, Inc.
        5674 Shattuck Avenue
        Oakland, CA 94609

Text design by Tracy Marie Powell.
Cover design by SHELBY DESIGNS & ILLUSTRATES.
Developmental and Copy Edit by Kayla Sussell.

Library of Congress Catalog Card Number: 98-66701

ISBN 1-57224-121-7

Printed in Canada on recycled paper.

New Harbinger Publications' Website address: www.newharbinger.com

First printing

Dealing with a chronic invisible illness that is not well understood carries with it a special challenge. It requires courage, perseverance, and inner strength. This book is dedicated to my worldwide extended FMily of all people with fibromyalgia and MPS, especially those members of my local support group and the Internet support group FIBROM-L. They have been my teachers as well as my students, and a constant source of inspiration to me. I hope that this book will fill some of their needs.

Contents

Foreword

In 1966, Devin Starlanyl and Mary Ellen Copeland coauthored *Fibromyalgia & Myofascial Pain Syndrome: A Survival Manual*. Both Dr. Starlanyl and Ms. Copeland have fibromyalgia. In addition to describing the symptoms of myofascial pain and fibromyalgia, the authors discussed the complex issues involved with various treatment choices. Their book was a savior for many people with these conditions.

My patients have repeatedly described to me how the book helped them to understand their condition and explain it to their families and friends. The *Manual* made it possible for laypersons and physicians to recognize that fibromyalgia is not a "wastebasket" diagnosis for people who just hurt a lot and don't seem to get better.

There are still far too few medical caregivers with expertise in treating the patient with fibromyalgia and/or Myofascial Pain Syndrome. Indeed, there are many caregivers who state that fibromyalgia does not really exist and is a psychological condition. Thus, many patients continue to be frustrated by their medical care and their families still do not take their condition seriously. Dr. Starlanyl addresses these issues in her new book and perhaps by so doing she will help to create changes for these unfortunate patients.

In this new book, *The Fibromyalgia Advocate*, Dr. Starlanyl reviews some of the more recent theories regarding these disorders. She also provides extensive referenced information for the patient's health care team. Her book will make it easier for people with FMS and/or MPS to help their health care teams become more competent.

Many people are disabled by these conditions. Part III of the book is devoted to illuminating the legal system that is supposed to protect the rights of disabled Americans and ensure some level of disability income. For those who have been disabled, it is important to understand the legal options and alternatives without having to rely completely on legal representation.

Before I read her first book, I met Dr. Starlanyl through the fibromyalgia listserve on the Internet. We had many discussions about fibromyalgia, myofascial pain, and various treatment options. More recently, Devin has become not only my friend and teacher, but also my patient. She is driven to help the people who are suffering from these conditions. She is also determined to help educate the medical profession so that those who suffer can be better served.

Hal Blatman, M.D.

Acknowledgments

This book was written in response to many requests for assistance. It also required many hands to compile all the information contained within these pages. Many of my FMily participated in this book by sharing their stories and their resources, for which I am grateful. I am also grateful for all the help that I have received, and that my publisher, New Harbinger, encouraged me in this endeavor.

In my life I have been blessed to count as friends some original thinkers who were trailblazers in the daunting and often intimidating field of medical research and theory. Some of this century's greatest doctors, including Hans Selye and David Simons, gave of their valuable time not only to teach me what they knew, but how they thought. My way has been illuminated by their brilliance, and I am forever in their debt. Our world is the poorer for the loss of one bright beacon, Janet Travell, who died last August after a full and meaningful life. My hope is that, in some small way, I will bring a small part of my teachers' light to others, so that those of us who tread the rocky path toward healing will not falter.

The perverse blessing of having FMS/MPS Complex has put me into contact with Paul St. Amand, Joanne Borg-Stein, Robert Gerwin, Hal Blatman, Ken Hoelscher, I. Jon Russell, David Nye, Wes Shankland, Robert Brossman, Jorge Flechas, Sam Yue, John Lowe, Michael Schneider, Darice Putterman, Richard van Why, and many other outstanding researchers and healers from whom I have learned so much, and continue to do so. They are out there for all of us, helping, teaching, guiding, and healing.

After you write a book, the hard work just begins. If this book is easy to understand, well organized, and enjoyable, the thanks go to Kayla Sussell, my editor, who has also become my teacher and friend. She made a formidable task easy to accomplish, and enjoyable for me too, and I have learned a great deal from her.

I also wish to thank my church family, my local support group, and the Internet group FIBROM-L, who have been patient with my absence during the last part of the writing.

Great thanks go to one of my own guardian angels, our hospital switchboard operator, Barbara Packard. At times, this woman was inundated with calls from the desperate who read my first book and thought, "Somebody understands!" and then tried to reach me. She balanced her devotion to healing with her concern for me, and through her care and unending kindness over the wire has personally saved a number of lives.

I thank the wonderful Brooks Memorial Library staff, especially the reference librarians, who came through for me again, above and beyond the call of duty, to supply me with many of the books, articles, and materials that I needed. I thank my doctors, Carolyn Taylor-Olsen and Craig Anderson, my nutritionist, Lynne August, and my therapists Julie Emonds and Debbie Feiner who enabled me to survive the ordeal of writing yet another book. Yes, I promise I will (try to) take it (relatively) easy (for a while).

Honors go to Jay Nickson, not only for setting up and operating my website, but also for untangling the snarl that can be created only in a computer operated by someone with FMS and MPS.

Day-to-day computer gremlins were defeated by my husband Rick, who is developing a greater understanding of the path I travel (along with a few trigger points), as well as more patience with my long run of medical projects, endless emails and phone calls, and my occasional attempts to travel in the name of medical education. The struggle to complete this book has brought us closer together.

I thank you all for allowing me to bring this book to life, and I thank God for bringing us together.

Introduction

If you have fibromyalgia (FMS), chronic Myofascial Pain Syndrome (MPS), or both (FMS/MPS Complex), you are unusually challenged. You have a chronic invisible disease that inflicts terrible wounds on you, but they are wounds that leave no scars. Because of your illness, you often need someone to run interference for you, an advocate who knows how to cut through bureaucratic red tape and save you some of your valuable time. This book will try to serve as such an advocate. It includes all of the latest information regarding these illnesses and provides stories from other patients to illustrate our need for advocacy. We must stand together to learn what we can do to improve the quality of our lives. You are not alone. Knowledge is power, especially in the case of chronic invisible disease.

There is a huge community of people with FMS and chronic MFS syndrome throughout the world that I call the "FMily." Most members of the FMily are either undiagnosed or mis-diagnosed. Nearly all are mis-treated, in the several senses of that word. We must not only struggle to overcome our illnesses, we must also try to educate our families, friends, and even our medical care teams, and do so in a manner that will not offend anyone. Our world lacks a support structure for chronic invisible illnesses, especially for illnesses that display varying symptoms. It is our job to create that structure, as well as to obtain justice, both for ourselves and for those who come after us.

There are some doctors and other health care workers who are well-informed and knowledgeable about both FMS and chronic MPS. Usually they are overburdened taking care of people who have been mistreated by others. If you are fortunate enough to be cared for by such, there are things you can do to help keep them from burning out. You will read about those ways in this book

You may find some doctors and other medical professionals who are willing and even eager to learn all they can about FMS and chronic MPS. They want to help you. Work with them. They are sparkling lights in a sea of dark indifference. Do what you can to nurture and encourage them.

Then there are the other kinds of doctors and other health care professionals we must encounter. Inappropriate medical treatment and physical therapy are among the most prevalent of the perpetuating factors for FMS and MPS. When these conditions are vigorously and appropriately treated at their onset, much pain and dysfunction can be prevented. Instead, the lack of training and the resultant ignorance of much of the medical establishment creates a massive drain on the health care system, as well as increasing the pain and despair of countless individuals and families. The despair is incalculable. Jobs, homes, and taxes are lost. Businesses go bankrupt. Families dissolve. Sick people are literally driven to suicide.

This book will try to give you the tools and medical references you need to deal with doctors and other health care providers who are not "FMS- or MPS-patient-friendly." There have been too many tears shed and, yes, too much blood spilt, because of willful ignorance; this must not be allowed to continue. My gloves have come off. It seems that many insurance company doctors and workers' compensation doctors have it in their interest to remain ignorant of the facts about these conditions. Money and self-interest are their bottom line. We must make it in their interest to become educated. When they begin to lose legal cases, and it hits them where they live—the pocketbook—they will have to start learning the facts about FMS and MPS in self-defense. That is the *only* way they will become knowledgeable about FMS and MPS.

The Current Medical "Climate"

I have heard some doctors say, "These are new conditions." In the Reference and Bibliography sections at the end of this book there are medical journal articles describing MPS that go back to the early 1940s (Travell, Rinzler and Herman 1942; Travell and Travell 1946). There is even an article describing FMS that was published in 1815 (Balfour 1815).

Then some of those doctors might say, "Your information is out of date." The References and Bibliography sections list current medical journal articles up to the month we went to press. All that skeptics and scoffers have to do is search the PubMed website files on the Internet to find a great many current medical journal articles on these and related subjects.

Some doctors say, "Fibromyalgia and Myofascial Pain Syndrome are the same." I have referenced medical journal articles by rheumatologists, physiatrists (physicians who specialize in physical medicine), family physicians, internists, neurologists, and chiropractors showing that FMS and MPS are *not* the same illness, and that understanding the difference between them is vital to their treatment. Travell and Simons explain the differences in detail in chapter 28 of their medical text, *Myofascial Pain and Dysfunction: The Trigger Point Manual Vol. II*, published in 1992. (In this book I will frequently reference Travell and Simons' works and often refer to them as the "Trigger Point Manuals.")

Some doctors even say, "I don't have time to read all this stuff." To those physicians, I say, "Doctors, you have no business treating these conditions if you don't understand the basic concepts. How can you justify taking money for what you do?"

Then, there are health care practitioners who *don't believe in* perpetuating factors such as reactive hypoglycemia. There are others who *don't believe in* pain medication for FMS and MPS. And there are the worst of the lot, those health care practitioners who *do not believe in*

FMS and chronic MPS at all. In the face of all the mounting evidence and all the medical journal articles written by respected practitioners, they cling stubbornly to their ignorance, while draining the substance and will of patients who are told to believe that their miseries are all their own fault.

These doctors hand out the diagnosis of "IAIYH" (It's All In Your Head) and dispense such cheerful homilies as "Put on a happy face," "Get on with your life," and "Don't dwell on it. It won't kill you." Or, "Lose some weight, and you'll be fine." Or, "Fibromyalgia? That just means achy muscles—I have them too sometimes. So what?" "Myofascial Pain Syndrome? It doesn't exist!" In this book, particularly in the References and Bibliography sections, you will find the facts to help you combat these and other doubters, but many will refuse to be educated. Don't waste your time or energy on them. They have abused their trust. They have broken their vow to "do no harm." Don't allow them to darken your lives any longer.

Some physical therapy and rehabilitation personnel say, "It doesn't matter what you have, we can treat it all the same." Perhaps some doctors, treating holistically, can do this. Cranio-sacral therapists can do this. In any case, they can work on some of the perpetuating factors. The two separate conditions of FMS and chronic MPS *must* be treated differently by conventional physical therapists. Travel and Simons have clearly demonstrated that repetitious exercise is inappropriate for people with active trigger points, yet countless patients still suffer through work hardening and weight training, often becoming totally disabled in the process. They sensitize their autonomic nervous systems, and it takes enormous resources of time, money, and patience, not to mention the pain that is suffered, to try to restore function. All of which could have been easily prevented by the people allegedly trained to help in the first place.

Becoming Your Own Health Care Manager

You hire health care workers to help you to optimize the quality of your life. To achieve that result, you must become the manager of your own health care team. It is up to you to see that your team members' efforts are coordinated. This book will try to help you do that. If you have FMS and/or MPS, you probably have already realized that life is not always fair. The condition will not change by itself, no matter how much you rant and grieve. You must endeavor to create an atmosphere of fairness. We must all strive to create justice, and to become agents of change.

Before you begin to assemble your own FMS/MPS health care team, or to assess and perhaps change the one you have, there are many things you need to know. I have tried to present the information as clearly and understandably as possible. Take it in slowly, at your own pace. It's time to take charge.

How to Use This Book

Part I starts with what you need to know about FMS and MPS—the basics. Some of the material in this section was covered in my first book, *Fibromyalgia & Chronic Myofascial Pain Syndrome: A Survival Guide* (Starlanyl and Copeland 1996). However, a great deal of new information has come to light since the publication of that book, and readers are advised not to skip this section because they may learn new and valuable information that will help with their treatment plans.

Part II begins with what you need to know to successfully manage your health care team. This is followed by information on and for your medical support team. It is by far the largest section of the book. That's because much of how you fare with both the legal world and your personal environment is in some measure based on how well informed you and your medical team are about your medical conditions.

Part III is about rights, responsibility, and advocacy. It informs you about the legal issues you will face when fighting for your rights, and provides you and your doctors with the kinds of information that you will need when you are doing battle with government agencies and other bureaucracies.

Part IV is also about rights, responsibility, and advocacy. But here the focus changes to your family and friends. What are their rights and responsibilities to you? What are yours to them? The last chapter deals with crises, conflicts, and special issues, such as pregnancy, menopause, the elderly, and on-the-job issues.

Part V is comprised of four appendixes and the References and Bibliography sections. Appendix A, the "Self-Diagnostic Guide to Trigger-Points," offers a way for you to track down some of the possible causes of your symptoms. Using the guide, you should be able to look up a symptom, and then find its possible cause. Appendixes B and C offer two different approaches to advocacy. Appendix B is a public policy statement on the use of opioids in the treatment of pain, and Appendix C is a petition regarding FMS/MPS that you might like to circulate among your friends and acquaintances for signatures. Appendix D is the Functional Inventory Assessment.

In some ways, the References and Bibliography section are among the most important parts of this book. Refer to them. Read them. Use them. They are your best tools when you must deal with health care personnel who don't believe the facts about these two medical conditions. The proofs are in the citations. In this book you will also learn how to obtain copies of medical references.

The purpose of this book is to help people with FMS, MPS, and other chronic invisible illnesses to advocate for themselves. In my last book, I made some people angry. I have had my character disparaged, as well as my work. If this book has the effect of empowering patients, I expect a lot more criticism. Medicine has become political, and writing always has been. Don't waste your time trying to defend me against physicians who don't want to give you the medications, or the physical or experimental therapy that might bring you some relief. Don't waste your energy trying to defend me from people who say I shouldn't be writing about melatonin, chromium, or guaifenesin. There are references that you can refer to and alternatives that you can access yourself. Don't let others' negativity get to you. Negativity is your worst enemy. I am on my path, and you don't have to defend me. I let God handle that kind of stuff.

—Devin J. Starlanyl

PART I

What You Need to Know About Fibromyalgia (FMS) and Myofascial Pain Syndrome (MPS)

Part I, comprised of chapters 1 through 5, is intended to provide the reader with an overview of the concepts that lie behind the diagnoses of FMS and MPS. Chapter 1, "The Basics," describes the symptoms of both and explains why they are two different conditions, although they are frequently found together in the same individual. Chapter 2, "The Neurotransmitters," offers an analysis of how these important biochemicals work, and describes how they are implicated in both FMS and MPS. For anyone who has either or both conditions, chapter 3, "Perpetuating Factors," is important reading. It may hold the key to improved health. Chapter 4, "Coexisting Conditions," briefly discusses a number of conditions that can coexist with and affect the course of FMS and MPS. Part I ending with chapter 5, "Chronic Pain Management," has detailed accounts of therapeutic procedures specifically designed to ease chronic pain conditions.

1

The Basics

For those of you who haven't read my first book, *Fibromyalgia & Chronic Myofascial Pain Syndrome: A Survival Manual* (Starlanyl and Copeland 1996), this chapter is intended to provide you with a brief refresher course and some new information.

Fibromyalgia Syndrome (FMS)

Fibromyalgia, a chronic invisible condition, has finally come "out of the closet." Contrary to popular opinion, it isn't a brand-new illness like AIDS; it has been known for some time. It was first described in the early eighteen hundreds by William Balfour, a surgeon at the University of Edinburgh (1815). For many years it was known by different names, including chronic rheumatism, myalgia, and fibrositis. For a while, as with many other belatedly recognized illnesses, some physicians thought that the condition's origin was primarily psychological.

In 1987, the American Medical Association (AMA) recognized FMS as a true physical illness and a major cause of disability. Now, eleven years later, it is still too often dismissed as the "newest fad disease." Most physicians still lack the training to diagnose and treat it. What the medical community now calls "fibromyalgia" is not well categorized into specific subsets in the rigorous manner that other conditions such as diabetes or multiple sclerosis are classified and studied.

It is incorrect, and a disservice to the patient, to label all soft tissue chronic pain conditions "fibromyalgia." Those of us who work with and understand FMS currently are seeing a number of identifiable subsets emerge. Fibromyalgia is a specific, chronic nondegenerative, nonprogressive, noninflammatory, truly systemic pain condition. It is not a disease that has a known cause and well-understood mechanisms for producing symptoms.

It is called a syndrome, which means it exhibits a specific set of signs and symptoms that take place together. This does not mean that fibromyalgia is any less serious or potentially disabling than an ordinary "disease." Rheumatoid arthritis, lupus, and other serious afflictions are also classified as syndromes. The only laboratory tests available for FMS are those that rule out other conditions. There is still no blood test that can accurately identify it.

Who Is Affected?

Fibromyalgia can occur at any age. Many doctors who are expert diagnosticians of FMS have identified FMS developing in toddlers. There are also those who develop FMS in their geriatric years. According to Bates and Grunwaldt (1958), the first trigger points of Myofascial Pain Syndrome (MPS) may appear during birth. Only about 20 percent of FMS patients have a known triggering event that initiated the first obvious "flare" of the syndrome (Greenfield, Fitzcharles and Esdaile 1992). About 25 percent of the FMS patients I see are men. This ratio differs considerably from what is reported in the literature (Wolfe, Ross, Anderson, et al. 1995). I think this may be due to FMS being underdiagnosed in males.

The Symptoms

Tender Points

For a diagnosis of fibromyalgia, the official research definition requires that eleven of eighteen specified *tender points* must be present in all four quadrants of your body—that is, the upper-right and upper-left and lower-right and lower-left parts. The official definition further requires that the individual must have had widespread, more or less continuous pain for at least three months. Tender points hurt when pressed, but they do not cause pain in any other part of the body. That is, they do not *refer* pain to other parts of the body in the way that trigger points do (see "Myofascial Trigger Points" later in this chapter).

Many doctors don't understand that the official definition of tender points is used only for research subjects. If you had fewer than "eleven of the eighteen" tender points, you would be excluded from a research study on fibromyalgia. However, this would not mean that you did not have fibromyalgia. Fortunately, many doctors don't adhere to the research definition. They will diagnose fibromyalgia in patients who demonstrate bodywide flu-like symptoms, multiple tender points (not trigger points), characteristic sleep disruption, and its resultant fatigue.

Tender points occur in pairs on various parts of the body. Because they are paired, the pain is usually distributed equally on both sides of the body. Tender points can vary from person to person, which may cause further problems with diagnosis. For example, in traumatic fibromyalgia, tender points are often clustered around an injury instead of, or in addition to, the eighteen "official" points. These clusters can also occur around a repetitive strain or a degenerative and/or inflammatory problem, such as arthritis. The doctor must be very careful to distinguish traumatic fibromyalgia from myofascial pain syndrome (MPS).

Fibromyalgia and MPS are two very different conditions, although they may coexist in one person.

Other Common Symptoms of FMS

Pain is frequently the most prominent symptom of FMS, but there are many others. Among the most common are the following:

- The thermal regulatory system may not work properly. You may have to get out of bed often during the night because of bladder irritability, which, in turn, may be caused by trigger points (discussed below). At those times, you may experience extreme thermal fluctuations. After getting back into bed, you may have to wait for your temperature to cool down before you can pull up the blanket again. It isn't uncommon for your "normal" body temperature to be lower than average.

- Spasticity (tightness) of the muscles is another symptom of FMS. This can constrict the peripheral blood vessels—those closest to the skin. This symptom, especially in wintertime, makes certain parts of our bodies—most often the buttocks and thighs—feel like cold slabs of meat to the touch. People with MPS also experience muscle tightness, but for a different reason.

- Skin mottling and finger- and toenail ridges are a symptom. Fingernails can break off, often in crescent-shaped pieces. If nails do grow, they sometimes curve under. Cuticles may overgrow, and yet the nails also may develop hangnails, which take a long time to heal. You may get bruises, but you can't remember where you got them, and they take forever to heal.

Sensitivity Amplification

Fibromyalgia is a sensitivity-amplification syndrome. This means that you may be hypersensitive to smells, sounds, lights, and vibrations. The noise emitted by fluorescent lights can drive you crazy. You may be unable to tolerate crowds or cities. Fibromyalgia sensitizes nerve endings, and the ends of the nerve receptors change shape. Because of these changes, the body may interpret touch, light, or sound as pain. The brain recognizes pain as a danger signal—an indication that something is wrong and needs attention—so it mobilizes its defenses. Then, when those defenses aren't used, anxiety results.

Sleep Disturbances

Sleep, or the lack of it, plays a crucial role in FMS. You may not get enough sleep, or the right kind of sleep. You may have insomnia of several types, or a host of other sleep-related problems. People with FMS often have the alpha-delta sleep anomaly. During delta sleep, bodies heal and many neurotransmitters are restored to health. As soon as you reach deep delta-level sleep, alpha waves, which characterize the awake state, intrude and either jolt you to awakening or to a lighter stage of sleep. You wake up feeling as if you've been run over by a truck. When you are deprived of sleep, the deep delta-level healing processes are cut short before they can do their work.

Clumsiness and FMS

Neurotransmitters are electro-biochemical agents that cross the synapses between the nerves (see chapter 2). They are the messengers that carry information back and forth between the body and the brain. Normally, neurotransmitters constantly inform the muscles about what they're supposed to be doing, so their actions can be modified, as needed; but this is one of the functions that is disrupted by FMS. Because of these disruptions, much of our muscle tension is improperly controlled, and clumsiness results.

A large part of mental and physical security depends on the ability to repeat appropriate and predictable actions. Healthy people think nothing of picking up a glass of water and bringing it to their lips. They know just how tightly to grip, how heavy the glass will feel, and how much speed is appropriate to accomplish drinking smoothly. Those of us with FMS lack proper sensory feedback. Our thumbs grasp with too little pressure, and our wrist muscles let go when flexed. To sit, walk, and stand gracefully, the entire musculature must be able to feel its own activity. We feel eternally clumsy.

The Myofascia

Myofascia is the thin, almost translucent film that wraps around muscle tissue. It gives shape to and supports all of the body's musculature. Improperly functioning myofascia is the cause of a lot of pain. If you want to see what it looks like, cut up a fresh chicken. It is the thin, sticky, somewhat filmy material that wraps around the muscle tissue. It also wraps around each muscle fiber, bundle of fibers, and the muscles themselves. Where the muscle cells end, layers of myofascia adhere together to form tendons and ligaments.

It appears that a tightening in the myofascia occurs in many cases of FMS and MPS. If both of these conditions are present, this tightening causes more than double the trouble—because when myofascial tissues lose their elasticity, the neurotransmitters' ability to communicate messages between the mind and body is damaged. When an area of the body is in pain, the myofascia in that area becomes rigid to prevent movement, in order to "splint" the painful area. Furthermore, with myofascial tightness, the muscles often feel swollen, as if they were encased in a skin several sizes too small.

Myofascial Trigger Points

Acute pain causes a neuromuscular response, and the muscles around the pain site tighten, "guarding" the hurt area. When muscles are in a state of sustained tension, they are working (even if you're not). A working muscle needs more nutrition and oxygen, and produces more waste, than a muscle at rest. This creates an area in the myofascia that becomes starved for food and oxygen, and loaded with toxic waste—that area is a trigger point.

Trigger points (TrPs) are extremely sore points occurring individually or in ropy bands throughout the body. They are often easier to feel along the arms and legs. If you stretch your muscle about two-thirds of the way out, you can often feel them. Sometimes the muscles get so tight that you can't feel the lumps, or even the tight bands. The muscle itself feels like "hardened concrete." Trigger points can occur in the myofascia, skin, ligaments, and bone lining, as well as in other tissues. They are quite common.

Myofascial trigger points can entrap the nerves, blood, and lymph vessels, causing a variety of symptoms that confuse doctors and patients alike. Often nerve damage is erroneously suspected, and many expensive, unnecessary (and often painful) tests are ordered.

We are finding that trigger points are formed of multiple microscopic areas called *active loci* (pronounced low-sigh) (Simons 1997). These loci cause the segments of the muscle fibers, called *sarcomeres,* to become distorted. Eventually, a contraction knot forms, as well as a taut band. I have recently seen what may be the first video of a myofascial trigger point. Robert Gerwin gave a talk at the Focus on Pain Seminar in San Antonio, March 12–15, 1998, in which he presented an ultrasound and EMG video. I saw the taut band twitch in response to stimulation.

When you have TrPs, your muscle strength becomes unreliable. You may also notice that when one part of your body is supported by another part while you are sleeping, the part being compressed goes numb. Some other symptoms of TrPs include the following:

- Stiffness • muscle tightness and weakness
- localized sweating • eye tearing • copious salivation • poor balance • dizziness • nausea
- tinnitus • goosebumps • runny nose
- buckling knees • weak ankles • illegible handwriting • staggering gait • headaches
- muscle cramps

Most specific pains commonly attributed to fibromyalgia are actually caused by TrPs. Trigger points seem to form throughout life as a response to the many things that happen to our bodies. They can be caused by a variety of events ranging from a surgical incision (as in abdominal surgery), to overuse, repetitive motion trauma, bruises, strains, joint problems, and so forth. Janet Travell (1983) believes that many of the aches and pains attributed to "old age" may actually be due to TrPs, and may be reversible.

The first time I opened the *Trigger Point Manuals* (Travell and Simons 1983; 1992) I was dumbfounded. After having been told for many years that the pain patterns I described did not and could not exist, seeing them clearly illustrated in a medical text brought on a flood of emotions. At first, I was so relieved I cried. I felt vindicated. Then, as the truth started to hit home, I began to get angry. Why hadn't I learned about myofascial trigger points in medical school? Janet Travell was John F. Kennedy's White House physician. She and her partner, David Simons, had created these wonderful texts. Why wasn't their work the cornerstone of a basic medical course? How many people were suffering needlessly? How could I get the word out to them?

Trigger Points and Dizziness

In her autobiography, *Office Hours Day and Night* (1968), Dr. Travell explains how dizziness, ringing of the ears, loss of balance, and other symptoms can all be caused by TrPs in the side of the neck, in the muscle group called the *sternocleidomastoid (SCM) complex.* This muscle group performs many functions, one of which is to hold up the head. Receptors in the SCM complex transmit nerve impulses to inform the brain of the position of the head and body in the surrounding space.

When there are TrPs present, the receptors lie. What they tell the brain is not what the eyes tell the brain. When head movement changes the SCM message, that is., when you turn around, or look up, you get dizzy. This, coupled with poor balance, can make it seem as if the walls are tilting. When people with FMS drive, we get the impression that we "bank" our turns at a steep angle, as if we were driving a motorcycle. Also, TrPs associated with the SCM muscle group can cause patterns of light and dark, such as tree shadows on a road, to create an almost seizure-like phenomenon. Looking at certain printed fabrics, such as plaids, stripes, and polka dots, can make us dizzy. Escalators also disturb us.

Trigger points often form as a result of other medical conditions. For example, a case of arthritis might be otherwise well managed, but the accompanying TrPs might be completely overlooked. That patient's pain load could be substantially lessened if the secondary TrPs were treated successfully. Diagnosis really becomes challenging when bodywide TrPs develop with overlapping referral zones (see "Active Trigger Points" below). This "spread" of TrPs gives the impression that the condition is progressive, but it isn't. It may be getting steadily worse, but with proper attention to perpetuating factors and appropriate treatment, the "progression" can be reversed.

Active Trigger Points

An active TrP not only hurts when it is pressed, like an FMS tender point, but it also "triggers" a *referred symptom pattern* to somewhere else in the body. The symptom is usually, but not always, pain. Sometimes the TrP is inside the pain pattern, and sometimes the pain pattern occurs elsewhere. Each specific TrP on the body has a referred pain or other symptom pattern that has been carefully observed and documented in many patients (Travell and Simons 1983).

This pain pattern is similar from patient to patient. Active TrPs often produce other symptoms, also usually in their referred pain zones. Such a TrP hurts whenever you use the muscle involved. When the point becomes very active, pain and other symptoms result, even when the muscle is at rest. The fact that these pain patterns are so similar from patient to patient really helps in making a diagnosis *if* the diagnostician is familiar with the patterns as described by Travell and Simons. That's why familiarity with TrPs and an ability to take a good medical history is so important. An educated doctor will know where to look for TrPs before the physical exam begins. A "latent" type of TrP also occurs.

Latent Trigger Points

A latent TrP doesn't hurt at all, unless it is pressed. You might not even know it's there, but your body does. It restricts movement, and weakens and prevents full lengthening of the affected muscle. If you press on a latent TrP, it will refer pain to another part of the body in its characteristic pattern. A latent TrP may be activated by overstretching, overuse, or chilling the muscle.

People who do little exercise have a greater chance of developing latent points. This is an important issue, because some people feel that by restricting their range of motion, they can get rid of their TrPs. Nothing could be further from the truth. Physical stress or trauma is not the only cause of TrPs. Trigger points also can develop as a result of emotional tensions. If you are constantly holding your muscles tight in the "fight-or-flight" stress response, this will change your body's habitual biological patterns. Trigger points are caused by the *biological* effects of long-term emotional abuse or mental trauma.

If TrPs are treated immediately and vigorously, and perpetuating factors (conditions that aggravate and perpetuate the TrPs) (see chapter 3) are avoided or remedied, the TrPs can be eliminated. Unfortunately, if TrPs are left untreated, are inappropriately treated, or muscle action is restricted to avoid pain, the TrP usually becomes latent. This means that it doesn't hurt anymore unless you press it, but the muscle can "give out" when stressed. If the muscle is pushed to work in spite of the pain, especially if perpetuating factors exist, active TrPs may develop secondary and satellite TrPs. (See "Progressive? It's Not What It Seems to Be" later in this chapter.)

Attachment Trigger Points

Trigger points as documented usually occur in the belly of the muscle. David Simons described a new type of TrP at the March 1998 San Antonio seminar. It is called an attachment trigger point (aTrP), and occurs where the muscle attaches to other tissue. These TrPs have not had their pain patterns mapped, and the work on them is so new that it has not yet been published.

FMS and MPS Are Different

Fibromyalgia (FMS) and Myofascial Pain Syndrome (MPS) are very different syndromes. However, the majority of physicians lump the two conditions together, probably because they see many patients who have both FMS and MPS, which I call FMS/MPS Complex. Unless doctors have a thorough knowledge of and familiarity with individual TrPs, they don't stand a chance of sorting out the different symptoms of the two different syndromes.

One interesting difference between the two conditions is that more women have FMS than men. Myofascial Pain Syndrome, however, affects men and women in equal numbers. One important difference is that in MPS, muscles located some distance from the trigger points have normal sensitivity, whereas in FMS, there is an overall flu-like achiness, and generalized sensitivity, but no trigger points.

Chronic Myofascial Pain Syndrome

Fibromyalgia is, among other things, a *systemic dysregulation of the neurotransmitters*, with many biochemical causes. There are other problems as well, but they are systemic in nature, such as the alpha-delta sleep anomaly discussed above. Myofascial Pain Syndrome, however, is a *neuromuscular* condition. It is caused by mechanical failures—the mechanics of physics, not biochemistry. Due to the nature of trigger points, some of the symptoms may seem to be systemic, but they are not. Initiating events, such as repetitive motion injury, trauma, and illness, can start a cascade of TrPs. There are many medical journal articles that explain why FMS and MPS are different, and why the difference is important. (See, for example, Borg-Stein and Stein (1996), Schneider (1995), Travell and Simons (1992).)

The FMS/MPS Complex

The cases of "traumatic fibromyalgia" that I have seen have all been FMS/MPS Complex, which generally started with trauma-generated trigger points. FMS/MPS Complex has not yet been noticed by the medical community. I have the perverse blessing of having the Complex in a rather severe form, so I have an insider's understanding thereof. People with FMS/MPS Complex face more than just the two sets of symptoms of both conditions.

Fibromyalgia and MPS not only occur together, they reinforce and amplify the symptoms of both. Because of this, physical therapy and all other forms of treatment must proceed very carefully. Any treatment tried will be both more complicated and less successful than if the patient had only one of the two syndromes. One study has already been done. Hong and Hsueh (1996) found that those with FMS *and* MPS experience more pain when they receive trigger point injections, that the trigger point injections have less effect, and that the effect often takes longer to develop and may not last as long than if the patients had MPS only. As more researchers and clinicians realize that this synergistic condition exists, more studies will be conducted, and more light will be shed.

In FMS/MPS, a chronic pain condition exists, which is characterized by the trigger points of MPS and many other different symptoms. All of these symptoms and trigger points are intensified by the pain amplification aspect of FMS. Furthermore, some of the treatments normally prescribed for FMS patients can damage MPS patients and the reverse is also true. In FMS, many different neurotransmitters may be affected in different combinations interacting in different ways in different patients. Other biochemicals in the body are affected to different degrees. Various hormones may also be involved.

For example, histamine (a neurotransmitter) is often an important factor when there are many allergic manifestations, but the possible combinations are endless. When the possible combinations of TrPs are calculated, it is easy to see why no two FMS/MPS Complex patients are alike. Fibromyalgia perpetuates MPS and the reverse is also true. The spiral of pain/contraction/pain/contraction continues until it is interrupted by relief in some form.

A lot can be done to relieve MPS and lighten the pain load. And there are many things that help FMS, as well. It's important for people with this combination of syndromes to take on the responsibility of managing their own treatment. It isn't easy, and it takes concentrated focus to change the habits of a lifetime. Getting as well as possible—optimizing your quality of life—takes commitment. What is done to or for you can help a lot, but getting better is primarily a function of what *you* do for yourself.

Cognitive Deficits

Studies in the field of fibromyalgic cognitive deficits are extremely new. Yet these symptoms are often the most difficult we have to deal with, and the most disabling. *Cognitive deficits* is the technical term for what many of us call "fibrofog" when we are communicating with each other on the Internet. To be in a fibrofog means that you feel as if your brain isn't fully engaged. In fibrofog, it is as if your body was a large electrical system, and some of the circuit breakers have shut down and many of the fuses have blown. Your brain may feel clouded or stuffed with cotton. It's extremely difficult to function.

You forget the names of nouns, especially, and your use of the word "thing" rises exponentially. Sentences like "It's not the thing itself, but it's the thingie on the thingie-do that causes the thing" don't convey a whole lot of meaning to most people. For those of us with FMS, however, we understand them all too well. We've been there. You begin "tongue-tripping"—having difficulty pronouncing simple everyday words. Sometimes, you say a word that begins with the same letter of the word you wanted to say, but it will be entirely inappropriate. These are just some of the "cognitive deficits" that can turn your life into an obstacle course.

The Causes of Fibrofog

From what I have been able to discover, fibrofog may have multiple causes. As with all too many of the symptoms of fibromyalgia, however, the variables come with complicated issues of credibility. Let's take a look at some of the possibilities.

Neurotransmitters

In the section called "Clumsiness" earlier in this chapter, neurotransmitters were described as the electro-biochemical agents that cross nerve synapses to function as messengers between the mind and body. Chapter 2 has a more complete discussion of the role that the neurotransmitters play in FMS. Right now let's consider the role they may play in what the medical world calls "cognitive deficits," and what we know as "fibrofog."

Think of the consequences if just a few neurotransmitters misbehave. Too much histamine can cause permeable membranes and swelling. (Some days it may feel as if your entire brain is swollen.) Too much acetylcholine can cause nerve transmissions to fire off, and you may feel as if you're in the middle of a true "brainstorm," with every nerve firing in different directions, and the resultant confusion leaving you incapable of finding your way home.

Adrenaline and noradrenaline can cause indecisiveness and a lack of initiative, as well as apathy, irritability, and anxiety. In fibrofog, unless you put out your clothes the night before, you may be unable to decide what to wear. Dopamine irregularities can cause emotional hyperactivity. Changing serotonin levels can cause rapid mood swings, with fluctuating perception and awareness ("fibroflux"), slow thought processes, and diminished drive. We know that serotonin depletion, a common affliction among people with FMS, can lead to learning dysfunction in rats (Mazer, Muneyyirci, Taheny, et al. 1997). Whether this is part of the human picture is not yet known.

Ever Stop to Think, and Forget to Start Again?

When you start "fibro-flipping," to be sure you wrote a phone number (or any numbered sequence) correctly, you need to check and recheck it many, many times, because you cannot remember whether you checked it or not. It's as if you forgot where you left your short-term memory. You begin conversations in the middle, not realizing that you forgot to verbalize the thoughts that led up to your statement, and the person with whom you are talking is mystified. Or, you can go into what I call "fugue" states—staring into space until your brain gets a chance to catch up, before you can resume your conversation (or task).

When sleep deprivation and chronic pain are added to this volatile mix, we may feel that we have "totally lost it." Certainly, when we are in fibrofog, we have difficulties communicating to others what is going on in our lives.

Trigger Points and Fibrofog

I have seen three people with active trigger points in their digastric muscles, which blocked the drainage channels in the head region. I instructed them to use moist heat packs, and then to "milk" the digastric muscles gently by applying gentle fingertip pressure from the jaw area down to the base of the throat. As the area became less sensitive, they were instructed to increase the pressure. When adequate trigger point massage of the digastric muscles was accomplished, their fibrofog disappeared. However, I don't know how common a contributory factor this is with cognitive deficits. The autonomic "proprioceptor" symptoms of some of the trigger points can cause dizziness, loss of balance, and other symptoms that add to the fibrofog effects (Starlanyl and Copeland 1996, 27).

Reactive Hypoglycemia

Many of us have reactive hypoglycemia as a coexisting condition and/or perpetuating factor. (See chapters 3 and 4 for more information on coexisting conditions and perpetuating factors.) This can be a major contributor to fibrofog (Hvidberg, Fanelli, Hershey, et al. 1996). It even affects regional blood flow in the brain (Powers, Hirsch and Cryer 1996). In my experience, this type of fibrofog disappears when the patient gets the hypoglycemia under control with diet. It resumes with a diet lapse, but goes away again once the diet is reinstated.

Childhood Neglect

We know that childhood neglect can have an impact on clarity of thought and brain function (Mackner, Starr and Black 1997). A history of childhood abuse is not unusual in the FMS patient. How much this is a contributory factor to fibrofog is unclear. As usual, we, as FMS patients, must first convince the researchers that the cognitive deficits are real. Only then will the true research in this field begin.

Flare

During a flare, current symptoms become more intense, and new symptoms frequently develop. Life veers out of control. Even the best organized support systems become strained,

Accidents and Fibrofog

For those of us for whom the initiating event of fibromyalgia was a motor vehicle accident, there is mounting evidence that such an accident can account for post-traumatic stress disorder, phobias, and mood disturbances (Kuch, Cox and Evans 1996). Even in the case of minor head injuries of other types, there may be evidence of lasting brain abnormalities (Stewart, Kaylor and Koutanis 1996; Ingebrigtsen, Romner, Waterloo, et al. 1996; De Renzi, Lucchelli, Muggia, et al. 1995). There are studies from the Society of Automotive Engineers publications, which are not normally read by physicians, demonstrating that low impact collisions can profoundly affect the body, even when the damage to the vehicle is minimal. Some relevant article titles can be found in the Bibliography.

and the person experiencing flare must direct his or her entire focus to survival. The best way to deal with flares is to prevent them, and your best preventative weapon is knowledge. When you find yourself in flare, it is a sign that you have perpetuating factors which are out of control. If you keep a record of what is happening in your life, you may be able to prevent the reoccurrence of flare in the future. The following Flare Indicator Form can be copied or used as a guideline for a form of your own creation.

Flare Indicator Form

I can tell when I'm going into flare by the following indicators:

- increased fatigue/pain/dizziness

- increased mental confusion

- greater carbohydrate craving

- greater emotional instability

- other: _____

- _____

- _____

These are the steps I can take to avoid or lessen impending/present flare:

- schedule more physical therapy appointments

- increase/change medications

- meditate

- watch my diet more carefully

- delete/modify/delegate tasks

- avoid negative influences/people/things

- other: _____

- _____

- _____

Progressive? It's Not What It Seems to Be

I frequently hear from people with FMS and/or MPS who insist that their conditions are "progressive." When I reply that these conditions are *not* progressive, they want to know why they keep getting worse. The fact that their conditions continue to worsen is often due to a combination of hidden or untreated perpetuating factors (see chapter 3), and to the resultant spread of trigger points.

"Progressive" means that the course of a disease inexorably advances in spite of treatment. With spreading trigger points, however, once you deal with the perpetuating factors, and the TrPs are appropriately treated, the advance of the TrPs can not only be stopped—it can be reversed. There will not be any permanent damage, nor an advancement of the disease. Of course, there is always the danger that if your spine has been kept in an unbalanced posture over several years, some extra bone calcification and/or degeneration may have occurred, and this is not reversible.

Secondary and Satellite Trigger Points

One way that TrPs spread occurs when secondary TrPs develop. This happens when a muscle is subject to stress because another muscle weakened by a TrP isn't doing its job. For example, it may start with a fall and an injury to the right hip, and TrPs may develop in the gluteus minimus muscle on the side of the hip. Then, that leg is favored and takes shorter strides. More weight is put on the left leg, and it is used for more duties. This means that when you climb stairs, for example, you lift your body with your left leg instead of your right, to spare your weakened muscle any extra weight load. Your back then takes on some of the burden of the weak hip.

The shifting weight and added stress may cause secondary TrPs to develop in the left hip and low back, as well as in the low back on the right side. Sometimes, the pain can go from one side one day to the other side the next day, depending on how you have been using your body.

Trigger points also spread by developing satellite TrPs. If the primary, or first, TrP is in the gluteus minimus, it has a large referral pattern, and satellite TrPs can spread all over in the referral zone. The myofascia tries to splint the painful part of your body, to prevent it from moving and causing you more pain, and, suddenly, you may have TrPs all along the outer side of your right thigh.

Muscles with TrPs are weakened, so if they are left untreated, or if there are other perpetuating factors, the satellite and secondary TrPs develop satellites and secondaries of their own. This can happen in the upper body as well as the lower, depending on what the initiating event has been.

The Initiating Event

The initiating event may have been a fall, a repetitive task, an infection, a disease, a pregnancy, or even a painful menstrual period. It may have been allergies or a flu, with congestion in the head and neck creating TrPs there. It could have been something obvious, such as an automobile accident, or a traumatic period in your life when your muscles were habitually kept clenched in a tight, defensive posture.

Some people develop satellites easily, and tend to start with TrPs developing all on one side. Other initiating events create secondaries, which often lead to an upper or lower body problem. Without proper medical/physical therapeutic intervention, and without attention to perpetuating factors, the TrPs can lead to severe and widespread MPS. Many physicians who are used to looking for MPS as a regional syndrome are unaware that it can come in this whole body form. Sadly, it does, and when it does, it is usually a symptom of a medical care system that has failed the patient. Somehow, someway, the patient didn't get the proper care to prevent this scenario from being enacted.

I have observed that if a healthy person gets an active TrP or two, and there are no perpetuating factors, and s/he gets appropriate therapy, the TrP will go away. I have also observed that if a person gets a TrP or two and s/he has the genetic tendency toward FMS, and perpetuating factors, without proper intervention FMS and eventual FMS/MPS

Complex *will* develop. If a person has FMS and develops a primary TrP, it is vital that s/he get immediate therapy for it. Otherwise, the FMS becomes a perpetuating factor for that TrP, and it will develop satellites and secondary TrPs of its own. Ultimately, this will result in bodywide FMS/MPS. I have seen MPS arrive first, and I have seen FMS arrive first. Often the signs of FMS are there, but go unremarked until an accident or illness or some other stressor initiates a TrP cascade.

Breaking Up Trigger Points

With proper intervention, trigger points can be broken up and eliminated. When the perpetuating factors are conditions such as FMS, which presently have no cure, however, your medical team, including its manager, *you,* must gear up for the challenge of optimizing the quality of your life. The best way to start this is to discover any perpetuating factors. These can be many and varied, such as sleep deprivation, pain, chronic illnesses, paradoxical breathing, and so forth. In chapter 3 we will take a look at them and see what can be done.

2

The Neurotransmitters

It is important to first understand that medical science doesn't know all there is to know about neurotransmitters. It is a rapidly expanding field of knowledge and new discoveries are being made almost daily. The following material may seem like a lot to learn because the information on neurotransmitters is written in "medicalese" (or "doctorspeak"), without explanations of the underlying basic contexts. I'll try to translate the medicalese because I want you to understand the concepts—they are important for an understanding of what is going on in your body and mind. I will try to keep the medical terms at a minimum. Also, you may have heard some of the terms in this chapter used about your medications. It is my hope that the information you will find here will help to make those terms more meaningful to you.

Neurotransmitters may be the driving force of the body's clocks. We now suspect that almost every cellular and body system has a chronobiological rhythm and clock. The body moves to carefully orchestrated sets upon sets of specific rhythms. For example, the brain has an electrical rhythm of about 8–12 cycles per second. The skeletal muscles have a 4- to 6-minute strength cycle. At this point, a little background data is required to understand the complexities of the interconnected neurotransmitter network.

For example, we may take a medication to reduce fever, although that medication may also be used for pain. Yet fever itself reduces the body's pain threshold. We may take a medication to alleviate pain, but that may also mute the body's normal "danger response" to pain. Similarly, if we take a medication to increase the neurotransmitter serotonin, our pain threshold may go up, but too much serotonin can produce numbness and loss of consciousness.

When we take a medication to affect one specific neurotransmitter, it can't help but affect many other biochemicals in the body. For example, tranquilizers may ease anxiety, but they also can cause slumping posture, muted awareness of reality, and diminish the attention span and the ability to concentrate. Nearly always, medications produce unintended consequences, commonly known as side effects, as well as intended effects. With that understanding firmly in mind, let us begin with some of the basics of the interconnected neurotransmitter network.

Muscle Types

Consider the two basic types of muscle: smooth muscle and striated muscle. *Smooth muscles* function independently of conscious orders on our part. They are under the direction of the autonomic nervous system (ANS). "Autonomic" sounds like "automatic" and, in this case, it usually is. The ANS does many things at once. It delivers messages to the heart, the gastrointestinal system, and the glands. The secretions of our glands, the movements of our gut (peristalsis), and the rate of our heartbeat are all under the control of the ANS.

Striated muscle is what we usually think of when we think of the term "muscle." Well-developed striated muscles made Arnold Schwartzenegger famous. "Striae" is the medical word for "parallel lines." These muscles are constantly in some form of contraction or flexion. They are either extended or contracted. They work in pairs or groups. They have what we call "tone."

The autonomic nervous system tells striated muscle to react to physical or other forms of stress. It can cause us to tense involuntarily, to prepare to fight, or to flee danger. It is also supposed to tell us to relax when the stress is over. Unfortunately, in fibromyalgia (FMS), it often forgets the second part and the striated muscles do not relax but remain constricted—that is, they stay tight—ready to deal with a stress that is no longer present.

Both striated and smooth muscles have fibers and bundles of fibers, all individually wrapped in myofascia (see chapter 1 for a discussion of the myofascia). Muscles are one of the body's major pain generators, and yet they are the least understood of the body's systems, and are often the most ignored by many physicians.

The Role of the Glands

Hormones are specialized biochemicals that are secreted by glands found in specific areas of the body. They are also manufactured in specialized cells, such as those in the gastrointestinal system. They are interregulated, with feedback loops in case one gland produces too much of a specific hormone. They are also under the control of the neurotransmitters.

We know that in fibromyalgia, there is a disrupted HPA axis. This means that the critical *balance* between the hypothalamus, pituitary, and adrenal glands is no longer operating properly. The balance between the hormones that these glands produce is an important key to the proper functioning of the body.

The HPA-Axis

The hypothalamus is a small gland that many scientists consider part of the brain. It is the sentinel of the body, and decides when the body is under attack. When it makes that decision, it then signals its neighbor, the pituitary gland, to prepare the body for action. The pituitary gland then sends a message to the adrenal glands. These are a pair of tiny glands perched on top of the kidneys. They look like little triangular caps. They are minuscule but mighty, influencing almost all of the body systems. They produce adrenaline and many other biochemicals that the body uses in stressful situations. All of these glands communicate by way of the neurotransmitters which are secreted by the nerve cells or neurons.

Neurons

The neuron, or nerve, is a highly specialized cell. It is also a sentry post, prepared to notice any change in its environment, and to relay that information from neuron to neuron until the information reaches its destination. Neurons are not physically connected. They transmit signals to other neurons by releasing an electrochemical, called a neurotransmitter, into the neural synapse—the gap between the two neurons. Neurons function as part of a collective called the "neural net." Each signal—or message—travels from a nerve to the brain by a series of neurotransmitter transfers.

We have known about a few of the neurotransmitters for quite some time, but many are not yet known to us. Some are suspected but not yet named. To be classified as a neurotransmitter, the substance must be created within the nerve cell. The actual neurotransmitters that jump the synapses and the nerve cells that manufacture these neurotransmitters often have the same names. Also, the same names are often given to receptors (see "Receptors," below). Neurotransmitters exist for a brief time only, when they are being used as messengers. That's for as long as it takes for the biochemical to be released by one neuron and taken up by another neuron, at a site called the "receptor."

Hormones exist *much* longer than neurotransmitters: they exist from the time they are released from a gland or specialized cell, during their circulation through the body, until they arrive at their designated receptor somewhere else in the body. Endocrine glands release their hormones into the circulatory system. There are also other types of hormones that act on the cells near their release point.

Receptors

There are often many types of receptors on a cell. Usually, the receptors are made of glycoproteins. This is important because glycoproteins are large compounds composed of carbohydrates and proteins. These glycoproteins interact with the carbohydrates we consume, and can affect our health adversely when they are not operating properly (see "Reactive Hypoglycemia" in chapter 3). It is important to understand this because some alternative therapies are based on this information.

Receptors that cause a response are called "agonists." Receptors that block a response are called "antagonists." If a *medication* works by causing or blocking the same response, it is also given the name of "agonist" or "antagonist." There are often many different receptors for the same neurotransmitter. These receptors are each responsible for specific actions of the neurotransmitter. For example, you may have to take a histamine 1 blocker for one symptom, and a histamine 2 blocker for another symptom. These receptors are given the same names as the neurotransmitters they receive, but are numbered according to the specific type of action of the neurotransmitter with which they are involved.

Medications for Neurotransmitters

Many medications, as well as other foreign chemicals such as toxins, either *block* the function or *enhance* the release of neurotransmitters. Medications can block neurotransmitters in the following three ways:

- They can "fill up" the receptors so that there are no places for the neurotransmitter to "land."

- They can change the cell membrane, by combining with the neurotransmitter and creating a new substance that will not fit into the receptor space.

- They can alter the "reuptake" (reabsorption) of the neurotransmitter by the neuron.

One class of medications frequently prescribed for FMS/MPS Complex is the SSRI. This stands for "specific serotonin reuptake inhibitor." This means that after a serotonin molecule has completed its task, rather than it being shunted on its way, or "reabsorbed," it stays in the space between the neurons (the synapse) to do its task again and again, in effect allowing more serotonin to service the body. It is a kind of recycling.

Many neurons can *store* neurotransmitters inside their cells. You may have heard of "calcium channel blockers." Calcium channels are tubes that bridge the double layer of the cell membrane. When the channels are open, the material inside the cell is free to mix with the material on the outside of the cell. When these channels are blocked, material inside the cell, such as a neurotransmitter, cannot reach the outside. There are other ways medications can block neurotransmitters, the explanation of which is outside the scope of this book.

Many neurotransmitters work in pairs, forming a balance. One will produce an effect, and the other will stop the same effect. The theory is that this balance keeps a single neurotransmitter from going out of control. In FMS, something happens to cause this regulating system to break down, and the balances are lost. If you are interested in learning more about these fascinating biochemicals, which affect our lives so profoundly, you will find a number of books on neurotransmitters in the References and Bibliography sections at the back of the book. I particularly recommend the work of Birkmeyer and Reiderer (1989) and Hardie (1991). These books assume at least a basic knowledge of medical terminology. Be prepared. At the least, you will need a medical dictionary and more than a little extra patience.

Knowing a little about some of these basic neurotransmitters will help you to understand why neurotransmitter dysregulation can be such an overwhelming problem. The definitions provided here are, of necessity, simplistic, but, I hope, they are comprehensible.

Histamine

Histamine is the neurotransmitter often associated with allergies—we are all familiar with antihistamines. If your cell membranes are broken by trauma, such as a bruise or cut, or exposure to heat or chemical toxins, histamine is released (Schedle, Samorapoompichit, Fureder, et al. 1998). Histamine causes the smooth muscle of the bronchial area to constrict, so we become short of breath. It relaxes small blood vessels, but constricts some large ones. It provokes a generalized dilation of the blood vessels in parts of the brain, as any of us who has ever had a "histamine headache" knows very well. Histamine also causes an increase in the permeability of the capillaries. Bruising can result, as well as leakage of intracellular components into the area outside the cells. It causes a drop in blood pressure, secretion of gastric juices, and may cause nausea and vomiting. When histamine levels become high, swelling, a runny nose, and red eyes result.

Acetylcholine

Acetylcholine is the neurotransmitter that slows the rate and force of cardiac contraction. It also increases the amount of mucus in the upper respiratory tract, the secretion of enzymes in the stomach, and the amount of sweating. High levels can cause the gut to contract to the point of cramping, and involuntary bowel movements. It can do much the same with the urinary system. If unregulated, it can play havoc with eye focus, as well as reduce the pressure in the eyeball. It is also involved with involuntary motion, speech and thought processes, and sensory impression. All of these operations are under the control of one type of acetylcholine receptor. There is another type of acetylcholine receptor that regulates the transmission of nerve impulses.

You may have heard the terms "cholinergic" or "anticholinergic" medications. These are medications that interact with the neurotransmitter acetylcholine. Often, toxins interact with acetylcholine. For example, botulism toxin works by preventing all cholinergic neurons from releasing their neurotransmitters. It is easy to see how the dysregulation of acetylcholine would compound some trigger point symptoms, and thus how FMS and Myofascial Pain Syndrome (MPS) work together to create a misery that is more than the sum of the two parts.

Noradrenaline and Adrenaline

Noradrenaline and *adrenaline* are two very similar neurotransmitters. Adrenaline is produced by the adrenal glands. There are specific cells in the gut, lungs, and heart that release noradrenaline. Both of these biochemicals are associated with energy consumption. Noradrenaline controls the blood pressure in the peripheral areas of the body, that is, the arms and legs. It also inhibits digestive activity. When noradrenaline is released, the hypothalamus directs the body to lower its temperature. The thalamus lowers the pain threshold. Think about what might happen if these are not properly regulated. Does it seem familiar?

Too high a level of these neurotransmitters causes hypertension (high blood pressure), insomnia, weight loss, irritability, agitation, restlessness, and anxiety. Too low a level causes low blood pressure, lack of decisiveness and initiative, and apathy. Adrenaline and noradrenaline have many other duties, including the regulation of the sphincters of the bladder and rectum, the uterine muscles, and the pilomotor muscles, which are responsible for "goose bumps" (literally a hair-raising experience). Adrenaline and noradrenaline also elevate blood glucose, but they slow its absorption by the striated muscles.

Noradrenaline is very much involved with pain. It increases our perception of pain, creates anxiety that contributes to the apprehension of pain, and adds to the overall stress reaction. The stress reaction enhances our consciousness of pain, which again increases our sensitivity to pain.

Dopamine

Dopamine is a neurotransmitter that controls motor activity. It is responsible for our muscle tone. Too much dopamine creates compulsive nervous movements, emotional

A recent finding, which may have implications in any condition where the neurotransmitters are not in balance, is that in mice, the maternal instinct is governed by norepinephrine and epinephrine (Thomas and Palmiter 1997b). I have observed a subset of people with fibromyalgia who want to be good parents, but seem to lack the parenting instinct. This may be the connection, but again, we don't yet know. There is another mouse study which indicates that norepinephrine has a role in motor functioning, learning, and memory (Thomas and Palmiter 1997a).

hyperactivity, lack of appetite, and muscle cramps that won't let go, especially at night. A lack of dopamine causes unremitting weariness, hypokinesia, diminished movement, and a hunched posture.

Serotonin

Serotonin is the neurotransmitter that has been the most studied in FMS. It is also called "5-hydroxytryptamine." When we have migraine attacks, serotonin is released, causing constriction of all major blood vessels. The visual disturbances heralding a migraine are due, at least partially, to the constriction of retinal blood vessels. (This may be part of the reason why some of us see "stars" when we cough.) This is followed by a longer period of rebound, when the blood vessels dilate, resulting in a throbbing headache and nausea. Serotonin is also influential in producing and regulating sleep, moods, and vomiting.

Serotonin is balanced with adrenaline/noradrenaline. During pregnancy, there is more serotonin in the body, which is one reason why some FMS symptoms may diminish at this time. Unfortunately, many myofascial trigger point symptoms worsen. The birth process is activated by serotonin. If we have too much adrenaline/noradrenaline, and not enough serotonin, the birth process may be delayed or slowed. There is a subset of women with FMS who have longer gestation periods. Low levels of serotonin may be part of the problem. We also know that low levels of serotonin are associated with suicidal behavior in depressed patients (Mann, Malone, Nielsen, et al. 1997).

Serotonin is responsible for increased sleep requirements, lack of motivation, weight gain, edema, and, during pregnancy, decreased mental activity. It is also responsible for coordinating the lowering of blood pressure, heart rate, and blood sugar level during sleep. If sleep becomes too deep, there is a feedback loop that releases noradrenaline.

Dreams are the result of noradrenaline acting on the brain. When dreams begin, blood pressure, heart rate, breathing, and muscle tone increase. This balance is one of the reasons people get less deep sleep as they age. In older people, REM (rapid eye movement, or shallow) sleep becomes much more frequent, to ensure that the brain gets enough oxygen and nutrients from arteries that have become more constricted due to aging. This is an excellent example of why we shouldn't view neurotransmitters too simplistically. Their functions are all interrelated.

Serotonin, or the lack thereof, can be behind obesity, lethargy, the balance of the pain threshold, lack of awareness, diarrhea or constipation, slow thought processes, loss of drive, slow circulation, a general, diffuse swelling of extremities, or blood clots.

GABA

GABA is short for "gamma-amino-n-butyric acid." This neurotransmitter affects the bioelectrical system in various areas of the central nervous system (CNS). If there is too little

GABA in the spinal cord, muscle spasticity, or tightness, results. A low amount of GABA not only produces a change in muscle tone, it can also cause convulsions, seizures, memory impairment, and thinking and emotional disorders.

Substance P

Substance P is a biochemical often mentioned in conjunction with fibromyalgia. It acts as a local neurotransmitter influencing the balance between the hypothalamus, pituitary, and adrenal glands—the HPA axis. Substance P regulates sensory mechanisms. It causes pain if applied to the cut ends of sensory neurons, so it may be responsible for some of our sharper "nerve" pains. It is also a vasodilator (which means that it causes the blood vessels to widen). It lowers blood pressure, causes smooth muscle contractions in the gut, causes constriction in the airways, and may increase mucus production.

Peptides

There are other biochemicals, called peptides, which are interrelated with some neurotransmitters. They are synthesized in the nerve cells. Some of these are the enkephalins, endorphins and dynorphins, which affect how we feel pain, and how much pain we feel. When considering neurotransmitter modification, it is important to remember that FMS doesn't mean a lack of neurotransmitters. There are many subsets of fibromyalgia. We aren't homogeneous. Some of us may have high levels of one neurotransmitter and low levels of others. In addition, the levels of neurotransmitters may vary, hour by hour and day by day. This is no area for "cookbook medicine." Each one of us requires specific care, and what that care is must be determined on a case-by-case basis.

3

Perpetuating Factors

This chapter may well be the most important part of this book for you. Your success in healing depends on your ability to identify as many perpetuating factors as you can, and then to effectively deal with them. No matter what you do to relieve trigger points (TrPs), if you have perpetuating factors, TrPs will return. If you have chronic Myofascial Pain Syndrome (MPS) or FMS/MPS Complex you *do* have perpetuating factors, and if you want to feel better, you cannot ignore them. They won't simply go away, and neither will your TrPs.

Don't let the number of possible perpetuating factors intimidate you. Become a detective. Think of perpetuating factors as the clues that will explain why you feel so awful. The key to getting better is to track down all the clues, and then eliminate them. In his monograph, *Myofascial Pain Syndrome Due to Trigger Points,* David Simons (1987) says that effective therapy for trigger points should last indefinitely—unless perpetuating factors are present. *Factors that perpetuate trigger points will necessarily perpetuate fibromyalgia (FMS).* It bears repeating that if you want to heal, you must identify all of your perpetuating factors and then deal with them.

Your first move should be to have your TrPs mapped by a physical therapist who *knows* Travell and Simons' medical texts (1983; 1992). Don't be fooled by someone who says, "Sure. I know trigger points. You have all eighteen." This person clearly cannot distinguish between the tender points of FMS and the trigger points of MPS. Such a person can do you a lot of harm.

Coexisting Conditions as Perpetuating Factors

Coexisting conditions (see chapter 4) can be important perpetuating factors. Fibromyalgia can be both a coexisting condition and a perpetuating factor for MPS and the reverse is also true. This means that to get better, you have to work on them both. One of the best ways to begin is to start with a complete and thorough physical examination. With your physician, make a list of all the possible perpetuating factors that you may have, and discuss any required testing. Then, get the tests done. Some hidden perpetuating factors such as cancer, emphysema, infestations, and infections can be serious and even life-threatening.

Biochemical Factors

People with FMS have unbalanced neuroendocrine systems. Fibromyalgia can start a cascade of neurotransmitter imbalances. Your doctor should be aware that people with FMS may need more specific testing than s/he normally uses. For example, people with FMS often score low-normal on thyroid tests, and the BT2 panel (Total T4, Free T4, Total T3, and TSH) is required to get a true picture of the condition of the thyroid. In some cases, even a thyroid antibody test may be needed. If you are fatigued and your doctor is considering DHEA supplementation, a twenty-four-hour cortisol test may *not* be useful, because your cortisol may fluctuate wildly through the night and day, although the average value may be fine.

As another example, the usual test for anemia may tell your doctor that you are fine, but if your ferratin is checked, it may be discovered that the iron you have is not available to your muscles. Just because standard testing shows normal values does not always mean that everything is fine. It may simply mean that the proper tests have not been run You may need slightly more specific testing to obtain accurate results.

Metabolic problems such as diabetes or reactive hypoglycemia (RHG) can perpetuate TrPs. In my experience, reactive hypoglycemia (RHG) is also very common in FMS. In my last book (Starlanyl and Copeland 1996), I discussed the work of Lynne August and R. Paul St. Amand, physicians who independently came to the conclusion that reactive hypoglycemia is a major perpetuating factor of FMS. There are others (Crofford, Engelberg and Demitrack 1996; Eisinger, Plantamura and Ayavou 1994; Travell and Simons 1983; Simons 1987) who have reached the same conclusion.

Reactive Hypoglycemia

People often tell me that they've been tested for hypoglycemia and they don't have it, but they still exhibit all of the symptoms. *Reactive hypoglycemia* (RHG) is not the same as *fasting hypoglycemia,* which is manifested by low blood sugar after fasting. Reactive hypoglycemia will not show up on a typical glucose tolerance test, which is the test normally given for diabetes. A specific test for reactive hypoglycemia exists, but it requires a carbohydrate challenge meal, as well as blood tests to measure not only blood sugar but also adrenaline surges. The testing would have to be continuous, however, because the adrenaline spikes and blood-sugar drops can come at any time, and fluctuate.

Reactive hypoglycemia takes place within two to three hours after a meal of excess carbohydrates, when there is a rapid release of carbohydrates into the small intestine, followed by rapid absorption of glucose into the bloodstream, and then by the production of a large amount of insulin. This condition is also called insulin tolerance, postprandial hypoglycemia and carbohydrate intolerance. Unfortunately, it is also a condition that many physicians "don't believe in."

One of the chief reasons we have an epidemic of obesity and RHG in our country today is the poor education about them that is provided in medical schools. Reactive hypoglycemia, unchecked, often leads to obesity and type II diabetes (Sears and Lawren 1995). I believe that the reason Type II diabetes and obesity are so prevalent in this country is due to the high carbohydrate diet we eat, and until people are on balanced diets like the "Zone diet," tailored to each individual, this trend will continue.

Standard glucose tolerance tests will not pick up reactive hypoglycemia, but specialized testing is not necessary since the treatment of choice is to stop carbohydrate bingeing and switch to balanced diets such as the Zone diet (Sears and Lawren 1995). This diet may have to be modified to fit each individual, but the Zone books, although not written expressly for people with FMS and MPS, work very well to help those of us who have reactive hypoglycemia as a perpetuating factor.

Researchers have found that reactive hypoglycemia is due to increased insulin sensitivity with inadequate glucagon secretion (Leonetti, Foniciello, Iozzo, et al. 1996). There have also been studies that show supplemental chromium can help patients with reactive hypoglycemia (Anderson, Polansky, Bryden, et al. 1987) and can even enhance glucagon secretion (McCarty 1996). Cognitive deficits may also be caused by hypoglycemia (McCrimmon, Deary, Huntly, et al. 1996).

FMS, FMS/MPS Complex, and RHG

Reactive hypoglycemia is common in people with FMS and FMS/MPS Complex. In FMS, it is enhanced by dysfunctional neurotransmitter regulation and other systemic problems. Growth hormone, for example, is important in the regulation of glucose (Cryer 1996), and yet it is often deficient when fibromyalgia is present (Crofford, Engleberg and Demitrack 1996). With FMS, we crave carbohydrates but can't use them efficiently because of an electrolytic imbalance and other biochemical imbalances in our bodies. We produce adrenaline even when our blood sugar doesn't fall.

In fibromyalgia, the conversion of glucose into energy is abnormal (Eisinger, Plantamura and Ayavou 1994). We crave carbohydrates, because we need their energy, but since our insulin level is high, we store the carbohydrates as fat, often around the belly area. Fortunately, by eating a balanced diet, we can teach our bodies to eliminate excess fat by using it for energy.

In chronic MPS, the process of eliminating TrPs can be hampered or even totally blocked by the presence of hypoglycemia (Simons 1987). Trigger point activity is aggravated and specific therapy response is reduced by this perpetuating factor. If you have chronic MPS, it is vital that you begin eating a balanced diet and eliminating excess carbohydrates, as soon as possible.

Symptoms of RHG

Reactive hypoglycemia can range from very mild to severe. Headaches may occur (usually in the front or top of the head), as well as dizziness, irritability, chronic fatigue, depression, nervousness, memory and concentration difficulties, nasal congestion, palpitations or heart pounding, hand tremors (especially if a long time elapses between meals), day or night sweats, anxiety in the pit of the stomach, leg cramps, numbness and tingling in the hands and/or feet, flushing, and craving for carbohydrates (especially sweets).

The hunger pangs experienced in reactive hypoglycemia can come in the form of acute stomach pain and nausea, often coupled with anxiety. Severe RHG can cause hypoxic symptoms such as visual disturbances, restlessness, and impaired speech and thinking. Some of these symptoms are caused by extra adrenaline. Fainting can also occur, but it is rare. Also, eating carbohydrates at night often causes insomnia, and people with FMS already have problems sleeping. People with RHG are often overweight, although this is not always the case. Usually, those who are overweight are unable to lose the extra weight. They develop a fat pad on the belly that won't go away no matter what they do.

Hormones and RHG

Hormones usually work as a pair, called an axis, consisting of two hormones with powerful but opposing physiological effects. The most important axis involved in RHG is the insulin-glucagon axis. Insulin drives blood sugar levels down, while glucagon raises them. If insulin is too high or glucagon too low, the result is low blood sugar. To be insulin-resistant means that insulin levels are elevated, but blood sugar levels remain high because the target cells no longer respond to insulin. This can promote diabetes.

Insulin

Insulin is a storage hormone. It takes excess glucose and excess amino acids from dietary carbohydrates and stores them as fat. Insulin drives down blood sugar. Glucagon is a mobilizing hormone. It releases stored carbohydrates as glucose and restores blood sugar levels. The release of insulin is stimulated by carbohydrates, especially high-glycemic carbohydrates such as bread and pasta. Glucagon is stimulated by dietary protein. Insulin also triggers an adrenaline response. Coffee, tea, and colas stimulate the release of adrenaline, as does nicotine, which is often why we use products containing caffeine and nicotine. We want to keep that adrenaline flowing. Then we lose the ability to turn it off. Exercise, however, decreases insulin production.

Serotonin

The neurotransmitter, serotonin, regulates the appetite for carbohydrate-rich foods. This is influenced by our response to darkness and light. Carbohydrate cravers frequently overeat only at certain times of the day. The rate of conversion of tryptophan to serotonin is affected by the proportion of carbohydrates in a person's diet. Since most people with FMS have a shortage of serotonin, we need to watch our carbohydrate intake very carefully.

The Effects of High Carbohydrate Diets

A high carbohydrate diet can lead to decreased neurotransmitter production. Also, elevated insulin during sleep blocks human growth hormone release (Daost and Daost 1996). When you have RHG, if you eat a lot of carbohydrates for lunch, by 3 PM you are probably ready for a nap, because excess carbohydrates will have generated an overproduction of insulin. As your blood sugar drops, your brain begins to tune out. Because a massive amount of carbohydrates drives insulin levels up and glucagon levels down, the fats stored in your body cannot be released. You will crave more carbohydrates because you will need the energy. This occurs in 50 percent of the population. In 25 percent, the normal response is blunted, so those folks can get away with consuming excess carbohydrates. But the remaining 25 percent of the population exhibits an extremely elevated insulin response to carbohydrates. *Many of these people have FMS or FMS/MPS Complex.* Note that the tendency to be hypoglycemic is inherited and is often accompanied by a family history of diabetes.

The often overlooked factor about eating carbohydrates is that they stimulate insulin production. Insulin enables blood sugar to move to our biochemical "factories" in the cells, where it is burned as fuel. If there is already an excess of insulin in the blood, and a high carbohydrate meal or snack is consumed, the excess carbohydrates are stored as fatty acids in fat cells. If you have excess insulin in your blood, when you need more fuel your brain will tell your body *not to use* the stored fats as fuel. You become hungry for fast energy, so you eat more carbohydrates. You not only gain weight as fat, but you are also prevented from losing this fat.

A Balanced Diet Will Heal RHG

Before you can begin to balance your diet, you must understand that there are only *three* basic types of nutrients:

- Protein—beef, fish, poultry, cottage cheese, and tofu are largely protein.

- Fats—butter, cream, and vegetable oils are all fats.

- Carbohydrates—vegetables, fruits, grains, pastas, and cereals are carbohydrates.

Weight loss on a high carbohydrate diet is mostly water and muscle loss. Any subsequent weight gain is fat gain. The more carbohydrates you eat, the earlier adrenaline is produced as your blood sugar goes down. The more carbohydrates you eat, the more extreme your blood sugar swings will be. The ideal ratio of protein to carbohydrates is 3 to 4. It is important to keep to this balance for every meal and snack, because there is a hormonal response every time you eat. The ratio of 30/40/30 provides an adequate protein, moderate carbohydrate, low-fat diet. The hormonal response from a balanced meal should last four to six hours. This means you shouldn't crave food during that time. If you do, you are out of balance.

Each time you eat either a meal or a snack, your food intake should match the 30/40/30 ratio, because you need that balanced hormonal response each time you eat. At the same time, you need to adjust your caloric intake and exercise so that it satisfies the needs of your body. *Mastering the Zone* by Barry Sears (1997) explains in detail why the ratio of 30/40/30 is the healthiest diet for many people. There are tables in the book to help you calculate your amount of total body fat and other information you need to identify your dietary needs.

When you first look at the 30/40/30 ratio, it might seem as though there is a lot of fat there. That's misleading. Thirty percent fat sounds high, but it is often represented by a few slivers of almonds, or one macadamia nut. For example, the fat content of one typical meal is given as four teaspoons of slivered almonds. You will be eating a lot less carbohydrate, and the fact that you are eating a balanced diet will enable you to utilize the food much more efficiently.

Sorry, but premium ice cream and rich sauces don't belong in this food plan. At first you should strictly limit alcohol and sugar (in any form, including honey and maple syrup). Until you achieve balance, avoid fruit juice, dried fruit, baked beans, black-eyed peas, lima beans, potatoes, corn/popcorn, bananas, barley, rice, pasta or other heavy starches, and caffeine. Carbohydrate-dense products, such as grains, pasta, and heavy starches, are more restricted than fruits and vegetables, especially fruits and vegetables with lots of fiber. The fiber slows the rate that the carbohydrate enters the blood stream, and thus moderates the insulin response.

This is one tough diet, because if you need it, you *really* crave carbohydrates. You have to try it for only a few days before your body lets you know, "Yes, this is what you must do!" because you are attacked by whopping headaches and extreme fatigue as soon as your body begins its struggle for balance. Your excess fat will start to break down, and release large amounts of toxic substances and waste material. It is not fun. But diet alone is the treatment that works.

Fat with your meals will decrease the flow of carbohydrates into the bloodstream and decrease your "carbocraving." But you must learn to eat *moderate* amounts of fat and to cut down on the amount of carbohydrates you eat. Eat protein as part of every meal because it helps use up the fat stored in your body, as well as providing energy. When starting a meal, it is wise to eat some protein as your first course. That allows its products to reach your brain first. Exercise regularly to decrease the amount of insulin in your blood.

If you become hungry and crave sugar two to three hours after a meal, this will tell you that you probably consumed too many carbohydrates at your last meal. Be sure to drink at least eight ounces of water or a sugar-free decaffeinated beverage with each meal or snack. Remember, the breakdown products of caffeine tend to increase insulin levels.

You are probably aware that sugar can ease the symptoms of RHG in the short term, so you will be tempted to cheat. If you don't cheat, in one month you will see considerable improvement. Within two months, the RHG symptoms should be gone. When all is in harmony, your body is your best doctor. Once you are in balance it will tell you a great deal, if you listen. Learn to eat like a gourmet. Eat slowly, chew thoughtfully, and enjoy each bite. Eat less, but eat mindfully, and you will be satisfied. You may have the bad habits of a lifetime to break, but if you succeed, you will live a longer and healthier life.

You will probably find that once you are on the diet for a while, and your energy levels have increased, you will be able to afford to modify your food intake now and then. Your body will inform you when you have gone too far by a recurrence of your reactive hypoglycemia. Note that supplemental chromium seems to ease the hypoglycemia symptoms for some people (Anderson, Polansky, Bryden, et al. 1987).

NSAIDs

Another biochemical perpetuating factor that you and your doctor should consider is the possibility that you may have a malabsorptive condition in the gut, especially if you have been taking NSAIDs (nonsteroidal anti-inflammatory drugs). This malabsorptive condition is worsened if you have any vitamin and mineral insufficiencies. You may need to add vitamins and/or minerals supplements to your diet.

Oxygen

Paradoxical breathing is a major perpetuating factor that is often overlooked. *Paradoxical breathing*, also called "reverse breathing," is shallow breathing, where the belly is kept flat for fashion's sake and the movements of breathing are performed only by the chest. This causes oxygen starvation. When you inhale, your belly *should* expand, and it should go in when you exhale. Focus on breathing correctly, "belly breathing," to fill your body with life-giving oxygen that will help you to heal.

Note that air hunger may be compounded if there is an overabundance of the neurotransmitter histamine due to allergies, and other neurotransmitters are creating extra mucus or constriction in the air passages. Anything that diminishes the available oxygen to the muscles can perpetuate TrPs. This type of perpetuating factor can be present in the form of a metabolic problem, such as hypoglycemia, a deficiency, such as anemia, or even a mechanical factor, such as tight or restrictive clothing.

Infections

Infections and infestations can weaken your body and reduce its ability to recover. When you are already struggling with FMS or MPS, facing yet another illness may seem insurmountable. If you get the flu, your coping skills become stressed to the breaking point. Do everything within reason to minimize your chances of developing additional medical problems, including bacterial, viral, and/or yeast infections, and protozoal or parasitic infestations. Remember that sleep deprivation lowers your immune system's abilities to deal with infection, and, by the way, is another major perpetuating factor.

Mechanical Factors

Poor posture and poor body mechanics develop when we're not looking. When you sit typing at a keyboard, your shoulders may try to creep up around your neck. You may forget how to stand up straight. Your chest muscles may become tight because it hurts to breathe, so you hunch down. This contracts the neck muscles, which then roll the shoulders forward. Then, we develop a head-forward posture. You can almost watch the trigger points developing satellite and secondary TrPs because of this posture. Often, the effects of poor posture are cumulative. For example, a physical therapist cannot release (loosen) the neck muscles until the chest muscles (and often the shoulder muscles) have first been released.

Posture

Good posture means good posture *all the time*. This means *no* slouching—even at night when you are relaxing or watching television. Right now, take note of your body. How balanced are you? What areas of your body are feeling stressed? You can learn to relax *mindfully*, and still be fully aware of your posture. You can even learn to sleep mindfully (up to a point). For those of us with MPS, sleep posture is particularly important.

When Travell and Simons wrote the Trigger Point Manuals, they included diagrams of where pillows should be placed to help prop the body while sleeping. Unfortunately, the books were written for the treatment of localized TrPs. If you read these medical texts, each chapter deals with trigger points of a muscle or muscle grouping. It is only the very last chapter of the second volume that mentions bodywide chronic MPS. Most doctors think that bodywide chronic MPS can't happen. If it's bodywide, it must be FMS. Most doctors are wrong. When the whole body is involved, with overlapping pain patterns, it is very difficult to diagnose (and much more difficult to live with).

When you have bodywide chronic MPS, you can't lie on the unaffected side. There *is* no unaffected side. With bodywide trigger points, we learn to do a kind of sleep dance: When sleeping on our backs, we place pillows under our knees, then when we turn to the side, we shift the pillows to between our knees, often without fully waking.

Good Posture in Bed

When you lie on your back, check that your toes don't point out to the sides. That's a sign of piriformis syndrome, and sleeping that way can rotate the muscles further inside your hip, thus perpetuating the TrPs. When you make the bed, allow enough room under the top sheet for your feet. If you feel pain in your soles with your first steps in the morning, roll up a large towel and put it under the bedcovers at the foot of the bed, to help keep your feet in a neutral position.

Also, when lying on your back, try to keep your arms placed so that your hands face palms inward, toward your body, rather than palms to the bed surface, which would roll your shoulders. If you're lying on your side, avoid having your chin tucked down toward your chest, so that your neck muscles will not contract. Be patient with yourself. It takes time and effort to develop new habits—but it's worth it.

Moving Around in Bed

Be aware of how you move when you are in bed. When you turn over, roll with your head flat on the pillow, and use your arms to help you turn. Don't lift your head and "lead with it" as you roll to your side. Practice this. Turning in bed incorrectly can be a great stressor to the sternocleidomastoid (SCM) muscles in your neck and head, and it is a common perpetuating factor. Ask your physical therapist to teach you

- how to turn in bed

- how to get up from lying down, and

- how to get up from sitting

without stressing your body. These movements are called "body mechanics." (If we don't learn the proper ways to move, our bodies will need mechanics.) You may also find that sore spots develop if you rest one part of your body on top of another part. The places just below the knees on the inner side of the legs can become very sore. They aren't TrPs, but they do hurt. (For a discussion about sleep interruptions as mechanical perpetuating factors, see the section on sleep in chapter 16.)

Restorative Sleep

You need sleep. Not just eight hours of sleep, but sufficient *restorative* sleep. To heal, you must wake up feeling that you have slept well and deeply, *not* as if trained elephants have spent the night flamenco dancing on your body. If you were awake many times during the night, if you had no dreams, or if you woke up more tired than you were when you went to sleep, you did *not* get restorative sleep. You and your doctor must work together to find out which medications or combination of medications will provide you with this blessing that so many people take for granted.

The Right Bed

What constitutes a comfortable bed is different for each one of us. Some require a firm mattress, a bed board, or a futon. Others need a waterbed or an air mattress. Some, as in the story of "The Princess and the Pea," find even a waterbed or an air mattress too hard. Finding the right pillow can also be a challenge. Because of neck trigger points, many of us have hardly any curvature in our necks. The standard cervical pillow doesn't work for us. Some people prefer a small pillow that is soft enough to allow them to mold it the way they want it. Some use a water pillow. Often, when we find a bed and a pillow that work well, our body changes, and we must begin the search again. It is a continuing trial and error procedure to find what works best.

Physical Traumas

Previous surgeries and previous physical traumas can create adhesions and weak areas that become targets for trigger point formation. As your body tries to compensate for extra tissue or lack of mobility in tissue, these areas become perpetuating factors. Any physical trauma can cause myofascial adhesions. I've observed that people with FMS tend to develop all sorts of tissue overgrowths as well. Trigger points that form in surgical scars often have a burning or prickling pain that can be avoided by intracutaneous trigger point injections of 0.5 percent procaine along the incision line before surgery (Travell and Simons 1983, 19).

> **Sleep-Aid Alert**
>
> I have found that there is a subset of us who react oddly to Benadryl, Ultram, Pamelor, Paxil, and some other medications that usually product drowsiness. We become wired, more alert rather than sleepy. Ten mg of Paxil helps me to fall asleep, but only if I take it in the morning. Otherwise it would keep me up all night. I shouldn't take Benadryl at all. I can explain what it does to me only in Eastern terms. It "rattles the chi." I don't like what it does at all. But, for those who can tolerate it, it is a marvelous, safe, and effective sleep aid. For the rest of us, taking these medications at night would become an additional perpetuating factor.

Behavioral Factors

Particular behaviors, whether voluntary or involuntary, can be perpetuating factors. Some perpetuating actions, such as chewing gum, may seem harmless, but you can pay for them with the formation of new TrPs. Breathing through your mouth, constantly using facial expressions such as squinting, wearing ill-fitting or rigid-soled shoes, and living with poorly designed furniture can all contribute to the stresses on your body. Consider the following list of behaviors:

- Do you carry a heavy shoulder bag?
- Do you smoke?
- Do you drink too much alcohol?

- Do you stay up too late and get up too early?

- Do you keep irregular hours?

- Do you work rotating shifts?

- Do you perform repetitious exercise or work?

- Do you procrastinate and then double your workload to catch up?

- Do you experience a great amount of stress and negativity in your life?

- Do you promise to do things for others and then half-kill yourself trying to fulfill your promises?

- Do you continually push yourself beyond your limits?

These are all behavioral stressors that you should try to change because they can be perpetuating factors that worsen your illness.

The Good Sport Syndrome

By nature, many of us are helping, giving people. We like to lend a hand, even when both of our own hands are tied behind our backs. This is the good-sport syndrome, which can be damaging to your health. We must learn how to cultivate a sense of enlightened self-interest. We tend to overextend ourselves when we feel well, and then we crash. Such extreme fluctuations are a clear warning of being out of balance, and being out of balance can only worsen your condition. I know this is one of my biggest perpetuating factors.

Asymmetrical Bodies

Physical imbalance can also be a perpetuating factor. Perhaps you were born with one leg shorter than the other, or one side of your pelvis smaller. You may have proportionally short upper arms, so that when you sit, you must tilt sideways to lean one side on an armrest. You may have short lower legs, so that most chairs automatically cut off the circulation of your hamstring muscles. Imbalance can even result from aging; our bodies can wear out unevenly, much as our teeth do.

Be sure that you and your physical therapist consider *both* sides of your body when doing stretching and bodywork. You may have active TrPs only on one side of your body, but both sides need work. The body is designed to be a functional whole. Remember that, and it will reward you with better performance.

Anything that causes you to hold your muscles in a tightened or unnatural condition for a period of time can also be a perpetuating factor. Anxiety, grief, chronic pain, depression, repetitive action, dental work, needle work, or constant use of a computer mouse are examples of stressors that perpetuate trigger points.

If you consistently look only in one direction, the muscles of your eyes may develop TrPs. When you are doing close work, be sure to look around you every once in a while. Look up and down, and then roll your eyes, stretching the eye muscles first up and then to each corner of the eye. Then roll your eyes clockwise and counterclockwise.

Obesity, Morton's foot, or FMS/MPS foot (see Starlanyl and Copeland 1996), overwork, immobility (even immobility caused by prolonged bedrest or casts), and inappropriate physical therapy are also common perpetuators of TrPs. Inappropriate physical therapy, such as work hardening, weight training, and attempting in any way to strengthen a muscle with active TrPs, is a form of malpractice. Travell and Simons have documented this in their texts (1983; 1992), and there is a growing volume of literature concerning myofascial trigger points, and yet this preventable perpetuating factor is more common than ever. There are intelligent and enterprising attorneys who are discovering the works of Travell and Simons, and I hope this book educates more. Sadly, it may only be after losing lawsuits that some doctors and physical therapists start learning about Myofascial Pain Syndrome. They will then have to face the formidable fact that many of them have been torturing patients for some time. That's tough to take, but nothing like what their patients have had to take. The abuse must end, and if it takes the courtroom to educate these "experts," so be it.

The Effects of Change

We are creatures of habit. As such, we don't tolerate change well. Even as slight a change as the switch from Standard Time to Daylight Savings Time can affect FMS and MPS temporarily. If you live in a time zone with seasonal changes, you may notice that your health declines in the spring and the fall, when there are more rapidly changing extremes of temperature, moisture, and barometric pressures. At all times, consider your clothing as part of your preventative medicine. Dress in layers and be especially mindful of drafts. Avoid sitting under air conditioners or heater ducts.

The Effects of Travel

When we travel, our ability to tolerate change is often sorely tested. New schedules, the immobility of travel itself, new foods, new surroundings, and being without your "life support team" can be devastating. They all add to sensory overload and your brain may not be able to keep up with the rapid new input. You may find yourself in flare after every trip. If you travel for a living, your job may be the number one perpetuating factor that you need to change.

Pollution

The increasing burden of pollution is a perpetuating factor that requires us all to work together to remedy. No matter how carefully we eat, move, and live, the growing amounts of toxins in the air, water, and soil affect our lives. As the Earth becomes less healthy, so shall we all. It is in your own self-interest to become an environmentalist, and to become aware of your impact on nature, and it on you. The story of life is a closed circle. Be mindful of it.

Think about these perpetuating factors and analyze those that have an impact on you. Then, think about ways to eliminate or minimize their influence.

Misinformation: The Hidden Perpetuating Factor

A great science fiction writer once said that you should never attribute to malice that which you can lay at the feet of ignorance. If ignorance is bliss, there is a vast number of

If Ignorance Is Bliss, Some Doctors Must Be Ecstatic.

Misinformation can be a real killer. You may have fought for years to educate your family and friends about the true nature of fibromyalgia. Then someone may come along with a newspaper article that says, "Fibromyalgia just means achy muscles, and if you put it out of your mind it will disappear of its own in a few weeks." A nationally syndicated doctor actually said this. He was still saying that even after I sent him an information packet. How many people has he damaged with his misinformation?

fibromyalgia "experts" wallowing in blissful delight, unaware of the misery that they are spreading. It's time to root them out. We've been victimized long enough, and I can't resist challenging the misleading and misguided messages of these minions of the Evil Empire. Like Jedi Knights, let's unleash our light sabers and banish phases like "It's All In Your Head." It is time for our dream of justice to become a reality. For that to come about, we must expose these "experts" for what they are. Consider the following examples of harmful misinformation:

> Fibromyalgia is stiffness and pain felt in the fibrous tissues, usually deep within the muscles. . . . It is common, especially in people past middle age, and usually clears up on its own. Hot baths and aspirin or other nonsteroidal anti-inflammatory drugs should help relieve pain.
>
> From *The American Medical Association Family Medical Guide* (1994, 579; CD ROM 1995)

This kind of misinformation creates what we sometimes call "Fibromyopia" on the Internet. It is common among doctors, employers, attorneys, Social Security Administration workers, insurance representatives, and, all too often, friends and relatives. It is caused by an inability to see beyond the fact that we *look* just fine. Such misinformation, in turn, leads to the IAIYH diagnosis ("It's All In Your Head"), which, in turn, causes no end of misery to those of us with FMS and MPS.

Some of the misinformation is more insidious. For example, the *Merck Manual* (1992) under "Fibromyalgia," lists "Myofascial Pain Syndrome; Fibromyositis" as subheadings (page 1369). In chapter 1 of this book and in my previous book (1996), I went to great lengths to explain that FMS and MPS are entirely different conditions, with different causes and different treatments. When I wrote Merck about this and cited many references from respected medical journals, they replied that *their* experts believed FMS and MPS to be the same condition. I like the *Merck Manual,* but I hope that they aren't as misinformed about other conditions. Doctors and researchers depend on them for the facts.

Another resource, my 1995 edition of *Stedman's Medical Dictionary,* doesn't even have the word "fibromyalgia" listed. It does list "fibrositis" (page 650) but defines it as an "inflammation of fibrous tissue." Is it any wonder that so many doctors are stumbling in the dark?

Trying to correct this misinformation can be tremendously frustrating. We aren't going to change the medical establishment overnight. But you should understand that every time you educate one more person, even in your own household, you are taking a stand. With every data sheet you hand out, you will strike a blow against ignorance. By helping someone else figure out what is going wrong with his or her body and mind, you may be saving a life. There are an awful lot of us with FMS and MPS out here.

Once you're armed with the facts in this book, you can do a little more Jedi Knight work of you own. Ask your friends and relatives to cut out such misinformed clippings and send them to you. Make sure they include the date, name, and address of the publication. Write to the publisher, indicating the misinformation and supplying the correction. Send a copy to the Fibromyalgia Network. Let's get these uneducated people out of the misinformation business. Together, we can make a difference.

Recent Examples of Misinformation

In the Dark Ages, misinformation was rampant. Gossip spread from mouth to mouth like the plague. In these days of the information superhighway, there is even more information, and it spreads like wildfire in a high wind.

The following examples of misinformation are from a web page called "Know Your Enemy," written by Moira A. Smith, one of our FIBROM-L FMily in Australia. Moira has kindly allowed their use here. Don't take them personally! Remember, they have been exposed on the Internet, and are now being exposed to you. Being exposed to any toxic substance may cause you to feel pretty bad, but it's so much better to know when there are toxins in your environment, so that you can protect yourself against them.

These are from the website "Chronic Pain Assessment and Treatment" by Alan Brandis, Ph.D., of Atlanta Area Psychological Associates PC.

- "... as painful as pain is, it has covert emotional bonuses and rewards...."

- "Taking medicine for pain can also be a factor that prolongs and maintains the chronic pain condition."

These are from the article "Pain Is a Blind Guide in Injury Management" by Kelly Patrick Flannigan, M.D., on website Summit Injury Management Inc. (This one is positively malignant!)

- "... recognize sickness as a social role."

- "[Pain] is the main reason for voluntary or physician-advised restriction of activity and occupation of the 'sick' role."

- "[In some] cases ... the physical disorder provides an incomplete explanation for the individual's occupation of the sick role ... this is particularly true when the person seems unable or unwilling to 'get well.'"

Some of the "abnormal or inappropriate illness behavior" listed here are "whole leg pain, tailbone pain, whole leg numbness, whole leg giving way, never free of pain, intolerance of

> In my opinion, the only reason the Arthritis Foundation is interested in FMS patients is because they are potential donation dollars. Let me explain. In my town, the Arthritis Support Group has about twelve people who attend per month. The FMS group usually has over a hundred. It doesn't take a genius to understand what is going on here.
>
> —A FMily member

> A few years ago after I was diagnosed with "fibrositis" and trying to explain to my family what was happening to me, a doctor had a short letter in his newspaper column about FMS. In it he stated that the pain was indeed real, but that the symptoms improved with time and would eventually clear up. I was so excited thinking things would soon improve.
>
> —A FMily member

treatments, ER visits." He mentions "bizarre, inconsistent, or physiologically impossible disorders of gait, posture or balance." This guy sounds like he never heard of trigger points. We pay for his ignorance, which he spreads around like an avid gardener fertilizing his crops. After I read this article, I felt violated and, somehow, dirty.

These are from the website "Chronic Pain Study" by T. J. Murray O. C., FRCPC, FACP.

- "Chronic pain does not respond well to analgesics and narcotics and is resistant to most traditional therapies for pain."

- "Although less than ten percent of all pain patients go on to become chronic, the chronic care patients account for three quarters of the overall costs of health care and compensation for pain. . . ."

This is supposed to be worthy of note? As if someone in pain for sixty years isn't going to spend more for care than someone who recovers after being in pain for three weeks? I believe that if the pain were adequately treated, the costs would be much less.

- ". . . overuse of analgesics and other medications often lead to dependence and addiction but little pain relief in these patients."

- "Signs of distress such as 'overly dramatic verbal expressions of pain,' 'hostility,' 'steady deterioration of symptoms,' and 'frequent emergency room attendance' will be interpreted as suggesting that 'complex psychosocial factors' are contributing to your pain, rather than an indication that the program is inappropriate for you." And, God forbid, that the *doctor* has made an error, and you are getting worse because of it!

- "Workers with chronic pain should be strongly urged to return to work almost immediately. . . ."

- "Pain alone is an insufficient cause to delay resumption of work."

This author fails to realize that a person experiencing the kind of mind-numbing pain we sometimes have would be a danger to self as well as others.

Reading these articles was hard. I was acutely aware of the damage they could do. Moira's website gave me an education about attitudes we are up against, and the proliferation of misinformation on the Internet concerning chronic invisible illnesses.

There is a danger to the "rehabilitation model" of pain management. This has been taken to extremes in many cases, backed up by quotes from medical references that are quite frightening and can be terribly damaging. This model suggests that because your pain persists longer than the six months allowed for tissue to heal, and has *no observable* cause, there must be "psychosocial" reasons for your "pain behavior" and your choosing to play the "sick role."

The thought that people are being told "pain behavior" rather than the pain itself is the problem is frightening. What Moira calls "Blame the Victim." On the surface, these articles seem to be sympathetic. What they are, in essence is *pathetic*. The principle of "Do No Harm" is violated once again, and so are we. As Moira puts it, ". . . don't expect to be prescribed adequate pain medication by these guys. . . . Instead, they will help you unlearn your "pain behaviors (grimacing, groaning etc.) so that you can become a psychological healthy adult once more, ready to resume your place in the economic system." Such instruction may make *them* feel better. But it erodes our self-esteem and our support systems, and does nothing to help us toward healing. I have one thing to tell these misguided doctors. *Get Real!* There! That sure made *me* feel better! Thank you, Moira, for exposing these people and giving us a chance to answer this attack on the quality of our lives. If you are connected to the World Wide Web, drop by her website at http://www.spirit.net.au/~masmith/pain/enemy.htm and say hello.

4

Coexisting Conditions

General Information

Uncommon presentations of common conditions are always more likely to occur than common presentations of uncommon conditions. It often seems that someone may have many different medical problems, and yet they all turn out to be part of the FMS/MPS Complex. For example, neither fibromyalgia (FMS) nor Myofascial Pain Syndrome (MPS) is inflammatory, but when trigger points (TrPs) cause sufficient contraction of the muscles so that bones are pulled out of alignment, the mechanical stress *can* cause secondary inflammation of the joint areas. Of course, other factors may be involved as well.

It is important for you to be familiar with some of the illnesses that frequently coexist with FMS and/or MPS. Both FMS and MPS often appear with another disorder, and enhance the symptoms of that disorder. If TrPs recur, in spite of appropriate therapy for known perpetuating factors, there is a hidden perpetuating factor. If in doubt, check it out.

This chapter on coexisting conditions is not meant to be complete. To list and explain all the conditions that can occur with FMS and MPS would be a book in itself, and a very large one at that. Some of the more common coexisting conditions, however, are presented here with very brief explanations.

Arthritis

Arthritis, in all its forms, is inflammatory and can cause the development of trigger points secondary to the arthritic inflammation. Arthritis will also worsen FMS. You may not be able to get rid of the arthritis, but obtaining appropriate therapy for the FMS and for the trigger points will lessen your pain load considerably.

Carpal Tunnel Syndrome

Carpal Tunnel Syndrome is a condition of wrist pain and soreness and weakness of the thumb, caused by pressure on the median nerve. It is often caused by repetitive motion stress. These same symptoms are frequently the result of subscapularis TrPs. Remember that TrPs can entrap nerves. Before considering any surgery for carpal tunnel, a check for shoulder, arm, and hand trigger points should be made.

Chronic Fatigue Immune Deficiency Syndrome

Chronic Fatigue Immune Deficiency Syndrome (CFIDS) is characterized by a history of extreme exhaustion that lasts at least six months, but it is much more than that. People with this condition often want to sleep all the time. Exhaustion can be brought on by the slightest effort. Aches and fever, sore throat, and an inability to concentrate are usually part of CFIDS, as well as Irritable Bowel Syndrome, frequent infections, and a dysfunctional HPA axis. CFIDS often begins with a severe flu-like illness. When the fever and aches diminish, they leave behind disabling fatigue, immune dysfunction, and a disrupted neuroendocrine system.

As with fibromyalgia, there are many subsets of CFIDS and, in some of these subsets, the two syndromes appear to overlap. It is wise to remember that research in these two conditions is in its infancy. More is unknown about them than is known. Many illnesses are classified together as part of a family of neurotransmitter disorders. However, not all neurotransmitter disorders are the same.

There is a group of patients that meets the general requirements for both fibromyalgia and chronic fatigue, but I have observed that chronic fatigue is often misdiagnosed in cases of FMS and/or MPS. Either the sleep disruption that results from the neurotransmitter problems of FMS or the extreme pain of MPS can cause the fatigue. Even one night of sleep loss will depress the immune system (Irwin, McClintick, Costlow, et al. 1996; Moldofsky 1995).

In cases of FMS and MPS, however, appropriate therapy results in the elimination of the fatigue. If researchers would become familiar with Travell and Simons' texts on MPS (1983; 1992), many of the symptoms classed together with FMS and CFIDS would be recognized as those of MPS. Then these symptoms could be properly treated, and patients and doctors would be better able to deal with the condition(s) that remain.

Depression

Depression can cause overwhelming sadness most of the time, as well as the inability to enjoy those things that once made life worth living. Someone suffering from depression might be overwhelmed by lethargy, confusion, poor memory, sleep problems, and appetite changes. It is natural to feel grief when you have a chronic pain problem, but that is not the same as major depression, which can be a life-threatening condition, especially when coupled with a chronic physical illness. It should never be taken lightly either by you or by your physician.

Diabetes Mellitus

Diabetes mellitus is a disorder of carbohydrate metabolism, where the body cannot create enough insulin, or use what insulin is made. It can occur abruptly in childhood, but the onset of the disease in adults (type II diabetes) is gradual. Some of the common symptoms are extreme thirst, itching, hunger, weakness, and production of a great deal of urine. I believe that type II diabetes is often a result of reactive hypoglycemia, which results from an inherited tendency as well as from a high carbohydrate diet (see "Reactive Hypoglycemia" in chapter 3).

HIV and AIDS

HIV and AIDS have swelled the ranks of people with FMS/MPS. One study found probable or definite FMS in 41 percent of HIV patients with musculoskeletal pain and 11 percent of *all* HIV-infected patients (Simms, Zerbini, Ferrante, et al. 1992).

In all the AIDS patients I've seen with probable FMS, MPS is present, as well. I have also found trigger points in every other AIDS patient I have seen. This is vitally important, as appropriate treatment of the TrPs can dramatically improve the quality of life for these patients. Anything that can accomplish this with so little effort must not be ignored.

Hypoglycemia

Hypoglycemia is generally defined as a deficiency of sugar in the blood. A type of hypoglycemia occurs in FMS where there is an insufficient amount of *usable* sugar in the blood. This is called reactive hypoglycemia, and it occurs in response to a high carbohydrate intake. There is no reason for your doctor to deny the existence of reactive hypoglycemia. Check out the following references (Anderson 1992; Anderson, Polansky, Bryden, et al. 1987; Cryer 1996, 1994, 1993; Eisinger, Plantamura and Ayavou 1994; Fernstrom 1994, 1991; Genter and Ipp 1994; Genter 1994; Hvidberg, Fanelli, Hershey, et al. 1996; Leonetti, Foniciello, Iozzo, et al. 1996; Leonetti, Morviducci, Giaccari, et al. 1992; McCarty 1996; McCrimmon, Deary, Huntly, et al. 1996; Piotrowski 1997; Reaven, Brand, Chen, et al. 1993; Rokas, Maurikakis, Iliopoulou, et al. 1992). Also see "Reactive Hypoglycemia" in chapter 3.

Hypothyroid

Being hypothyroid can cause people to be more susceptible to developing trigger points. Thyroid hormones influence growth, energy production, and energy consumption. Low-normal thyroid often escapes detection because "low normal" is not a worrisome condition, but when it is coupled with FMS and/or MPS, the added burden is one you don't need. Some current research shows that many patents with FMS respond to T3 (Triiodothyronine) thyroid supplements (see "New and Experimental Treatments" in chapter 9). Many hypothyroid symptoms are the same as the symptoms of FMS and/or MPS, and combine to multiply the effects. Hypothyroid patients are usually cold most of the time, especially in their hands and feet. Some are intolerant of heat as well, and don't sweat normally. These patients are stiff and ache all over, and often experience substantial hair loss.

Hypermobility

Hypermobility is characterized by joint relaxation that allows the muscles to stretch beyond their normal range of motion. If you have this problem, stretching techniques should be avoided. Often, TrPs are found in muscles that cross hypermobile joints. If you suspect you are "double-jointed" or hypermobile, discuss this with your physician and your physical therapist. Your physical therapist must be careful never to "stretch through a joint."

Lupus Myositis

Lupus myositis, also called discoid lupus, is a disorder that is confined to the skin. There is a scaling, red-pink or brown rash, often taking the shape of a butterfly on the face, although it is not limited to that area. This rash is very photosensitive, and these patients must avoid the sun. Some FMS patients also have this "butterfly rash," although it may result from the "toxic acid sweat" that is a symptom of FMS.

Systemic Lupus Erythematosus

Systemic Lupus Erythematosus (SLE) can attack many organ systems. It is a connective tissue disorder and like rheumatoid arthritis it is considered an autoimmune disorder. This means that your body attacks itself. Neither FMS nor MPS is an autoimmune condition. SLE can also cause a butterfly rash, but all of the connective tissue can be involved as well, not just the skin. There can be involvement with any of many organ systems, producing a host of symptoms. It isn't unusual for people with FMS to test positive for SLE.

Multiple Chemical Sensitivities

Multiple chemical sensitivities may have a tendency to develop with FMS. The immune system's weakening, which is caused by lack of sleep, is probably crucial here, along with what is called the "leaky gut syndrome." We often take many medications, such as NSAIDS (nonsteroidal anti-inflammatory drugs), that cause our gastric lining to become more permeable. This allows larger than normal foreign proteins to enter the body, which then develops antigens to combat the foreign proteins. The patient becomes sensitized to one chemical after an exposure.

Then, other foods and environmental irritants that were previously tolerated begin to provoke allergic or sensitivity reactions. The signs and symptoms are many and varied. They include fatigue, headaches, muscle aches, coughing, watery eyes, and tremors. If this condition advances to the state where nearly everything is intolerable to the patient, it is considered multiple chemical sensitivity. At this state, the patient may be unable to tolerate clothing and many foods, and may need to drink specifically filtered water. Today, many support groups and resources are forming as multiple chemical sensitivity becomes more identifiable and well-known. For specific information, contact the National Coalition for the Chemically Injured at 2499 Virginia Avenue, Suite C501, Washington, DC 20037.

Multiple Sclerosis

Multiple sclerosis (MS) is caused by the breakdown of certain central nervous system (CNS) tissues that occur in multiple, random sites. The fatty sheath that surrounds some of the nerves is called myelin. In MS, this sheath becomes damaged and neurotransmitter information is lost or scrambled. There is cellular overgrowth at the damaged sites, and hardened or "sclerotic" areas result. Multiple sclerosis is not related to FMS or MPS, but, as MS causes symptoms, those symptoms may initiate and perpetuate trigger points. These will aggravate FMS. Using a wheelchair, or other relative immobility, will perpetuate TrPs.

Post-Polio Syndrome

Post-Polio Syndrome is also called Post-Polio Muscular Atrophy (PPMA). It occurs many years after recovery from an initial episode of polio. Post-Polio Muscular Atrophy causes muscle weakness and recurrent paralysis, which can lead to respiratory paralysis, with slowly progressing muscle wasting. It is often mistaken for FMS, but life-threatening respiratory complications of Post-Polio Syndrome may develop, so, clearly, a proper diagnosis is essential.

Raynaud's Phenomenon

Raynaud's phenomenon is a condition where the fingers and/or toes turn white, then blue, and then red. This can occur during periods of cold or emotional stress. Numbness, tingling, and burning may also be present at these times. Raynaud's phenomenon is common in both FMS and MPS. The dilation of the blood vessels is governed by neurotransmitters, and in FMS this is dysfunctional. Some TrPs cause blood and lymph vessel entrapment. These various conditions can work together to multiply your misery.

Reflex Sympathetic Dystrophy Syndrome

Reflex Sympathetic Dystrophy Syndrome, also called RSDS or causalgia, is a disorder of the sympathetic nervous system that causes irregular blood supply to the affected area, which can be the hand, foot, knee, hip, or shoulder. It causes severe pain, often burning in nature. It often follows an injury, including surgery. In many cases there is no apparent cause. FMS and/or MPS is often misdiagnosed as RSDS.

Seasonal Affective Disorder

Seasonal Affective Disorder (SAD) is moderated by light. In northern areas in the winter, people with SAD become sleepy and easily fatigued, and have little ambition or drive. These feelings disappear in the summer, or when vacationing

Trigger Points Run Amok

My trigger point specialist, Hal Blatman, feels that RSDS is caused by trigger points running amok and hypersensitizing the sympathetic nervous system. He divides the RSDS patients into "hot" and "cold," depending on their symptoms. The "hot" patients get medications to calm the pain, and treatment for trigger points. The cold form receives more focus on TrP work. He is often able to save the tissue structures and restore function with these treatments.

in areas of greater sunshine. Light therapy often works well for this. Seasonal affective disorder may belong to the family of neurotransmitter disorders. About one-quarter of my local FMS/MPS group has SAD.

Temporomandibular Joint (TMJ) Problems

Temporomandibular joint (TMJ) problems are symptoms, not an illness, and often occur as a result of TrPs. There is severe pain in the area of the jaw joint, with a clicking, crunching noise of the jaw that accompanies chewing. This is often accompanied by ringing and/or itching of the ears. Sometimes there is some hearing loss. Temporomandibular joint dysfunction often starts the trigger point cascade that eventually can cover your whole body. If the TrPs aren't promptly treated, the bite will be off balance and the joint of the jaw may begin to deteriorate.

Yeast Infections

Yeast infections often coexist with FMS and MPS. One of the best books I have found explaining this, as well as the chronic fatigue connection, is *From Fatigued to Fantastic* by Jacob Teitelbaum (1996). Any infection can become a perpetuating factor of TrPs. Fungi are opportunistic organisms. That means they will take over any area that is made comfortable for them. A body with an impaired immune system is a prime target for fungi. It is common medical knowledge that any infection will adversely affect someone already struggling with other chronic conditions. Why the medical establishment has resisted the fact that chronic yeast infection will also impact on someone with FMS and/or MPS is beyond my comprehension.

Vulvodynia

Vulvodynia, or vulvar pain, is pain that some women experience in their external sexual parts, although often there are sharp pains in the vaginal area as well. Some of this may be due to trigger points, and some to causes as yet unknown. It is important to know that there is help. Contact the Vulvar Pain Foundation, Post Office Drawer 177, Graham, NC 27253, or call (336) 256-0704.

Conclusion

There are many more conditions that coexist with FMS and MPS. Remember that they all may be considered perpetuating factors for both FMS and MPS, and co-contributors to your body's burdens. Whatever you and your medical team can do to alleviate those burdens will raise your quality of life.

5

Chronic Pain Management

Chronic Pain: The Invisible Dragon

When we are children we are allowed to express ourselves when we feel pain, but as we mature, we are taught to disregard it as much as we can. We are led to believe that pain somehow lessens us. The way that pain is treated in television and movies adds to this altered perception.

Yet if medical practitioners were more truthful, perhaps we couldn't bear it. How would you feel if your dentist, instead of saying, "This will hurt a little," actually said, "This will probably hurt a lot. In fact, knowing what I know, if I were in your shoes, I'd run out of here right now." We'd probably all be wearing artificial choppers by age twenty-five.

Pain is an integral part of the body/mind connection. It can become an interface of such misery and despair that it can turn into a kind of black hole which destroys your whole personality and devours the quality of your life in the process. There is growing scientific evidence that prolonged pain is an aggressive, physically destructive disease. With chronic pain, harmful biochemical changes take place in the body that can even interfere with gene expression (Dubner 1991a; Dubner 1991b; Liebeskind 1991).

We know that in fibromyalgia (FMS) there are deficiencies in the ability to modulate pain (Lautenbacher and Rollman 1997). This means that many of the ways a healthy body has to moderate pain signals (once the initiating pain source has been dealt with) are not available to those with FMS.

Chronic nonmalignant pain is any noncancerous pain that lasts more than six months. It is persistent and relentless. The body reacts differently to chronic pain states than to acute

Nothing Is Impossible for Those Who Don't Have to Do It.

Recently, my husband and I saw the movie *Starship Troopers*. There is a scene where one of the female leads has her shoulder pierced by a "bug" claw. The bugs are the size of a medium dragon (or a small tank). Once the claw (and the bug) have been removed, the heroine continues to perform heroic actions. She isn't slowed down one bit by pain. My husband insisted, "No way! Nobody with that kind of injury can keep on going like nothing happened." I replied, "You still don't understand FMS/MPS Complex at all." Life goes on.

pain, including producing *less* in the way of natural opioids. "Chronic pain ... may be considered a disease state" (Gritchnik and Ferrante 1991). One study, in 1996, stated that chronic nonmalignant pain costs the American economy $40 billion a year (Sheehan, McKay, Ryan, et al. 1996). By now, it probably costs a lot more. Why aren't we doing more to prevent it?

In the United States, as in many other countries, chronic pain conditions are not adequately treated. This gives rise to needless suffering and the growing popularity of the "Kevorkian system" of pain control. According to one study on successfully completed suicides motivated by chronic pain (Fishbain, Goldberg, Rosomoff, et al. 1991), the needs of chronic pain sufferers are *not* adequately met. As one researcher put it, "Long-term outcome for the majority of patients with fibromyalgia is sufficiently disappointing so that most patients can be considered to have 'resistant' disease" (Wilke 1995).

Chronic pain can destroy the quality of life, as well as life itself. Pain costs employers millions of dollars a year in missed work, below-par performances, expensive hospitalizations and trips to the ER, suicide attempts, depressions, and overdoses on drugs and alcohol. What's it going to take to educate the personnel of the medical establishment?

Chronic Pain and the Medical Establishment

Medical tools to treat chronic pain successfully are available. Unfortunately, the road to these tools is strewn with obstacles placed there by people fortunate enough to be ignorant of the devastation chronic pain causes. We must remove those obstacles. It is remarkable how difficult it is to train doctors so that they have a working knowledge of Myofascial Pain Syndrome (MPS), and yet many *patients* can see the trigger points in other patients. Members of a support group will say, "Her doctor says she has fibromyalgia, but she has trigger points. Just look at the way she moves her shoulders!"

In medicine, there is a natural aversion to the study of chronic pain. Most doctors—and the medical establishment as a whole—feel that they have failed us if we don't get well in a predictable fashion. Chronic pain patients—and terminal patients—are often ignored. We're written off. We don't fit into the health care system. We are their failures. This often makes *us* feel like failures. The very people who require the most support from the medical system are those who generally get the least support.

In order to provide adequate pain control, doctors (and others in the medical establishment) must become trained in the realities of FMS and MPS. Most patients with FMS/MPS Complex will have to remain on pain medication to optimize the quality of their lives. Yet some doctors still adamantly refuse to prescribe pain medication for their patients. And their patients get worse and worse.

Yet evidence shows that, if the proper interventions are put into place while FMS and MPS are developing, the full-blown stages can be avoided. "Early and effective intervention in focal pain states could reduce the chances of developing full-blown FMS" (Burckhardt, Clark, Campbell, et al. 1995). We know from Travell and Simons that adequate trigger point treatment prevents full-blown MPS. Unfortunately, most people do not get the care they require. Again, I have to blame this on the inadequacies of medical education. It's common knowledge that only a small percentage of medical schools require chronic pain management—or any pain management at all—as part of the curriculum.

Diagnostic Uncertainty

Chronic pain is often poorly treated and undertreated because of diagnostic uncertainty. Insurance companies and legal systems demand objective proof before they will reimburse for treatment. But pain perception is sensory—not measurable. At least, not yet. Janet Travell teaches that, above all, doctors must believe that their patients hurt as much and in the ways that they say they do. She states that to take a good medical history, the physician must first be willing to believe what the patient says. And some things must be believed in—taken on good faith—before they can actually be seen.

Dr. Travell tells a story about a surgeon suffering from nerve entrapment. She treated him and he told her, "How strange it is that until you treated me, I *never* saw a patient with nerve entrapment due to trigger points." Since his own treatment, he encounters patients with nerve entrapment caused by trigger points frequently.

Natural Checks and Balances

The body has many ways to enhance or dampen pain in its own system of checks and balances. Emotion, attention, and motivation can affect the perception of pain. Anxiety and apprehension may enhance and intensify pain (Yunus 1992). One of the mechanisms that seems to take place with fibromyalgia is that the pain perception system in the body becomes hypersensitive to stimuli, such as pain. (Sorensen, Graven-Neilsen, Henriksson, et al. 1998; McDermid, Rollman, McCain 1996). It can even become so hyperexcitable that it reacts to normally nonpainful stimuli by feeling pain. This is called allodynia.

Allodynia causes the central nervous system (CNS) to change its response pattern, with the result that nonnoxious substances and stimuli cause pain. It is thought that at least part of this is due to excess substance P, a peptide, in the spinal fluid (Russell 1996). Presently, there is a new class of drugs in clinical trials. Called substance P antagonists, they are powerful anti-inflammatories, which offer hope for better pain control in the future (Sjolund, Sollevi, Segerdahl, et al. 1997).

Sometimes, Only a Poem Can Express the Feeling.

I wrote to Dr. Kevorkian and sent him information about FMS and MPS, but have to date received no acknowledgment. I can understand why someone thinks longingly of suicide when pain becomes unbearable. I've been there. At those times, my entire being seems to be reflected in the T. S. Eliot line, "I should have been a pair of ragged claws scuttling across silent seas."

Drugs and Pain

Drugs can be diverted to illegal purposes, true. And addiction can happen, although it is rare, especially once doctors learn precisely what addiction is (see chapter 8, "Medications: Perceptions and Realities"). It's time for courageous doctors to face the truth and to reexamine their knowledge of and attitude toward drug addiction, and then to change their ways. It's time for enlightened doctors to say, "Yes, we've been needlessly cruel to our patients because we didn't understand. Now we are ready to treat you the way you deserve."

At the 1998 San Antonio Focus on Pain Seminar, I. Jon Russell said that fibromyalgia could be considered "chronic, widespread allodynia." ("Fibromyalgia Syndrome: New Insights from the Clinic and the Laboratory." Presented March 13, 1998.) Pain can be protective, but not when it can't be turned off. It is not protective when it is the response to a stimulus that is not dangerous or harmful to the body.

Untreated or inadequately treated pain can have profoundly negative physiological effects on the body, including the release of stress hormones, impaired immune responses, altered respiratory patterns, and cough suppression (Hitchcock, Ferrell and McCaffery 1994). On the other hand, aggressive prevention and treatment of pain have demonstrated significant positive health benefits for patients (Reidenberg and Portenoy 1994; Jones 1996).

The Origins of Chronic Pain

Pain was created by nature as a vital danger signal—a warning of damage. The brain gives pain priority over other senses and feelings, blotting out the rest of the world, and making it very hard for those of us who are told to "learn to live with it." Today, finally, a few medical schools have begun to teach that pain is another vital sign to be charted, not something to belittle (McCaffrey and Ferrell 1997; Portenoy, Dole, Joseph, et al. 1997).

Patients often find the nervous system confusing because there are so many ways it can be "divided up" and categorized. One way to understand the nervous system is to study it in two parts—the central nervous system, which basically consists of the spinal cord and the brain, and the peripheral nervous system, which are all the nerves that lie outside the brain and spinal cord.

Pain is a dynamic phenomenon that can cause both transient and long-lasting changes to take place in both the peripheral and the central nervous systems. We once thought that the entire nervous system stayed constant and didn't change. A given stimuli would produce a certain reaction. Now we know that the nervous system can change its settings. This ability to adapt and remold itself is called "plasticity," which is similar to the use of the term "plastic" in plastic surgery. The implications of nervous system plasticity are changing the face of pain management, and none too quickly at that (McQuay and Dickenson 1990).

Types of Chronic Pain

Most people are not aware that there are many different types of chronic pain. People with FMS and MPS experience pain resulting from a variety of different mechanisms (Sorensen, Bengtsson, Ahlner, et al. 1997). Some researchers think that people with FMS/MPS have a reduced ability to filter out pain, both at the spinal cord and the brain.

People with FMS also have a neuromuscular hyperexcitability, which increases the pain load. Not only do we have central nervous system hypersensitization due to plasticity, but our peripheral nervous system—the nerves that go all the way out to the skin—also becomes irritated (Bennett and Jacobsen 1994). We also have a problem with decreased collagen cross-linkage which means, in essence, that our nerve ends are raw and often screaming for attention (Sprott, Muller and Heine 1997).

N-methyl-D-aspartate (NMDA) receptors are involved in some of the pain mechanisms of fibromyalgia. They can cause hypersensitivity to pain, as well as allodynia. This suggests a central sensitization present in FMS, and that tender points represent secondary hyperalgesia (Sorensen, Bengtsson, Backman, et al. 1995).

Pain and Patients' Behavior

Often, patients unwittingly contribute to the undertreatment of their own pain. Men, especially, don't want to be thought of as wimps crying for help. But nobody wants to be thought of as a "problem patient," always complaining. No one wants to be seen as a malingerer, demonstrating "drug-seeking" behavior. Most patients try to "tough it out" until they can no longer bear the pain.

Legislation for Chronic Pain Care

There have been many attempts to legislate chronic pain care, but, as stated previously, they've been stalled by the opposition of insurance companies and other health care providers. Also, the providers of pain control have often focused on the terminally ill, but studies show that even the terminally ill are inadequately medicated and are also subject to needless suffering (Angell 1982; Charap 1978; Foley 1985; Marks and Sachar 1973). We differ from terminal patients in one respect. We don't die from the source of the pain, directly. Our lives become an endurance marathon instead.

Deafferentation Pain Syndrome

Deafferentation pain syndrome is very common in FMS/MPS Complex. *Deafferentation* is a general term describing a condition of the peripheral nervous system. Damage or disease of a nerve leads to loss of capacity to conduct input information. The damage or disease can be caused by viral or other toxins, or from trauma. Pain can also result from nerve damage. The nerve tries to repair itself, but the result is a tangle of nerve fibrils. This also happens when the growth and reinnervation of the skin or other tissue is blocked by an obstacle. The growing nerve end forms a mass called a neuroma, which itself causes chemical and mechanical sensitivity resulting in unusual electrical generating patterns.

Reinnervation means the restoration of nerve control to a denerved area, either spontaneously or after parts of the neural net have rejoined. The *neural net* is the name given to the network of nerves throughout the body. You can think of the neural net as the very first Internet, literally. Tightened, constricted myofascia can create an obstacle to repairing nerve endings, as can concentrated chemical toxins in the area. (See "Alternate Tryptophan Pathway" below.)

Neuromas

Neuromas can be microscopic or macroscopic. They cause a specific pain that feels like a jabbing, electrical burning. Skin may become sore from the pressure of clothing. A small number of patients develop neuropathic pain after correction of severe hypoglycemia. This pain is present even at rest, and worsens with movement. In this condition, nerve cells broaden their receptive fields and they respond to normally nonpainful sensations as if they were painful stimuli.

The Alternate Tryptophan Pathway

An alternate tryptophan metabolic pathway may be the root cause of one kind of FMS pain (Russell 1996). *Tryptophan* is a biochemical the body uses to build muscles, among other things. It also is a "precursor" of serotonin. That means the body takes tryptophan and makes serotonin out of it. Tryptophan, an amino acid, doesn't *have* to build muscles or serotonin. Instead, it sometimes can be sidetracked onto something called the "kynurenine pathway" to produce a biochemical called "quinolinic acid." If too much is sidetracked, not only will the body be short of serotonin, but there will be an overabundance of quinolinic acid, which is a nerve *toxin* (Heyes, Achim, Wiley, et al. 1996). We know that quinolinic acid formation increases if there is acute immune system stimulation (Saito, Crowley, Markey, et al. 1993), which fits in with what we know about FMS.

More tryptophan is diverted to make quinolinic acid in women, particularly during premenstrual stages, as well as during periods of alcohol intake. The "pathway" from tryptophan to quinolinic acid also gets more frequent use during immune system activation (Heyes, Chen, Major, et al. 1997). This alternate pathway operates in the brain, blood, and systemic tissue. Is this still another cause of "fibrofog"? (Shear, Dong, Haik-Creguer, et al. 1998).

It even looks as if quinolinic acid may be implicated in AIDS dementia complex (Saito 1995). Presently, I am observing a small subset of people with FMS and seizure-like activity. I have never seen FMS and seizures connected, but there *is* a study that shows a connection to quinolinic acid and seizure disorders (Schwarcz, Speciale and French 1987).

I have observed that foods that are high in serotonin, such as turkey and peanuts, can make some of us feel worse, even though we have low serotonin levels. Those of us with FMS also feel worse if we take L-tryptophan. This would follow logically if this subset of fibromyalgics have biochemistries utilizing the kynurenine pathway.

I have discussed these possible connections with I. Jon Russell, who is not only an M.D. and Ph.D, but also able to mobilize research efforts and to translate complex biochemistry into terms that patients can understand. We live in exciting times, and remember, this is all experimental. This alternate tryptophan pathway research may point to a new class of pain reliever for FMS in the future. Some researchers are already working on this (Wu, Salituro and Schwarcz 1997).

Trigger Points as Pain Initiators

Active trigger points (TrPs) hurt all the time. Individual TrPs can be difficult to live with, but they often respond immediately to specific therapy. If you already have a ropy, taut band of TrPs that you can feel, they will be harder to eradicate. Once a primary TrP has developed satellites and secondaries, it's even harder to get rid of them. In cases of chronic Myofascial Pain Syndrome, with bodywide TrPs and overlapping referral patterns, life can become a true challenge. What eases one TrP may adversely affect another. This is especially true if fibromyalgia is also involved.

As stated in chapter 1, fibromyalgia amplifies the pain and other symptoms of myofascial trigger points. FMS/MPS Complex is not to be taken lightly. Neither are individual trigger points. "A swimmer may drown from a muscle cramp produced by a myofascial trigger point. Myofascial pain has driven some patients to suicide. . . . Myofascial back pain is a major, unrecognized source of industrial disability" (Travell and Simons 1983, 18). It is important to remember that Travell and Simons are writing about individual trigger points. When dealing with Myofascial Pain Syndrome, the pain is magnified many times.

> **I Need to Back Up My Hard Drive But I Can't Get It in Reverse.**
>
> While writing this book, my sacroiliac became rigid and my upper body became immobile. I needed a lot of extra physical therapy and pain control to relax those muscles from all the sitting at the computer I had to do. I used three different chairs while working, and kept switching from one to the other to deal with the pain.

Assessing Trigger Points

Fixation of joints by muscular rigidity caused by trigger points leads to inflexibility. The results can be "frozen shoulder" and other joint motion restrictions. Effective treatment of something as complex as chronic MPS takes time. There is no magic wand. Don't allow yourself to become discouraged. Think about how long it took for your body to get into this state. Of course, if you're already in such pain that your circuits are overloaded, you may not be able to tell what makes it worse. But if you review your regular physical activities, you may discover some clues about the kinds of changes to make to get some pain relief. Whatever the treatment, the severity of your condition can be assessed in the following manner:

- Phase 1: Constant pain from severely active trigger points

- Phase 2: Pain from less irritable trigger points that is felt only when you move

- Phase 3: Trigger points that cause no pain, only weakness

When the trigger points are extremely irritable, almost any activity makes them worse. Travell and Simons say that if you hurt for more than a few seconds after you exercise, you should avoid that exercise (1983, 94).

In Phase 1, about the only thing your body can tolerate is moist heat and gentle, passive stretches. Ask your physical therapist what movements are likely to abuse the affected muscles. Write down any activities that cause referred pain. Report this to your physical therapist and doctor. If these movements are unnecessary, unlearn the bad habit. If the task is unnecessary, don't do it anymore. If it is necessary, find an alternate way to do it.

In Phase 2, there is the great danger that because you hurt when you move, you will stop moving. It is vitally important that, with the guidance of trained myotherapists, you learn how to move and stretch. You also must continue to deal with your perpetuating factors.

In Phase 3, there are only latent trigger points, but these can sometimes be the most dangerous. They don't hurt, so they are often ignored. But they are like land mines, waiting to go off. They also may cause unexpected weakness, such as buckling ankles, and lessened range of motion. As we get older, we tend to have more latent trigger points.

Exercise and Trigger Points

Exercise should be as carefully considered as a prescription. You need the right dose, the right timing, and the right kind. You must never exercise when your muscles are tired or cold. As trigger points are inactivated, begin carefully graded exercises to increase your strength and endurance. Your physical therapist will be your guide in this. If mild exercise soreness disappears after the first day, you can repeat it on the second day. If it persists to the second day, postpone any more exercise until the third day. *If soreness persists on the third day, your exercise* routine *must be changed.* This protocol is true for any treatment, such as massage or electrical stimulation. Stretching that involves rolling the head around in all directions is hazardous, and likely to activate trigger points. Nonrepetitious exercise is best.

Treatments for Chronic Pain

Unfortunately, most pain management clinics spend a lot of time helping people learn to live with their pain when, frequently, some of it can be eliminated. Once identified, trigger points—those lumps of fascia and waste materials—can be broken up, or at least minimized. Many doctors don't know how to check for them, but some physical therapists do. When you find someone who knows how to work with TrPs, you will have to give a good medical history, but it may be difficult to do that if all you can tell your doctor or physical therapist is that you hurt "all over." You may feel that way, but that won't help in the treatment of specific TrPs.

Think about it. Does the tip of your nose hurt? Your fingernails? How about your elbow? If it hurts, when does it hurt, and how? There are many words to describe pain. It can burn, pulse, throb, stab, pinch, and so on. See page 112 of *Fibromyalgia & Chronic Myofascial Pain Syndrome* (Starlanyl and Copeland 1966) for more terms to describe your pain accurately. The more precise your language is, the more easily your doctor or physical therapist will identify the cause of your pain. It will also help if you keep a pain record.

Use the following "Symptom Mapping Creature Chart" to "map" the pain you experience as a visual record and fill in the five parameters below the illustration to describe the pain verbally. Here's how to do it:

1. Make a number of copies of the illustrated chart so that you can map your pain symptoms for several weeks.

2. Using colored pencils, draw your body's pain patterns on the figures in the chart. Use blue for generalized pain, yellow for numbness or tingling, red for burning feelings, green for cramps, and purple for tightness.

3. Each time you draw a map of your pain, be sure to fill in the details regarding the duration, quality, aggravating factors, and so forth. Keep these records and compare them frequently so that you can periodically track your progress as you are treated.

Symptom Mapping Creature Chart

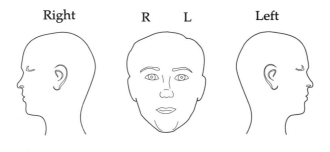

Right   R   L   Left

Name _____

Blue = pain   Yellow = numbness, tingling   Red = burning   Green = cramping   Purple = tightness

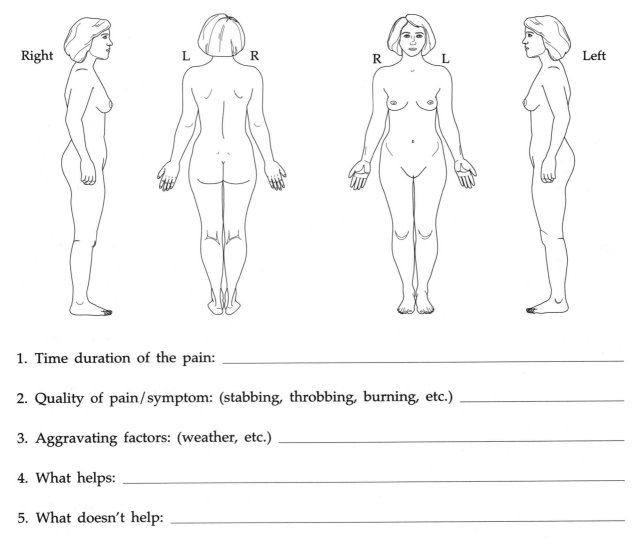

Right   L   R   R   L   Left

1. Time duration of the pain: _____

2. Quality of pain/symptom: (stabbing, throbbing, burning, etc.) _____

3. Aggravating factors: (weather, etc.) _____

4. What helps: _____

5. What doesn't help: _____

(Modified from a chart created by Hal Blatman, M.D.)

When you find someone who knows how to work with trigger points, follow this sequence:

- First, identify active and latent TrPs.

- Second, estimate their importance in the quality of your life. Those TrPs that interfere with vital functions, such as breathing and sleep, and those that cause the most debilitating effects, such as migraine and dizziness, should be treated first. Remember, many TrP-referred pain zones may overlap each other.

- Third, develop a treatment plan for the major trigger points, using a treatment sequence that respects their interactions.

After any kind of treatment, soak in a hot tub bath and take it easy. Your body will have been working hard. Don't plan on traveling, sightseeing, going to the movies, or shopping. Allow your muscles to rest and recover more normal function. Avoid strenuous swimming, but lazy stretching in a warm pool can be very helpful.

Treating Perpetuating Factors

If a trigger point recurs after effective treatments, there are hidden perpetuating factors. If the pain recurs but the TrP is gone, look for another cause, including cancer and other systemic diseases. Delayed-onset muscle soreness, which appears a day or two after doing too much physically, is a function of FMS and not of trigger points.

Your doctor may need your help in finding your perpetuating factors—those factors that reinforce, aggravate, and continue the conditions that sustain the trigger point (see chapter 3). It bears repeating that FMS is one of the most common perpetuating factors of MPS. Your doctor and physical therapist can uncover such factors as skeletal defects, but you can help them by becoming more aware of how you move through your life.

You can provide your health care team with specific data concerning your daily routines, including sleep positions, work conditions, and family dynamics. You may observe that certain repetitive motions give rise to strain and stress on certain muscles, which can result in specific trigger points. Make a careful evaluation of your movements, postures, and so on. Ask your health team for assistance in observing your body.

Eliminate multiple causes of pain. For example, you may have good control of rheumatoid arthritis, but the resulting trigger points may have been left untreated. "Perpetuating factors act clinically like the missing link that converts an acute single muscle syndrome into a chronic pain syndrome. These factors may be systemic or mechanical" (Simons and Simons 1989). As a rule, one stress activates a trigger point and another perpetuates it. If you have a poor response or no response to specific trigger point therapy, it's a good indication that you have significant perpetuating factors. Your therapist may have tried to treat the secondary trigger points and not the primaries.

Nutrition

You may have an enzyme dysfunction caused by nutritional inadequacies, such as insufficient B vitamins and/or an insufficiency of essential minerals. You also might have a metabolic and/or endocrine dysfunction (hypoglycemia, anemia, low electrolytic levels, subclinical hypothyroidism, estrogen deficiency), chronic infection or infestation, or psychological stress. A well-balanced diet may not be enough to ensure adequate nutrition, especially in conjunction with other perpetuating factors. You may be experiencing a loss of nutrients through improper food preparation, increased metabolic requirements, or impaired absorption.

Foot Problems

The foot shape called Morton's foot is a common trigger point perpetuating factor. The most common type of Morton's foot has a relatively short first metatarsal and a long second metatarsal. (The metatarsals are the bones in the foot that correspond approximately to the knuckles in the hand.) There is often a long web between the second and third toes. Calluses are likely to develop in a characteristic pattern.

I have observed a similar foot type I call the FMS/MPS foot. This is a foot that is wide in front, narrow in back, and often has a high arch. There is usually a large space between the big toe and second toe. A variation of this occurs with a flat arch. Finding comfortable shoes for this type of foot is difficult for women, because most women's shoes are manufactured with pointed narrow fronts and wider heels.

Both of these foot shapes can cause excessive pronation, or turning out of the foot. Pronation often causes and perpetuates trigger points. Pain from these foot shapes may be eased by the use of the Travell shoe insert. (See Starlanyl and Copeland 1996, page 61, if you wish to see pictures of these foot shapes and of the shoe insert.) Although finding shoes that fit is a challenge, it is possible to live with both of these foot configurations, and I do. In addition to the shoe insert, Janet Travell has some pointers about how to go about looking for comfortable shoes (Travell and Simons 1992, 517).

Check your shoes for the following characteristics:

- The toes should not curve away or point.

- The top of the shoe must be loose, so the toes have enough room.

- The sole must be flexible at the heads of metatarsals.

- Get rid of shoes and slippers with rigid soles. It's difficult for people with these foot shapes to wear ice skates or other types of rigid-soled shoes.

- The heel must fit well, be firm, and must be flat. Check for excessive wear on the outer side of the heel and on the inner edge of the sole.

- Make sure your shoes have good arch support.

- If you have Morton's foot or the FMS/MPS foot, use the Travell shoe insert (see Starlanyl and Copeland 1996, 61).

Hypermobility

Hypermobility syndrome is a condition in which the joints can overstretch. This is a perpetuating factor, and people with hypermobility must be very careful when doing physical therapy. About five percent of all adults have hypermobility. It often accompanies flat feet, mitral valve prolapse (the mitral valve is a heart valve), weakness of the abdominal and pelvic floor, and elastic skin that develops stretch marks easily. There is also a greater tendency for the muscles to rotate, causing imbalances and trigger points (Travell and Simons 1983).

Head-Forward Posture

Another common perpetuating factor is the head-forward posture. If you have this posture, your head juts forward when you try to stand straight. This causes a round-shouldered slump, which activates trigger points in the pectoral and cervical muscles, the SCM, and the jaw area. This can lead to the "dowager's hump" deformity in older years. See your physical therapist for exercise advice if you think that this is happening to you.

Paradoxical Breathing

A very common perpetuating factor that is often overlooked is paradoxical breathing. It is covered in chapter 3, but it is so important I will go over it again here. When you breathe in, your belly should expand outward. As you exhale, your belly should flatten. If you do the reverse, you are asking for trigger points. Your body will quickly develop air hunger from insufficient oxygen. If you lie on your back on a flat surface, you may find it easier to check whether you are breathing in this improper way.

Repetitious Exercise

Repetitious exercise and inappropriate physical therapy are some of the most common trigger point perpetuating factors. Weight training is *not* appropriate for someone with active trigger points. Many forms of "treatment" are up to you. For example, the following behaviors can help a great deal:

- Vary tasks to avoid using the same muscle group.

- Avoid immobility.

- Slow your working pace to the point where your muscles are comfortable. (See chapter 9 for natural pain-relieving options.)

- After any kind of treatment, you can usually expect some soreness as your muscles try to recover more healthy positions.

Trigger Point Injections

Trigger point injection methods are covered in Travell and Simons' *Myofascial Pain and Dysfunction: The Trigger Point Manuals* (1983; 1992). Each specific trigger point injection technique is described in detail. This is important, as each TrP must be treated in a specific manner due to the type of musculature involved. Patients with FMS may not find the injections as effective as those who have MPS do. The injections may hurt more, and their effects will last for a shorter period of time. Stretched and injected muscles are likely to be sore for two to three days following treatment. Strenuous activities should be avoided for the period of muscle soreness, including shopping, gardening, and traveling.

Medicinal Pain Relief

You need a doctor who understands pain, and a pharmacist to match. Physical dependence is the body's natural adaptation to some types of medication. If you stop taking the medication, you get a withdrawal effect. This is dependence, *not* addiction. *Addiction is the psychological craving for a drug in order to experience altered states of consciousness.* People with chronic pain conditions and no history of drug abuse should not be denied adequate pain control because of the misunderstanding that they will become addicted. You have a great deal of pain. Don't compound it by adding unnecessary guilt (see chapter 8).

Opioids

Normally, physical and/or emotional trauma releases the body's own painkillers—the *endorphins,* which are naturally occurring opioids. *Opioids* are central nervous system analgesics (painkillers). They are called opioids because originally they were derived from the opium poppy. Opioids moderate pain perceptions in the thalamus and cortex. They suppress both the perception of and reaction to pain. Opioids are painkillers.

There are many types of opioid receptors in the body. Morphine fits the body's opioid receptors exceptionally well, shutting off the pain. But most patients are terrified of using opioids because of their fear of becoming addled or addicted. With proper management, however, opioids, including morphine, needn't be sedating, mind-fogging, or addictive. Opioids do trigger the depression of the respiration center of the brain, but it is a transient state. It is not appropriate to use opioids as sedatives unless the insomnia is caused by pain.

NSAIDS

NSAIDS, or nonsteroidal anti-inflammatories, are often used as analgesics, even though neither FMS nor MPS is an inflammatory condition. These can have side effects such as hypoglycemia. We are still discovering the more adverse effects of NSAIDS (Gardner and Simpkin 1991), and yet they are often recommended by doctors because they are easily obtained, over-the-counter medications. This book does not discuss non-opioid analgesics in any depth, because the advocacy problem is not as urgent. The greatest problem lies in the use, or rather, the non-use, of opioid analgesics for chronic pain.

Posttraumatic Hyperirritability Syndrome (PTHS)

This condition is often mistaken for multiple chemical sensitivity. That's because with this condition, you become sensitive to *everything:* light, sound, touch, chemicals (even very mild ones such as those in tomato juice), smells—all can be "translated" as pain by the body. Usually, patients with PTHS have experienced a major trauma of some kind. There is frequently a history of an auto accident or a fall that was sufficient to cause unconsciousness (although it is now recognized that there is a form of mild concussion in which consciousness is not lost). This trauma affects the sensory pathways of the CNS to create an extended form of allodynia.

Some people with this syndrome cannot stand the odors from a telephone, or from their clothing, and they must wash their clothes in vinegar and water, or baking soda and water. They must wait for months for their natural cotton clothing to "outgas." Each bout of an "allodynic flare" brings with it an increase in sensitivity to subsequent stimuli. These cases must be treated *very* carefully. All identifiable TrPs must be inactivated as gently as possible, and all perpetuating factors must be corrected. This condition can be extremely debilitating, as it often necessitates the complete isolation of the patient from the outside (and normal inside) world.

Headaches Due to Myofascial Trigger Points

There are many possible causes of headache. For those with the hyperaroused autonomic nervous system of FMS, sensitivity to noise, cold, heat, and light only adds to our headache woes. Allergies, fatigue, hormonal imbalances, reactive hypoglycemia, congestion, vasomotor rhinitis, and neurotransmitter dysregulation can also be factors in producing headaches. By far, however, the most common cause of headaches is referred pain from myofascial trigger points. All of the above-mentioned factors frequently activate and/or perpetuate TrPs.

Poorly fitting glasses or improperly corrected vision can also contribute to headaches. This is especially tiresome if your vision is changing constantly due to extrinsic TrPs. TrPs around the eyes are also likely to be involved. Get into the habit of doing acupressure work on your face and neck for brief periods, whenever you have the time.

Because TrPs can entrap blood and lymph vessels as well as nerves, TrP pain is often confused with neurological, rheumatic, or inflammatory pain, especially with some of the more bizarre autonomic nervous system symptoms that can occur. Trigger point headache pain is often variable, and may change with body position or muscular activity. It may be so severe at times that you can't function or even think clearly. Trigger points refer pain elsewhere in the body in specific patterns, so it is important to become familiar with the pattern and any possible accompanying symptoms, as well as with the location of the instigating TrP. All of these TrPs are documented in *Myofascial Pain and Dysfunction: The Trigger Point Manuals*, Vols. I and II (Travell and Simons 1983; 1992).

Frontalis TrPs

The frontalis muscle is one part of the broad musculo-fibrous layer of the occipito-frontalis muscle, which stretches across the forehead, top, and back of the skull. The frontalis portion is—you guessed it—in the front. Trigger points in the frontalis muscle remain local, causing pain over the forehead and often radiating up over the scalp. When you press on these TrPs, they scream at you, "Here I Am!" You usually feel like screaming right back at them, "Go Away!" These TrPs are often activated by overwork, especially in tense people who habitually use a lot of facial expressions.

Occipitalis TrPs

Occipitalis TrPs cause local pain over the area of the rest of the skull, and also refer pain to the back of the head, through the skull, and to the back of the eyeball. Often, you can feel the lumps and bumps of these TrPs with your fingers. They may become so severe that you cannot bear the weight of the back of your head on a pillow. Trigger points in the head and neck region respond to moist heat, unless there is nerve entrapment. For nerve entrapment, ice helps. Massage is beneficial, as well as Cranio-Sacral Release (CSR) and Spray and Stretch (S&S) (see Starlanyl and Copeland (1996, 248), but you also must check for perpetuating factors such as stress, eye strain, and overwork.

Temporalis TrPs

Temporalis TrPs occur in a line a little beyond the outer edge of the eye to just behind the tip of the ear. Each temporalis TrP refers pain in a different pattern. The one closest to the eye refers pain over the eyebrow, straight up the side of the head, and to the front upper teeth. Trigger points further back along the line to the ear refer pain to different teeth. The further back the TrP, the further back the tooth or teeth. They also refer pain upwards of their position, causing headache.

Extrinsic Eye Muscle TrPs

Trigger points in the extrinsic eye muscles are a frequent contributor to headaches. For vision to be clear, both eyes must take the same picture at the same time, and all the muscles of each eye must work together in harmony. Trigger points in any of these muscles can cause a misalignment. Double vision, blurry vision, and/or changing vision can result if these muscles are being contracted at different tensions.

To find out if you have TrPs in your extrinsic eye muscles, place one hand on the top of your head, right above your forehead. Then, keeping your head still, raise your eyes up and try to look at your hand. This shouldn't hurt. If it does, it is likely that you have TrPs in those eye muscles. A good exercise for TrPs in this area is to move your eyeballs back and forth from one upper corner to the other, but be sure to do this gently. This movement may activate the TrPs and *cause* a headache. This doesn't mean you shouldn't do the exercise—in fact, it is a warning to tell you how badly these eye-muscle stretches are needed. Start slowly, and go gently, but keep at it. It is important to remember to vary your gaze frequently. When you are doing close work, look up and into the distance every once in a while.

Masseter Muscle TrPs

Check for TrPs in the masseter muscles along the lower border of your jaw just after the "corner." These TrPs, which are by no means the only possible ones in the masseter muscles, refer pain along the line of the eyebrows, as well as to an area along the side of the lower jaw, contributing to headaches.

Lateral Pterygoid Muscle TrPs

Trigger points in the lateral pterygoid muscle are found in the jaw about an inch in front of the center of the outer ear. Another set of TrPs is often found about an inch below those. These TrPs refer pain in front of the ear and pain deep in the TMJ and maxillary sinuses. Both of these, especially sinus pain, can add to headache misery.

There is a TrP in the back of the digastric muscle that sometimes refers pain to the back of the skull. To use acupressure on the digastric muscles, lean into your thumbs with your elbows bent on a table in front of you. Start the acupressure at the area under your chin, and press. Continue working with your thumbs in a line under the jaw, all the way back to the ear.

This TrP also radiates pain to the upper part of the sternocleidomastoid (SCM), which is an exceedingly complex muscle that is discussed later in this section. The spillover pain can be in the front of the throat under the chin along the jaw line, and can be much worse under the ear. It can continue to extend upward and backward, in a diagonal, nearly to the back of the head.

Neck Muscle TrPs

In the neck, as in many other parts of the body, TrPs can occur in many layers of muscles. The splenius capitis muscles are wide bands that run from the back of the skull at the sides to the upper vertebrae. Trigger points here feel like sore areas on either side of the back of the head, directly under the skull. These TrPs transmit pain to the top of the head.

Splenius cervicis muscles are thinner muscles connecting the vertebrae. Trigger points in the upper splenius cervicis muscles send pain to the back of the head that diffuses throughout the skull, creating intense pain behind the eyeballs. These TrPs can cause blurring of near vision in the eye on the same side as the TrP. Trigger points in the lower splenius cervicis muscles are found on either side of the neck, just below where the neck joins the trunk, above the shoulder blades. Referred pain flows down to the shoulder, collarbone, and angle of the neck. You may not be able to rotate your neck due to pain.

Posterior Cervical TrPs

There are several types of posterior cervical muscles. A TrP in the semispinalis cervicis, which is alongside the spine right below the skull, creates pain up the back of the head toward the top. A TrP in the semispinalis capitis muscle just above the base of the skull, on the back of the side of the head, creates a headache that feels as if you are wearing half a headband bound very tightly, with the highest pain intensity in the temple and over the eye. If you have TrPs on both sides, the pain can be incapacitating. A TrP in between these two other TrPs sends pain up to the base of the skull. It may also cause neck pain, spilling over to the top of the collarbone and the upper inward border of the shoulder blade. Posterior cervical TrPs below the skull can also produce pain in the hands and feet on both sides, or in the body below the shoulder on the same side as the TrP.

Suboccipital TrPs

Place your hand alongside your head, with the heel of your hand directly under your ear, resting against the square of your jaw. Your outstretched fingers should be wrapping diagonally around to the back of your head. You can find suboccipital TrPs on a diagonal line (the higher side is toward the back of the skull) under your palm. These TrPs initiate deep head pain that radiates from the back of your head to the cavity of your eye. The pain seems to penetrate inside your skull, because these muscles are deeply placed, just below the base of the skull on the side.

Multifidi Muscle TrPs

Multifidi run along the entire spine. Neck multifidi are often headache inducers. These muscles are short and deep, and go from one vertebra to another. Pain is transmitted in different patterns depending on which multifidi muscle has TrPs. Activation is usually caused by prolonged bending of the neck doing close work, by stooped posture, or by gross trauma. If you have trigger points in the multifidi of your neck vertebrae, pressure from your pillow at night can be intolerable. In addition to pain, there can also be tingling, numbness, or burning pain over the back of your head on the same side as the TrPs. This is an indication that the TrPs are causing nerve entrapment. Check to see that your workstation is ergonomically correct. *Don't slump.* Avoid tight hats and headbands, heavy eyeglasses, heavy overcoats and tight collars. To relieve these symptoms, sit in a hot shower while you stretch your neck muscles downward.

Trapezius Muscle TrPs

The trapezius muscle may have TrPs in many locations. There is one spot that sends pain up the same side of the neck and head, in a hook shape. Follow a line about an inch behind your ear down the side of your neck above the collarbone about halfway to the start of the shoulder. There is often spillover pain in the neck region, beneath the ear, as well as under the eyebrow. This is a major source of tension headache and neck aches. There can also be a mild pain at the top of head, in the lower back teeth, and in the outer ear. One or both ears can burn, turn red, or lose all color as blood vessels dilate or contract in response to this TrP.

Sternocleidomastoid (SCM) Muscle TrPs

The sternocleidomastoid (SCM) muscle connects to the head, but separates into two parts. One part connects to the collarbone, and one to the breastbone. TrPs in the breastbone (sternal) part, in the front, can refer pain to the top or back of the head, and over the eye (among other places). Midlevel TrPs can send pain arcing across the cheek and jaw, over the eyebrow ridge, and deep inside the eye, as well as pain to the ear on the same side. TrPs in the upper sternal SCM cause pain behind but not close to the ear, and to the back of the head. SCM TrPs also affect the eyes and sinuses, and can cause tearing, reddening, or drooping of the eye, as well as an inability to raise the upper eyelid. They can also cause visual disturbances. Patterns from window blinds and escalator treads can cause an out-of-control seizure-like feeling. Stripes, checks, and polka dots can be a problem—as can anything with strongly contrasting light and dark spaces. You may experience dizziness, runny nose, and sinus congestion on the involved side, as well as a ringing in the ear and deafness. The SCM is the "big cheese" when it comes to TrPs in the head and neck, but unlike a cheese, it seldom stands alone. Be sure to check for other TrPs.

Clavicular TrPs

Trigger points in the collarbone (clavicular) area cause a frontal headache and an earache. Middle TrPs in this area also cause pain to the front of the head, which can extend across the forehead to the other side. Anything that hyperextends the neck, such as sleeping on two pillows, can aggravate these TrPs. Mechanical stresses such as doing overhead work, writing on a blackboard, or hanging curtains, also aggravates these TrPs.

For more information on headaches and TrPs and for diagrams see my video "Chronic Myofascial Pain Syndrome: The Trigger Point Guide," which is available from New Harbinger Publications. See also *Fibromyalgia and Chronic Myofascial Pain Syndrome: A Survival Manual* by Devin J. Starlanyl, M.D., and Mary Ellen Copeland, M.A., M.S., New Harbinger Publications, Oakland, Ca, USA, (800) 748-6273: Canada (800) 561-8583.

PART II

Your FMS/MPS Health Care Team

To take charge of your health care team, you need to know how to choose and organize the people who will be on it. You need to know how to listen and how to be heard. Chapter 6 discusses the various issues you will have to deal with to assemble your team. Chapter 7 provides you with data sheets for each specific member of your team. These sheets are formatted for ease of copying and are well referenced. If your team members read the information contained in these sheets, there will be no excuse for them "not to believe" you when you describe your symptoms. Chapter 8 deals with obtaining pain relief and specifically with the use of opioids. Chapter 9 offers an extended discussion of alternate treatment options and methods. You are your own best health care team manager and, as such, you want to know about whatever is available to help you optimize the quality of your life.

6

Becoming Your Own Health Care Manager

If you ran a large corporation, you would want a well-educated manager who was in the best possible shape and well-informed about all aspects of the job. Well, *you* are the perfect manager for your health care team and the intention of this chapter is to supply you with some new managerial skills. It's time to put some time and effort into getting your manager into the best possible shape.

Educate Yourself

No one knows more about the state of your body and mind than you do. However, it may be necessary for you to learn to listen to your body and then to integrate body and mind. The ways to do this are described in my first book, *Fibromyalgia & Chronic Myofascial Syndrome: A Survival Manual* (Starlanyl and Copeland 1996). Because we have more than enough ground to cover in this book, and I want to avoid duplication, I refer you to it.

Your local librarian is an excellent resource for self-education efforts. No matter how rural your location, you can obtain information through an interlibrary loan. Speak to your reference librarian about this. The medical references listed in the Reference and Bibliography sections in the back of this book are available this way, at little or no cost. The books in the Advocate's Reading List (located at the end of the Bibliography) are also available through interlibrary loan. If you find them helpful, suggest that your library purchase them. Usually, libraries have forms for suggestions for purchase. These books will then be available to help other people in your locality. Your educational program will be continuously ongoing, for life itself is an educational process.

To be truly self-empowered you must learn to talk to your caregivers as equals. Respect yourself and respect what you know. By so doing, you will reduce the pain and frustration of not communicating effectively and increase the probability of being completely understood. Also, you will better understand the limitations each member of your team may have. Good communication can help avoid patient and caregiver burnout and hostility, both of which are often the result of misunderstandings.

You have already taken an important first step. By reading this book, and the book that preceded it, you are developing a greater understanding of your medical conditions. By educating your family, friends, and co-workers, you are raising the general educational level of the public about fibromyalgia (FMS) and Myofascial Pain Syndrome (MPS). This doesn't mean that you have all or even most of the answers. None of us does. It does mean that you are able to ask the right questions that will lead to even deeper understanding.

Support Groups

Visit your local FMS/MPS Support Group, and think about whether it could be a positive force in your life. Be careful. There are some groups claiming to be support groups that are actually venting grounds. That is, the people in the group do little more than moan and groan about what a lousy hand life dealt them. A little venting is good for the soul and the health of everyone. But if the entire discussion is centered on moaning and groaning, it will drag you down into the depths of negativity. *Avoid negative groups.*

If such a group is your only local option, consider starting a group on your own. It could be just three or four people who gather to talk about how things are going—not just the negative things. You could decide to swap easy-to-prepare, healthy recipes, or to exercise together. You might want to share books, videos, and magazines. Whatever your needs are, you can be sure there are other people with those same needs. Find them. If there are a number of people who are interested in joining your support group, and you would like to use a public space to meet, many hospitals and public libraries offer large meeting rooms to such groups at a nominal fee.

If you have access to a computer, connect to the Internet for up-to-date information from all over the country. There are also many local, regional, and national fibromyalgia resource organizations that publish newsletters (see Resources).

Above all, don't lose your identity to your illness. Remember that you are more than just your condition. Give yourself time to do things unrelated to your FMS or MPS. Get away from it when you can. Take the time to develop other interests. There's no time limit on your education. One step at a time will take you there, and your journey will be far more pleasant if you stop to watch the birds and butterflies along the way.

If you do start your own support group, the following chart will give you an idea of how little information is needed to maintain a support group list.

Support Group Form

Support Group Meeting Times: _____

Support Group Meeting Address: _____

Support Team Membership List:

Name _____   Phone _____

Address _____

Name _____   Phone _____

Address _____

Name _____   Phone _____

Address _____

Name _____   Phone _____

Address _____

Name _____   Phone _____

Address _____

Name _____   Phone _____

Address _____

Assembling Your Team

It isn't easy to put together a "user-friendly" health care team. Sometimes we have little choice, due to the constraints of our health insurance or HMO regulations (see chapter 12). You might not know where to turn, since there is so much medical "misinformation" about FMS and MPS around. Check your local support group for referrals. This book will supply you with the data sheets to educate specific members of your health care team. The remainder of this chapter will give you some pointers on how to go about finding these team members.

Each of us is a unique individual with a unique set of needs. We each require a different assortment of advisors on our health care team. We all need a primary care physician and nearly all of us need a physical therapist of some kind (see chapter 7). Both the primary care physician and the physical therapist must know the difference between fibromyalgia (FMS) and Myofascial Pain Syndrome (MPS). In addition, they must be able to accept *you* as the manager of your health care team. They must be able to listen well and hear you when you speak, and you must be able to trust them. They are your advisors.

"I've learned far more about FMS while caring for FMS patients in my practice than I learned during my entire medical training (including three years of rheumatology practice). Look for a physician who'll listen to you and work with you to find the answers."

—Emergency Room doctor

Physical Therapy

To find a physical therapist, first call your local hospital and ask to speak to someone in the physical therapy department. You may find it's easier to get insurance coverage for physical therapy if it takes place at the hospital. Ask if the department has someone who treats trigger points and is familiar with Travell and Simons' *Trigger Point Manuals* (1983; 1992). Inquire whether they have a registered trigger point therapist, called a "myotherapist." If they do, ask to talk with that physical therapist.

You will probably have to wait until that physical therapist is free, so leave your number for a call back. *Remain available until you get the call back.* When the therapist calls, talk to her/him and listen well to the answers to your questions. If you can, take notes during the phone conversation. Does the physical therapist understand FMS and MPS? How does s/he treat trigger points (TrPs)? Does s/he know the difference between the trigger points of MPS and the tender points of FMS? Find out a little about the therapist. Ask if electrical stimulation is available (see Starlanyl and Copeland 1996). Inquire about other forms of physical therapy that might be available at that hospital. If the answers are satisfactory to you, then make a *trial* appointment. If you don't like the way the appointment goes, remember, you are in charge. You don't have to return for another appointment if it doesn't feel absolutely right to you, and you are free to continue searching for a physical therapist with whom you can work well.

When you visit your local support group, be sure to ask the people there about their doctors and health team members. Ask about their physical therapists, both in the hospital and in private settings. It's important to get several references. Different people have different needs. If the hospital near you doesn't have a physical therapist who knows how to work with TrPs, look in your phone book. See who is listed and what they do. Take the time to do some phone interviews. See who you can find that way. Check "Agencies and Organizations" in the Resources section at the back of this book for TrP-therapist information. Explore the alternative types of physical therapy described in my previous book. Your support group might consider inviting several therapists to demonstrate their specialty. Once you find a good physical therapist, that person may be able to give you good advice on building the rest of your health care team.

Dealing with Your Doctor

Unfortunately, you can't go by specialty when it comes to FMS and MPS. If there is a physiatrist (a doctor who specializes in physical medicine and rehabilitation) or rheumatologist in town, by all means go for an interview. Find out how well they understand these conditions. It will be a bonus if the doctor is pleasant and you get along, but be sure that your needs and you are taken seriously. See how willing they are about accepting and reading reasonable amounts of information that you will supply to them.

Confrontation, even when gentle, can be stressful. You may not know the medical terms you think you need to explain what is happening, or what you need. Or you may become temporarily inarticulate. If you are worried about that possibility, bring notes with you to refer to during the interview. It is important to remember that you don't have to use the same language your doctor would use to describe your condition. Never make the assumption that you aren't supposed to say anything. The physician needs your feedback. Talk about what worries you about your condition.

Medical people often don't deal well with chronic conditions. The ups and downs of FMS/MPS may be very confusing to them, and they may feel guilty that you are not doing better. They need to understand that your symptoms will vary from day to day, and from hour to hour. Often your response to treatment will be delayed. Medical care teams can become frustrated with the absence of a long-term response. It's important that they know we sometimes need the short-term reprieve that *any* type of therapy gives to us. Until the perpetuating factors are tracked down and dealt with as much as possible, you will still need relief from pain, and this means physical therapy as well as medications. Your doctor must be willing to help track down those perpetuating factors to ensure that you can create the best possible life for yourself (see chapter 10 on rights and responsibilities).

Gatekeepers

Be on the alert for a "gatekeeper." These are the people who control access to physicians, the secretaries or assistants. (Note that the term "gatekeeper" is also used in the Health Maintenance Organization [HMO] setting. There, however, gatekeepers do not work for doctors but for the HMOs.) Many doctors have gatekeepers, and they serve a necessary function. It is impossible for a doctor to work efficiently if people keep interrupting all hours of the day and night every day of the week. This really happens. Good doctors are busy. Sometimes, however, the gatekeeper may make incorrect or unauthorized decisions. Make sure that your messages get through to your doctor, or find out why they don't. Be open and honest with your doctor. If something about the way the office is run worries you, talk to your doctor about it.

Doctors don't have an easy life. The hours are long, and the daily demands are far beyond what many people ever have to face. Much of the work is tedious and unrewarding. It is not at all as television would have you believe. Doctors are human too; they have their limits. They, like their patients, also have rights and needs (see chapter 10).

I know a lot of doctors and most of them are noble, compassionate, and work hard at the task of providing their patients with the best possible care. Why, then, do I continually meet people who "hate doctors," "don't trust doctors," or are "afraid of doctors"? Some of this may be an acquired emotional response that was learned through stress and pain. Is some of it communication difficulty? Perhaps. This book will try to give you the tools to fix that. Have too many of your doctors taken the medical course called "God 101"? Avoid

---

**Sometimes
We Win One.**

After struggling to educate any/everyone in the medical community here in Tallahassee, I found this man who actually knows what he talks about! His experience with TMJD led him to the world of fibromyalgia, and he has done considerable research. The most delightful of all was his message to medical professionals that it is not AIYH! That it requires a team approach. I asked how on earth we could get this taught in medical schools. I think my question kinda caught him unaware. He did assure me, though, that it is being taught at the school of dentistry at UF in Gainesville.

—FMily member

Working for the Patient—Not the HMO

A special doctor I met through the Internet told me that he works for the patient, not the insurance company or the patient's employer, and it was important that all parties know this. He believes that his most important task with FMS/MPS patients is as an educator. He helps the patient who is lost to find some direction. I'm always delighted when I can send someone to him, because I know that they will get the best care.

those doctors like the plague that they are. Maybe they'll get the idea—when enough of their patients leave.

There are many good doctors out there, and the ranks of those who are educated in FMS and MPS are growing. We must find them, and reward them with our loyalty. Eventually, I hope to organize a corporation to set up an FMS and MPS doctor-database on the Internet. Things are changing for us, because we are forcing the change. The road to health will become easier for us and those who come after us, only if we all help clear the debris from the road.

Checklist for Your Doctors

You probably already have a primary care physician. If you are happy with your doctor, that's great. Build your health care team around her/him. If you aren't satisfied, you need to find out why. Sometimes it isn't obvious. Ask yourself the following questions:

- Is your doctor knowledgeable and sympathetic to those with FMS/MPS, or does s/he exhibit the MEGO response (My Eyes Glaze Over) whenever you mention one of those conditions?
- Does s/he "tune you out" when you mention certain symptoms?
- Does your doctor think that FMS or MPS is primarily a "psychological" problem?
- Does your doctor listen well, or does s/he keep one hand on the doorknob and eyes on the clock?
- Does s/he believe you?
- Will your doctor schedule extra time to talk with you at your request?
- Will your doctor be your advocate?
- Do you trust your doctor?
- Does your doctor know that your condition is treatable?
- Does your doctor understand that, right now, FMS is not curable?
- Do you feel free to talk about all of your symptoms with your doctor?
- Do you ever have the feeling that your doctor dreads seeing your name on his/her list of appointments?
- How does the office staff treat you when you call?
- Do you have access to your doctor?
- Do you worry whether your doctor gets your messages?

- Do you think your doctor ignores your messages?
- Does the doctor/staff treat you as if you were a drug addict when you request pain relief?
- Do you and your doctor differ on what constitutes a good quality of life for you?
- Do you feel that your doctor is unwilling to experiment to find the best combination of medications and therapies for you?
- Does your doctor encourage you to try new treatments?
- Can you always ask why, or why not?
- Will your doctor accept your input about new treatments? Will s/he read material (within reason) about your condition that you bring to the office?
- Do you feel that your doctor understands the pressures and strains that FMS and/or MPS puts you and your family through?
- Does your doctor follow up on agreed testing, therapies and medications?

> **My Doctor Didn't Want to Make Me an Addict, So He Just Crippled Me.**
>
> On the Internet, the phrase "I'm teaching a course in FMS" often means "I have a new doctor." Some people are unhappy with their doctor, but dread the thought of going through the "training" process with someone new. We call that "Doctor Fatigue."

The Office Visit Form on page 78 will help you prepare for your office visit, as well as help to ensure that your visit is efficient and meaningful for both you and your doctor. You may want to have your doctor copy this form when you leave the office, or send a copy to her/him later if you need more time to complete it.

Active Listening: The Essential Attribute

Doctors who don't listen to you and/or don't believe you will often blame you for your symptoms. This can destroy what little self-esteem you have left. Sometimes, a misunderstanding becomes magnified with time. Have you communicated your needs clearly to your doctor? Do you know what your needs are?

Scared Listening

Don't be a victim of "scared listening." Some of us become so stressed about the office visit that we don't hear a word that is said. If this describes your behavior, perhaps you need to spend some time visualizing a successful visit to the doctor. You may need to learn more about successful communication. There are a number of excellent books available that can help you learn how to deal with high-stress encounters of such a personal nature. Check the Advocate's Reading List at the end of the Bibliography for *The Tao of Conversation* (Kahn 1995), *Resolving Conflict* (Scott 1990), and *An End to Panic* (Zuercher-White 1995).

Office Visit Form

Date _____ Visit to: _____

Major reason for visit: _____

Major symptoms: _____
(see Symptom Mapping Creature Chart [page 59] if applicable)

Aggravating (perpetuating) factors: _____

Questions I need answered: _____

What I have tried: _____

_____

Effects: _____

Doctor/therapist comments: _____

_____

Anything else I can try to help? _____

_____

Suggested therapy/medication _____
(see Medication/Therapy Chart)

_____

Expected results: _____

Possible side effects: _____

Any signs/symptoms for which I should call: _____

_____

Any follow-up scheduling needed: _____

Comments: _____

FMS and Communication Problems

Remind your doctor that with FMS, there may be memory and cognitive deficits. Most FMS and/or MPS patients will have worse penmanship that most doctors. Many doctors will encourage you to keep a written record of the problems and questions that occur to you between visits. During a visit, you may feel mentally confused, forgetful, and want it to be over as soon as possible.

Write Your Questions Beforehand

You may feel you that your doctor has sent you signals that it would be better not to ask too many questions during a visit. In that case, write down your questions succinctly and bring them to the office with you. If you don't write well, ask someone to help you frame your questions clearly, or bring a tape recorder along. This will ensure that you don't forget anything. Bring your notes with you. When you go to the doctor, ask him/her to make a copy of your notes, so that you can keep the original, along with the doctor's recommendations. This will help your doctor keep a record, as well. Consider bringing another person to accompany you to help you communicate. That person might remember something you forget.

The Office Visit Form will enable you to keep detailed records of everything that happens during your office visits to your health team members.

Visualize

Visualize things as they are explained to you. If you don't understand, ask for a printed handout or an explanation. Inquire about demonstrations or drawings of specific procedures. There may be booklets or brochures available. If you are unsure of what is being said, rephrase it and repeat it back to the doctor in this way: "You said that such and such might help, and that you want me to do the following—is that right?"

Don't Be Afraid to Change Doctors

If your doctor does not meet your needs, is it realistic to think that a doctor *can* meet your needs? If it is, consider a change. Ask about where you might find a good doctor. Ask the people at your support group, your friends, your co-workers, your church members. You don't need a doctor who could win a popularity contest. You need someone who is willing to help you find what you need. The "my doctor says I have to grin and bear it, so that's all there is to it" approach doesn't cut it anymore.

Common Sense Isn't

My suggestion is to look for a physician who is informed about FMS, or is willing to be informed. I also think there may be many medical students who graduate each year who don't know as much about it as I do. I know that any time my kids (both of whom have FMS) are seen by any doctor/resident/student in a clinic, I ask if he/she is familiar with FMS, and if not, I inform them about some of the basic issues.

—FMily member

Keep Records

I use a fax modem to communicate with my doctor. I find it avoids misunderstanding if everything is written down. I also keep a record of the communication, so I can follow up on it. My doctor includes the fax in my record, so it saves her time. It also eliminates one long message that the front desk would have to handle.

—FMily member

Self-Esteem Issues

Avoid doctors who cause you to doubt yourself or to lose your self-esteem. If you have negative thoughts after each doctor appointment, try to figure out why. Have your needs been met? Did your doctor understand what you wanted? You've probably been told, "You don't look sick, so why should you feel sick?" Remember, medicine is a service occupation. You hire a doctor and staff to help in your care. You are their employer. Lack of self-esteem is an important perpetuating factor for FMS and MPS. You must learn to respect yourself, and demand the respect of others. Your doctor *must* respect you. You are never going to communicate successfully with someone who refuses to listen. There is an old Russian proverb that says when you dance with a bear, you had better let the bear lead. Perhaps it's time for you to decide to stop dancing with the bear.

Be Reasonable

Your doctor has many patients. Don't expect a cure. **Don't** expect hand-holding. That's what support groups and friends and family are for. Don't waste your doctor's time. I have spent more than an hour with one patient on the phone, without accomplishing anything but hand-holding. She felt better, having made contact, but she had no questions. She was just doing poorly that day. So was I. I had hundreds of e-mails and other correspondence to deal with, as well as other tasks. If doctors are good, they are busy. You are the doctor's employer, and the doctor is your employee, and you both deserve each other's respect.

7

What Your Doctors Should Know: Information for Medical Specialists

How to Use These Data Sheets

In this chapter you will find separate data sheets for many specific specialists who might be on your health care team. To avoid duplication, the first section of this chapter contains the information that *everyone* on your health care team should have. You, as the manager of your team, must decide who on the team needs which data sheets. When you have made your decision, copy the following section, "What Everyone on Your Health Care Team Should Know," and then copy the relevant pages for your specialist. Be sure to provide the specialist with *both* sets of data sheets on your next visit. Remember to copy and include specific information on "Reactive Hypoglycemia" from chapter 3, or "Headaches Due to Myofascial Trigger Points from chapter 5 if they apply to your symptoms.

Of course, it is not necessary for you to see all of these specialists. Indeed, I hope you require very few of them. In some cases, your general practitioner will be able to serve as your primary care physician. In other cases, you might have a family practice specialist, an internist, a physiatrist, or a rheumatologist for your primary care physician. Your doctor could be an M.D., D.O., D.C., N.D., or homeopath. Mix and match the data sheets as your specific needs dictate. Read them all, one at a time. You may learn a great deal. You may want to discuss a particular data sheet and what it means with the team member who receives it, perhaps on a later date. Or you may decide to forward some data sheets to team members and ask them to review the material beforehand, because you wish to discuss it on your next visit.

I specifically did not include data sheets for physiatrists (doctors who specialize in physical medicine and rehabilitation), endocrinologists, or rheumatologists. By now, they should know about FMS and MPS. In the best of all possible worlds, they do. As you know, however, this is not the best of all possible worlds. If necessary, give these specialists "What Your Primary Care Physician Should Know" in addition to "What Everyone on Your Health Care Team Should Know," and see how they react. Sometimes, it is all a specialist can do to keep up with developments in her/his area of knowledge. Aspects of FMS and/or MPS are relevant to all medical disciplines, so become an educator. Your team members will thank your for it (or they don't belong on your team).

Note that the information on trigger points (TrPs) in many of these data sheets comes from the script of my video, "Chronic Myofascial Pain Syndrome: A Guide to the Trigger Points." This video can be obtained by writing to: New Harbinger Publications, 5674 Shattuck Avenue, Oakland, CA 94609. Phone: (800) 748-6273, or (510) 652-0215.

What Everyone on Your Health Care Team Should Know

You may have seen some patients with fibromyalgia (FMS) and Myofascial Pain Syndrome (MPS), and you may see more of them. It is important that you understand the concepts behind the diagnosis of each of these conditions. Fibromyalgia is a systemic, biochemical condition with tender points that hurt in specific areas (Russell 1996). Myofascial Pain Syndrome is a mechanical, physical condition with nodules and ropy bands that not only hurt, but also cause muscular weakness, decreased range of motion, and referred pain. In some cases there are autonomic concomitants (Travell and Simons 1992; 1983). Each of these syndromes is an authentic and well-documented medical condition. They are very different from each other, although they frequently occur together and are often confused. People with FMS and/or MPS may look very healthy and are often discriminated against for having an "invisible" chronic pain condition. Understanding how these syndromes work may provide the answer to some of your more "challenging" patients. Listen carefully and you may learn a lot from these people.

If you doubt the validity of FMS, MPS, perpetuating factors like reactive hypoglycemia, or the cognitive deficits that can accompany FMS, ask your patient to let you look over the References and the extensive Bibliography section at the back of this book. It is to your advantage to become as educated as possible on these topics.

Fibromyalgia

Fibromyalgia is a specific systemic dysregulation of the neuroendocrine system. It is the most common cause of widespread pain (Bennett 1995a). It is not just a term for achy muscles; it is a diagnosis of inclusion, not exclusion. It has, among other things, a disrupted hypothalamus-pituitary-adrenal- (HPA) axis. It is nonprogressive (although it may seem to be progressive), nondegenerative, and noninflammatory. It is responsible for diffuse body-wide pain, tender points that hurt but don't refer pain elsewhere in the body, and sleep disturbances. The central nervous system can be profoundly affected. In FMS, studies indicate that there are biochemical abnormalities requiring metabolic adjustment (Eisinger, Plantamura and Ayavou 1994; Samborski, Stratz, Schochat, et al. 1996). The "eleven out of eighteen" tender points "test" for FMS is intended to be used to identify only those FMS patients who meet the criteria for inclusion in research studies. It was never intended for use in clinical settings. (Scudds 1998).

Also, in people with FMS, there are neurohormonal changes that can significantly diminish the normal repair of muscle tissues (Neeck and Riedel 1994). This must be taken into account when prescribing exercise. Most FMS patients experience chronic sleep deprivation (Branco, Atalaia and Paiva 1994) and thus lose all of the benefits that deep delta-level sleep brings to healthy individuals.

FMS/MPS Patients

Some physicians consider those who have FMS and MPS to be "difficult" patients. However, these patients usually have experienced extreme frustration trying to get doctors to listen to them and take their symptoms seriously. Previous encounters with such frustration may cause them to seem hostile or moody. They are probably in great pain, and past experiences with the medical establishment may have included ridicule and abuse. When dysregulated neurotransmitters (which control mood) and chronic sleep deprivation are added to this volatile mix, you cannot expect to find a cheerful, happy person.

Be patient. If you listen well and take their symptoms seriously, they will find you very reassuring. Under the pain, there are people desperate for knowledge and understanding. These are people who want only to get on the road to recovery. Counsel patience to them as well. It took a long time for their bodies to get to this shape and there are no "quick fixes."

Inflammation

It is important to keep in mind that neither FMS nor MPS is inflammatory, although secondary inflammation of the joints may sometimes occur in long-standing untreated MPS. This occurs because contracted muscles harboring trigger points (TrPs) can pull bones slightly out of alignment. NSAIDS make handy analgesics, but they do contain components that are unnecessary for noninflammatory conditions. Furthermore, NSAIDS often disrupt the deepest stage of sleep and can contribute to permeable gastric mucosa. Your patient probably already suffers from severe sleep disruption and may also have multiple allergies and chemical sensitivities.

Pain

Pain is a perpetuating factor, and you need to work closely with your patient to find a medication that will relieve pain without causing undue side effects. There are studies showing that people with FMS have aberrant central pain mechanisms (Bendtsen, Norregaard, Jensen, et al. 1997) and abnormalities in regional blood flow to some areas of the brain which are associated with low pain thresholds (Mountz, Bradley, Modell, et al. 1995). The pain stimulus itself may contribute to long-lasting changes in central nervous system excitability (Dubner 1991a). Sleep deprivation is also a perpetuating factor and a medication will be needed for this, as well. Care must be taken to address all perpetuating factors with a combination of diet, physical therapy, exercise, mindwork, and medication. Your patient will need a lot of help at first, while the perpetuating factors are brought under control. Don't expect results overnight. It took a long time for your patient to get in this position, and it will be a long, slow path to healing.

The Patient's Credibility

Believe what your patient tells you. Both fibromyalgia and myofascial pain syndrome are verified medical conditions (Wolfe, Smythe, Yunus, et al. 1990; Bennett 1987; Travell and Simons 1992; 1983). There are no acceptable reasons for disbelief, and there are many therapies and treatments. In specific cases, some therapies work better than others. Communicate with the others on your patient's medical team. You may be able to help unravel a veritable Gordian knot of symptoms.

Therapies

Begin therapies slowly. Due to the variations in FMS (many neurotransmitters are affected to different degrees) and MPS (there are many different trigger points), your patient will need time and attention. Initially, the patient may be able to tolerate nothing more than moist heat and passive stretching, with many pain medications needed. Because bodywork promotes the release of trapped toxins and wastes, feelings of fatigue and nausea may arise. These are indications that the patient must go slowly. At first, bodywork may not be tolerable more than once a week. The body must be given time to detox, with gentle, brief, nonrepetitive stretching (when tolerated). Once restorative sleep has been regained, with adequate pain control and a proper diet, healing may proceed much faster (Moldofsky 1994).

Medication

Once you have found medications that adequately control your patient's pain symptoms, please don't withhold those medications. There is at present no cure for FMS. Once you find medications and therapies that successfully deal with the factors that are perpetuating your patient's symptoms, it is appropriate to allow them to remain on those medications and therapies, or the symptoms will reoccur (Andersen and Leikersfeldt 1996; Fishbain, Goldberg, Rosomoff, et al. 1991; Garcia and Altman 1997a).

Proper medication can give your patient the "breathing space" needed for body and mind to return to healthier states. Only after the perpetuating factors have been brought under control, the body has been detoxed, and the autonomic nervous system has returned from its hyperirritable state should you begin decreasing the dosages of the medications— one at a time—as the patient begins to feel that s/he can make do with less support.

There are many interrelated imbalances in many neurotransmitter and hormone systems in FMS (Russell 1996; Crofford, Engleberg and Demitrack 1996; Bennett, Cook, Clark, et al. 1997). The doctor as well as the patient must be patient while the perpetuating factors are identified, and methods (medicinal and nonmedicinal) are found that will treat them adequately.

Myofascial Pain Syndrome (MPS)

Chronic Myofascial Pain Syndrome (MPS) is a *musculoskeletal chronic pain syndrome.* It is nonprogressive (although it may seem so), nondegenerative, and noninflammatory. It is composed of many trigger points (TrPs), which refer pain and other symptoms in very precise patterns in specific regions of the body. It seems progressive because each TrP can develop satellite and secondary TrPs, which can form secondaries and satellites of their own. With treatment of TrPs and the underlying perpetuating factors, however, the TrPs can be "reversed" and minimized or eliminated.

Two excellent medical texts on MPS are available: *Myofascial Pain and Dysfunction: The Trigger Point Manual, Volume I: The Upper Body* (Travell and Simons 1983) and *Myofascial Pain and Dysfunction: The Trigger Point Manual, Volume II: The Lower Body* (Travell and Simons 1992). These texts locate and illustrate the referred pain patterns, and tell what causes them and how to relieve them.

FMS and MPS

FMS and MPS are separate and unique conditions that can form a synergistic, mutually perpetuating FMS/MPS Complex. This is a condition of interconnected symptom spirals that become increasingly worse until the spiral is interrupted. That is, the pain causes muscle contraction which causes more pain which causes more contraction, and so forth.

Sometimes, due to myofascial splinting, the patient's muscles can feel like hardened cement. Each hard lump is a contraction knot. This consists of contracted sarcomeres. The ropy, taut band that forms is most probably created by compensating elongated sarcomeres. They produce a palpable tension to educated fingers (Simons 1997).

Trigger Point (TrP) Pain

Trigger point pain is rarely symmetrical. If perpetuating factors exist, secondary TrPs may develop in muscles that must compensate for those muscles that have already been weakened by primary TrPs. In addition, satellite TrPs can occur in the pain referral zones of the primary TrPs. These secondary and satellite TrPs can then form secondaries and satellites of their own, giving the impression that the condition is progressive.

The patient usually presents with complaints from the most recently activated TrP. When this is eliminated, the pain pattern may shift to an earlier TrP, which also must be inactivated. Trigger points are *directly* activated by acute overload, overwork fatigue, direct trauma, and chilling. They are also activated *indirectly* by other TrPs, visceral disease, arthritic joints, and emotional distress. Active TrPs vary from hour to hour and day to day. The signs and symptoms of TrP activity long outlast the precipitating event.

The chronic stress of the resultant sustained contraction, or excessive fatigue during repeated contractions, may cause a vulnerable region of the muscle to become strained, repeating this same process. One factor often initiates a TrP and another perpetuates it. Expect allodynia or hyperesthesia. Allodynia is a noxious response to a nonnoxious stimuli, like feeling pain from light, cold, heat, touch, vibration, or sound. Hyperesthesia is an amplified sensation, especially of pain.

Nerve Entrapment

When a nerve passes through a muscle between taut bands of myofascia, or when a nerve lies between the taut band and bone, the unrelenting pressure exerted on the nerve can produce *neuropraxia,* loss of nerve conduction, but only in the region of compression. The patient often has two causes of pain: aching pain, which is referred from the TrPs in the muscle, and the painful effects of nerve compression—numbness, tingling hypoesthesia, and, sometimes, hyperesthesia.

Patients suffering from nerve entrapment prefer cold on the painful region. Patients with myofascial muscle pain prefer heat and report that cold aggravates their pain. Limitation of range of motion is worse in the morning, and recurs after periods of immobility or overactivity during the day.

Therapies

A muscle with active trigger points cannot be strengthened. The TrPs must be deactivated first. This can be accomplished by careful galvanic electrical stimulation, spray and stretch techniques using Travell and Simons' methods (1992; 1983), trigger point acupressure, and other modalities. These therapies often work well in concert. Work hardening and weight training will do nothing but create more pain and disability.

Perpetuating Factors of Trigger Points

Common TrP perpetuating factors are skeletal asymmetry and disproportion • nutritional inadequacies • reactive hypoglycemia • paradoxical breathing • pain • impaired sleep • conditions impairing muscle metabolism • head-forward posture • chronic infections • habits such as chronic gum chewing • other TrPs • visceral disease • arthritic joints • FMS and other chronic illnesses • vitamin and mineral insufficiency • adhesions • previous surgeries • previous traumas • allergies • poor posture • poor body mechanics • poor coping behaviors • lifestyle • smoking • alcohol consumption • stress • Morton's foot • FMS/MPS foot • short upper arms • short lower legs • unequal leg length • hypothyroid • psychological stress • ill-fitting shoes • ill-fitting furniture and car seats • hypermobility • repetitious exercise and work • overwork • immobility • inappropriate physical therapy.

Scars and TrPs

Trigger points that refer burning, prickling, or lightning-like jabs of pain are frequently found in cutaneous scars. Scar TrP deactivation often can be accomplished by intracutaneous injection with 0.5 percent procaine or by repeated application of topical anesthetic. Trigger points may also be found in joint capsules and ligaments.

Autonomic Reactions and TrPs

Some trigger points may produce autonomic reactions, such as sweating, blanching, dizziness, and nausea. These autonomic responses may be relieved by treating the trigger point. To become adept at the diagnosis and treatment of trigger points, you must become familiar with referral patterns and autonomic concomitants, as well as the trigger points (Simons 1987). Keep in mind, however, that autonomic effect zones are not necessarily the same as pain referral zones. Trigger point sites can vary slightly from patient to patient. Many muscles have multiple TrP locations. The major factor in TrP pain is always mechanical, even if it was triggered by stress.

Each patient has a unique combination of neurotransmitter disruption and connective tissue disturbance. All patients need professionals who are willing to work with us until an acceptable symptom relief level is reached. For a clear and brief synopsis of myofascial trigger points, contact the Gebauer Company at 9419 St. Catherine Avenue, Cleveland, OH 44104, (800) 321-9348, and ask for the free monograph *Myofascial Pain Syndrome Due to Trigger Points* by David Simons, M.D.

For more information on FMS and/or MPS, you may contact Devin Starlanyl at her website. This site will provide you with an email address.

http://www.sover.net/~devstar

References

Andersen, S. and G. Leikersfeldt. 1996. Management of chronic non-malignant pain. *Br J Clin Pract* 50(6):324–330.

Bendtsen, L., J. Norregaard, R. Jensen and J. Olesen. 1997. Evidence of qualitatively altered nociception in patients with fibromyalgia. *Arth Rheum* 40(1):98–102.

Bennett, R. M. 1995. Fibromyalgia the commonest cause of widespread pain. *Comp Ther* 21(6):269–275.

———. 1987. Fibromyalgia *JAMA* 257(20):2802–2803.

Bennett, R. M., D. M. Cook, S. R. Clark, C. S. Burckhardt and S. M. Campbell. 1997. Hypothalamic-pituitary-insulin-like growth factor-I axis dysfunction in patients with fibromyalgia. *J Rheumatol* 24(7):1384–1389.

Branco, J., A. Atalaia and T. Paiva. 1994 . Sleep cycles and alpha-delta sleep in fibromyalgia syndrome. *J Rheumatol* 21(6):1113–1117.

Crofford, L. J., N. C. Engleberg and M. A. Demitrack. 1996. Neurohormonal perturbations in fibromyalgia. *Baillieres Clin Rheumatol* 10(2):365–378.

Dubner, R. 1991. Basic mechanisms of pain associated with deep tissues. *Can J Physiol Pharmacol* 69(5):607–609.

Eisinger, J., A. Plantamura and T. Ayavou. 1994. Glycolysis abnormalities in fibromyalgia. *J Am Col Nutri* 13(2)144–148.

Fishbain, D. A., M. Goldberg, R. S. Rosomoff and H. Rosomoff. 1991. Completed suicide in chronic pain. *Clin J Pain* 7(1):29–36.

Garcia, J. and R. Altman. 1997. Chronic pain states: pathophysiology and medical therapy. *Semin Arth Rheum* 27(1):1–16.

Moldofsky, H. F. 1994. Chronological influences on fibromyalgia syndrome. Theoretical and therapeutic influences. *Ballieres Clin Rheumatol* 8(4):801–810.

Mountz, J. M., L. A. Bradley, J. G. Modell, R. W. Alexander, M. Triana-Alexander, L. A. Aaron, K. E. Stewart, G. S. Alarcon and J. D. Mountz. 1995. Fibromyalgia in women. Abnormalities of regional cerebral blood flow in the thalamus and the caudate nucleus are associated with low pain threshold levels. *Arthritis Rheum* 38:926–938.

Neeck, G. and W. Reidel. 1994. Neuromediator and hormonal perturbations in fibromyalgia syndrome: results of chronic stress? *Ballieres Clin Rheumatol* 8(4):763–775.

Russell, I. J. 1996. Neurochemical pathogenesis of fibromyalgia syndrome. 1996. *J Musculoskel Pain* 4(1/2):61–92.

Samborski, W., T. Stratz, T. Schochat, P. Mennet and W. Muller. 1996. Biochemical changes in fibromyalgia. *Z Rheumatol* 55(3):168–173 (German).

Scudds, R. A. 1998. Lecture: Fibromyalgia and Myofascial Pain: Differential Diagnosis and Differences. Travell Seminar: Focus on Pain 1998, San Antonio, TX, March 13–15.

Simons, D. G. 1997. Myofascial trigger points: the critical experiment. *J Musculoskel Pain* 5(4):113–118

Travell, J. G. and D. G. Simons. 1992. *Myofascial Pain and Dysfunction: The Trigger Point Manual, Volume II: The Lower Body.* Baltimore: Williams and Wilkins.

———. 1983. *Myofascial Pain and Dysfunction: The Trigger Point Manual, Volume I: The Upper Body.* Baltimore: Williams and Wilkins (revision in process).

Wolfe, F., H. A. Smythe, M. B. Yunus, R. M. Bennett, C. Bombardier, D. L. Goldenberg, P. Tugwell, S. M. Campbell, M. Ables, P. Clark, et al. 1990. The American College of Rheumatology 1990 Criteria for the Classification of Fibromyalgia. Report of the Multicenter Criteria Committee. *Arth Rheum* 33(2):160–172.

What Your Primary Care Physician Should Know

By Devin Starlanyl, M.D., and Ken Hoelscher, M.D.

Please read the preceding section "What Everyone on Your Health Care Team Should Know."

Who Gets Fibromyalgia and Myofascial Pain Syndrome?

People of any age can get FMS/MPS, even children. Infant colic is often caused by trigger points (TrPs) that can be relieved with gentle Spray and Stretch and Cranio-Sacral Release. Fibromyalgia (FMS) in youth usually starts with a flu-like illness, and then manifests as "growing pains," which can also be a manifestation of TrPs. Only 25 percent of all patients with FMS are men. There is no gender bias in Myofascial Pain Syndrome (MPS).

If you catch FMS/MPS early, and can teach your young patients how to handle it, you can give them a good chance at life. Undiagnosed, children with developing FMS and/or MPS are often shunted aside as "behavior problems." Once you find the right combination of medications, physical therapy, and coping skills, your patient can avoid many of the absences from school that would otherwise occur. There is a chapter on FMS/MPS in young people in my first book (Starlanyl and Copeland 1996), and I have noted common childhood trigger points (TrPs) in my video, as they are noted in the medical texts *Myofascial Pain and Dysfunction: The Trigger Point Manuals, Volume I* and *Volume II* by Travell and Simons (1992; 1983).

Physiological Information

Any patient with diffuse bodywide aches of long duration, coupled with a sleeping disorder (inability to stay asleep, very light sleep, and/or inability to get restorative sleep) should be evaluated for fibromyalgia (FMS). Those sleep problems indicate the presence of the alpha-delta sleep anomaly, which is common in FMS. Patients with specific patterns of referred pain (trigger points), indications of blood vessel, lymph, or nerve entrapment or proprioceptive disturbances should be evaluated for Myofascial Pain Syndrome (MPS).

Once you become familiar with the concepts behind the diagnoses of FMS and MPS, your diagnostic skills will become sharper and you will more easily be able to separate the two conditions, even when they co-exist in the same patient. It is important to understand the differences, as this changes treatment strategies (Borg-Stein and Stein 1996).

Tender Points of FMS Hurt in Place

These tender points are often found in the official "eighteen locations." In cases of traumatic FMS, they may be clustered near trauma sites (including degenerative changes such as those from OA or DDD, or surgical incisions).

Muhammad Yunus, M.D., has found that, when testing for tender points of fibromyalgia, a good indicator of proper pressure is that when you use your thumb to press, you notice a blanching of the fingernail. This produces 4 kg of pressure (Yunus 1988).

Trigger Points of MPS Refer Pain to Other Parts of the Body

Trigger points (TrPs) may be active or latent. Latent TrPs restrict movement and cause muscle weakness, but don't cause pain until they are activated by immobility, stress, or one of many possible perpetuating factors. Be gentle when checking for TrPs. Pressing TrPs can aggravate them and cause pain, which can stay with your patient for days. Individual TrPs can be difficult to live with, but they often respond immediately to specific therapy.

It is not unusual in cases of FMS/MPS Complex for the muscles to feel as hard as cement. You may be unable to palpate the TrPs or tender points, or even to feel the ropy bands. Often, it is easier to palpate ropy bands in the forearm if the arm is extended three-quarters of the way. Once galvanic muscle stimulation, Spray and Stretch, and other physical therapy modalities have been used to break up the myofascial splinting, and all the perpetuating factors have been brought under control, you will be able to palpate the TrPs.

Perpetuating Factors

If an altered HPA axis, altered metabolism, and reactive hypoglycemia have conspired to create obesity, or if there is extreme muscle guarding, rely on your patient's history to give you an indication of the pattern of possible TrPs. As you know, a careful history is the most important part of the physical exam. Check for perpetuating factors. The most common perpetuating factors of TrPs are the following conditions: fibromyalgia, impaired sleep, reactive hypoglycemia, paradoxical breathing, hypothyroid, skeletal asymmetry and disproportion. Also consider nutritional inadequacies, anything that impairs muscle metabolism, exposure to toxins, chronic infections, psychological factors, allergies, and inappropriate physical therapy and stress.

Exercise

I have seen too many patients with active TrPs who were put into weight-training and work-hardening programs, which changed them from injured people into totally disabled people. Listen to your patient. Because of their healthy appearance, FMS patients are frequently denied the support that other handicapped patients take for granted. Ask your patient to set realistic vocational, social, and recreational goals.

Prescribing exercise should be considered as carefully as writing a prescription. You need the right dose, the right timing, and the right kind. It's not uncommon for patients to feel nausea or a dramatic increase in muscle aches, especially headaches, and/or exhaustion after any physical therapy has moved a large amount of toxins and wastes from their constricted muscles. Warn patients to take it easy after physical therapy.

Some people blame FMS on deconditioning. This has been shown to be a fallacy. Everyone who is physically deconditioned does not get FMS. Conversely, some extremely athletic people have developed FMS as a result of traumas received while they were in peak physical condition.

As TrPs are inactivated, the patient should begin carefully graded exercises to increase strength and endurance. You need to work with a good physical therapist who is knowledgeable about both FMS and MPS. Initially, the patient may be able to tolerate only one short session once a week. The body needs time to process released toxins and waste. There is good evidence that continuing to exercise in spite of pain simply aggravates the abnormal pain filter (Bennett 1997).

Pain

What eases one TrP may adversely affect another. This is especially true in FMS/MPS Complex. Fibromyalgia amplifies the pain and other symptoms of myofascial trigger points. FMS/MPS Complex is not to be taken lightly. Neither are individual trigger points. As Travell and Simons say, "A swimmer may drown from a muscle cramp produced by a myofascial trigger point. Myofascial pain has driven some patients to suicide. Myofascial back pain is a major, unrecognized source of industrial disability" (1983, 18).

Pain is a large factor in FMS and MPS and is also a major perpetuating factor for both conditions. Furthermore, FMS sensitivity amplifies the pain of MPS. The general diffuse aching that is characteristic of FMS should not be confused with the specific trigger point sites and other symptomology of MPS.

If TrPs recur after effective treatments, there are hidden perpetuating factors. If the pain recurs but the TrP is gone, look for another cause, including cancer and other systemic diseases. Delayed-onset muscle soreness, which appears a day or two following overexertion, is a function of FMS and not of TrPs.

Above all, doctors must believe that their patients hurt as much as they say they do. To take a good history, the physician must first be willing to believe the patient. Undiagnosed FMS/MPS pain can be all-consuming, and even though the patient may look fine, many patients have been driven to suicide. Three FMS patients have made the news in the last three years because they chose the "Kevorkian option." Chronic pain can kill (Liebeskind 1991; Fishbain, Goldberg, Rosomoff, et al. 1991).

Psychological Information

Your patients may become confused or extremely stressed during office visits. They may have been misdiagnosed previously, perhaps several times. Furthermore, they may have been accused of malingering or of being neurotic psychosomatics. On the Internet, we call it the "It's All In Your Head" syndrome, or IAIYH. If you do have such patients, they should ask a family member or a trusted friend to accompany them to your office.

Depression

Depression is often a result of chronic pain syndromes. This is especially true when patients have had a long period of undiagnosed illness, or when their doctors and family have repeatedly said to them, "It's all in your head." Of course, it is also true that some patients do have emotional problems, and these can worsen the physical symptoms of MPS. Often, the constant effort of dealing with their so-called "untreatable pain" has reduced physical activity, limited social activities, impaired sleep, caused loss or change of family role, and perhaps been responsible for loss or change of job.

Think about it. Suppose you had lost your ability to practice medicine because you could no longer trust your fine motor control, and your ankles buckled. Suppose pain had become your constant companion and you felt confused and inarticulate most of the time. Yet through it all you continued to look just fine, and no one believed your account of your symptoms. How would you feel? Depressed? Misunderstood?

Acute pain that diminishes in the course of a natural healing process is generally manageable psychologically, but recurrent or persistent pain caused by an unrecognized cause threatens future function and well-being. It can lead to frustration, depression, and progressive disability. When patients mistakenly believe that they must live with and endure undiagnosed TrP pain because they have been told it is arthritis, they restrict their activities to avoid the pain. Then, their TrPs become latent. Patients must learn that TrPs are responsive to proper treatment. Conversations with patients should be about empowerment, not invalidation.

If relevant, order tests to identify coexisting conditions that might be contributing factors. Look for indications of reactive hypoglycemia. It is very common in FMS/MPS Complex. Take the time to talk with your patient. Take the time to *listen*. If you ask the right questions, you'll find out what you need to know.

Therapies

TENS units are not the best electrical unit for breaking up trigger points, because they don't create the necessary muscle contraction. Microstim, neuromuscular electrical stimulation, and galvanic stimulation work well. Home units are available with a prescription.

Trigger point injections can be part of an overall therapy regimen, but they do not stand alone. You must use myotherapy with them, and you must still identify and deal with the perpetuating factors. Stretched and injected muscles are likely to be sore for two to three days following treatment. Strenuous activities should be avoided while the muscles are sore, including shopping, gardening, and traveling. Patients with FMS/MPS Complex may not find injections as effective as will patients with just MPS. The injections may hurt more, and their effects may last for shorter periods of time. See the Travell and Simons *Trigger Point Manuals* (1992; 1983). Each specific trigger point injection technique is described in detail in those books.

If you get a chance to attend a seminar on FMS and/or MPS, do so. I'm sure you will find it worth your time:

- Contact Robert Gerwin, M.D., for information on Travell Myofascial Pain Seminars at (301) 656-0220.

- Contact Mary Maloney, P.T., at (203) 723-0533, for information on trigger point seminars.

- Contact Richard van Why, R.N., M.Div., M.L.S., for information on FMS regional seminars at (301) 698-0932.

- *Myofascial Pain and Disjunction: The Trigger Point Manual Volume I* and *Volume II* by Travell and Simons (1983; 1992) should be in your library and in your hospital library. The causes, perpetuators, and remedies for trigger points are all there. Keep the manuals on your desk and refer to them often. Think of them as an investment. Nowhere else can you get such a return on your time and money. The hard work has been done by Travell and Simons, and the answers are there.

- The *Journal of Musculoskeletal Pain* is an excellent source of new information, and don't neglect the *Fibromyalgia Network Newsletter*. It is a quick read, and summarizes much of the current ongoing research. It also provides you with a patient's-eye view of FMS, with tips on coping mechanisms.

The treatment of FMS/MPS can be a "throw away your crutches and walk" kind of experience that is all too rare in a physician's life. It is not that unusual to have an undiagnosed patient come to you on crutches, or even in a wheelchair, and within a few months of treatment to see that patient walk again.

References

Bennett, R. M. 1997. *Fibromyalgia Network Newsletter*. (July, p. 5) P. O. Box 31750. Tucson, AZ 85751-1750.

Borg-Stein, J. and J. Stein. 1996. Trigger points and tender points: one and the same? Does injection treatment help? *Rheum Dis Clin N Am* 22 (2):305–322.

Consensus Document on Fibromyalgia: The Copenhagen Declaration. 1992. Published in *Lancet*, vol. 340, Sept. 12, 1992, and *J Musculoskel Pain* 1(3/4) 1993.

Fishbain, D. A., M. Goldberg, R. S. Rosomoff and H. Rosomoff. 1991. Completed suicide in chronic pain. *Clin J Pain* 7(1):29–36.

Liebeskind, J. C. 1991. Pain can kill. *Pain* 44(1):3–4.

Starlanyl, D. J. and M. E. Copeland. 1996. *Fibromyalgia & Chronic Myofascial Pain Syndrome: A Survival Manual*. Oakland: New Harbinger Publications.

Travell, J. G. and D. G. Simons. 1992. *Myofascial Pain and Dysfunction: The Trigger Point Manual, Volume II: The Lower Body*. Baltimore: Williams and Wilkins.

———. 1983. *Myofascial Pain and Dysfunction: The Trigger Point Manual, Volume I: The Upper Body*. Baltimore: Williams and Wilkins (revision in process).

Yunus, M. B. 1988. Diagnosis, etiology and management of fibromyalgia syndrome: An update. *Compr Ther* 14(4):8-20.

What Your Cardiologist Should Know

Please read "What Everyone on Your Health Care Team Should Know."

There are many symptoms that can lead the person with fibromyalgia (FMS) and/or Myofascial Pain Syndrome (MPS) to your door. Chronic myofascial pain syndrome can mimic many cardiovascular problems (Travell and Simons 1983). You need to be familiar with the following myofascial trigger points (TrPs).

Myofascial Trigger Points

Scalene muscle TrPs can also cause nerve, blood vessel, or lymph entrapment. All three major scalene muscles can refer pain to the front and back of the body in a widespread pattern. In the front, they cause a persistent aching pain over the chest and down the front and back of the arm to the forearm. The chest feels "tight." On the left side, this pain may be mistaken for angina. Shallow pain also can be referred to the inner-upper border of the shoulder blade. There may be signs showing obstruction of veins and arteries and compression of the motor and sensory nerves of the arm. Sleep is often disturbed by pain from these TrPs. Your patient may have to sleep sitting up or propped up on pillows. There may be numbness, tingling, and odd sensations in the fourth and fifth fingers and in the little finger side of the hand and forearm.

Pectoralis major TrPs cause pain under the sternum. They also can transmit pain to the front of the chest and breast, extending down to the little finger side of the arm to the fourth and fifth fingers. Trigger points on the right side can produce arrhythmias. Trigger points on the left side often mimic heart-attack pain.

Trigger points of the pectoralis can occur in any of the muscle layers, in any place, but they are most common in particular areas. In the area of the collarbone, TrPs cause local pain. They also refer pain over the front of the shoulder muscle. In the breastbone area, TrPs are likely to broadcast intermittent, intense pain to the front of the chest and down the inner aspect of the arm. This can include a feeling of chest tightness, which is often mistaken for angina.

Trigger points of the pectoralis also can radiate pain to the inside top of the forearm, as well as to the little finger side of the hand, including the last two or more fingers. If you find arrhythmias and no other sign of heart problems, check for TrPs, especially in the right pectoralis major muscle between the fifth and sixth ribs. Chest pain that persists after a heart attack is frequently caused by these TrPs. Trigger points in the cardiac area can be relieved by the proper use of fluori-methane vapocoolant (Travell and Simons 1983).

Levator scapulae TrPs can cause shortness of breath (Neoh 1995). If your patient has a stiff neck as well, look for these TrPs.

Pectoralis minor TrPs send pain over the front of the chest and shoulder. Pain may run down the inner side of the arm, and include the last three fingers. Pain from a left side pectoralis minor TrP can mimic angina. These TrPs can entrap the axillary artery, as well as the brachial plexus nerve. The radial pulse can disappear as you move the arm to different positions. Numbness and odd sensations in the fourth and fifth fingers are common.

Overburdening these muscles can cause TrPs. They also can begin during a heart attack or other visceral disease. Some of these TrPs can entrap lymph vessels, which causes breast swelling. When coronary artery disease and TrPs coexist, myofascial constriction from the trigger points can cause further narrowing of the arteries.

Sternalis TrPs cause a deep ache under the breastbone, extending over the entire region of the breastbone and below. This can cover the upper chest and front of the shoulder on the same side, including the underarm and upper arm on the little finger side to the elbow. This produces an ache that feels like a heart attack or angina, and is independent of body movement. Trigger points can occur anywhere within the sternalis, but they are often found in the upper two-thirds and to the left of center at mid-sternal level.

Serratus anterior TrPs are responsible for the feeling of a "side stitch," as well as shortness of breath. There is referred pain to the side and to the back of the chest. This includes the lower interior border of the shoulder blade, and sometimes runs down the inner area of the arm, hand, and the last two fingers. There may be air hunger, with panting or mouth breathing. In severe cases, there is chest pain even at rest. The nerve going to the serratus anterior muscle may be entrapped because of scalene muscle TrPs.

Serratus posterior inferior TrPs produce an unusual ache radiating over and around the muscle.

Iliocostalis thoracis TrPs at mid-chest level send pain upward toward the shoulder as well as sideways toward the chest wall. Trigger points on the left side in this area cause pain that is often mistaken for angina.

Neurotransmitter Dysfunction

The dysregulation of neurotransmitters can lead to a drop in hemoglobin oxygenation during sleep (Alvarez Lario, Alonso Valdivieso, Alegre Lopez, et al. 1996). Part of this problem may be traced to constricted bronchi caused by neurotransmitter dysregulation. This can also contribute to excess mucus, which is often thicker than normal. These problems may be aggravated by coexisting allergies and/or asthma. In fibromyalgia, neurotransmitter dysfunction often has a direct impact on the cardiovascular system. Research has shown that chronic dyspnea is common in people with chronic primary fibromyalgia, but it is not due to cardiac or pulmonary causes (Caidahl, Lurie, Bake, et al. 1989). Respiratory pressures are low, but spirometric values have been reported as normal (Lurie, Caidahl and Johansson 1990).

Coexisting Conditions

Raynaud's syndrome is a common coexisting condition (Bennett 1991). Neurally mediated hypotension is often a frightening and potentially dangerous companion to FMS (Bou-Holaigah, Calkins, Flynn, et al. 1997; Clauw 1995). Look for symptoms of orthostatic sympathetic derangement (Martinez-Lavin, Hermosillo, Mendoza, et al. 1997). There is also an increase in mitral valve prolapse (Pellegrino, Van Fossen, Gordon, et al. 1989). Expect dyspnea (Weiss, Kreck and Albert 1998; Caidahl, Lurie, Bake, et al. 1989). The combination of these and other symptoms can be frightening, and add to your patient's stress. Check everything out, but reassure your patient that these are common problems with FMS.

References

Alvarez Lario B., J. L. Alonso Valdivieso, L. J. Alegre Lopez, S. C. Martel Soteres, J. L. Viejo Banuelos and A. Maranon Cabello. 1996. Fall in hemoglobin oxygenation in the arterial blood of fibromyalgia patients during sleep. *Am J Med* 101:54–60.

Bennett, R. M. 1991. Symptoms of Raynaud's syndrome in patients with fibromyalgia. A study utilizing the Nielsen test, digital photopleysmography, and measurements of platelet alpha 2-adrenergic receptors. *Arth Rheum* 34(3):264–269.

Bou-Holaigah, I., H. Calkins, J. A. Flynn, C. Tunin, H. C. Chang, J. S. Kan and P. C. Rowe. 1997. Provocation of hypotension and pain during upright tilt table testing in adults with fibromyalgia. *Clin Exp Rheumatol* 15(3):239–246.

Caidahl, K., M. Lurie, B. Bake, G. Johansson, and H. Wetterqvist. 1989. Dyspnoea in chronic primary fibromyalgia. *J Intern Med* 226(4):265–270.

Clauw, D. J. 1995. Tilt table testing as a measure of dysautonomia in fibromyalgia. *J Musculoskel Pain* 3(Suppl 1):10 (Abstract).

Lurie, M., K. Caidahl, and K. Johansson. 1990. Respiratory function in chronic fibromyalgia. *Scand J Rehabil Med* 22(3):151–155.

Martinez-Lavin, M., A. G. Hermosillo, C. Mendoza, R. Ortiz, J. C. Cajigas, C. Pineda, A. Nava and M. Vallejo. 1997. Orthostatic sympathetic derangement in subjects with fibromyalgia. *J Rheumatol* 24(4):714–718.

Neoh, C-A. 1995. Subjective shortness of breath and trigger points of levator scapular muscles. *J Musculoskel Pain* 3(Suppl 1):27 (Abstract).

Pellegrino, M. J., D. Van Fossen, C. Gordon, J. M. Ryan and G. W. Waylonis. 1989. Prevalence of mitral valve prolapse in fibromyalgia: a pilot investigation. *Arch Phys Med Rehabil* 70(7):541–543.

Travell, J. G. and D. G. Simons. 1983. *Myofascial Pain and Dysfunction: The Trigger Point Manual, Volume I: The Upper Body.* Baltimore: Williams and Wilkins (revision in process).

Weiss, D. J., T. Kreck and R. K. Albert. 1998. Dyspnea resulting from fibromyalgia. *Chest* 113(1):246–249.

What Your Chiropractor Should Know

Please read "What Everyone on Your Health Care Team Should Know," "What Your Primary Care Physician Should Know," and "What Your Physical Therapist Should Know."

Studies show that as a chiropractor, you are in position to help the patient with fibromyalgia (FMS) and/or Myofascial Pain Syndrome (MPS) in a fundamental way (Ferguson 1995; Hawk, Long and Azad 1997; Schneider 1992). It is vital that you understand the differences between FMS and MPS (Schneider 1995). Chiropractic has proven cost-effective for low-back and neck pain (Skargren, Oberg, Carlsson et al. 1997). In this specific area, a D.C. often has the edge over other medical practitioners, because Travell and Simons' work has been well understood and greatly utilized in the chiropractic field. If you are not familiar with *Myofascial Pain and Dysfunction: The Trigger Point Manual, Volume I* and *Volume II* (1992; 1983), I urge you to become so. These texts will revolutionize your practice.

Trigger Points and Chiropractors

One of the best ways to help people with FMS is to recognize that chronic MPS, or at least multiple trigger points (TrPs), are often basic perpetuating factors of FMS. Once you have checked for body asymmetry, head-forward position, paradoxical breathing, Morton's foot, and other TrP perpetuators, look for gastric malabsorption, hypothyroid, and reactive hypoglycemia. Adrenal stress is common, as are sleep disturbances and high levels of histamine. Vitamin and mineral insufficiencies are also common. Check for rotation of muscles, especially the iliacus. There are guidelines for the release of upper body trigger points (Mock 1997). There are also specific guidelines for individual muscles and muscle groups (Nilsson, Christensen and Hartvigsen 1997; Rask 1984; Saggini, Giamberardino, Gatteschi, et al. 1996). Be aware that some TrPs mimic respiratory and other systemic conditions (Neoh 1995).

Frequently, manual adjustment aggravates TrPs, especially if there is nerve entrapment. Activator adjustment is often well tolerated. Remember that your patient may hurt for some time after the adjustment regardless of your skill, and that any pain will be amplified by FMS. Traction does not seem to provide lasting relief. Electrical galvanic stimulation, with or without ultrasound, however, can be both diagnostic and serve to break up TrPs. It is important to remember that until the TrPs are broken up and the perpetuating factors dealt with, the contracted muscles will continue to pull the bones out of alignment (Schneider and Cohen 1992).

Ultrasound and Galvanic Stimulation

Ever since Dr. Willard Travell, Janet Travell's father, discovered that interrupted rhythmic electrical discharge produces a vigorous exercise of the muscle if it is directed properly, we've known that electromagnetics have a lot to do with tightness of the muscle. Alternate muscular contraction and relaxation increases blood flow through the muscles. Sustained contraction decreases blood flow. It is not unreasonable to expect that muscle stimulation and pulsed ultrasound can help break up myofascial trigger points. I have always found them very effective.

The use of ultrasound and high voltage pulsed galvanic stimulation to break up TrPs has been suggested in the literature. Travell and Simons theorized that "rhythmical contractions may increase local blood flow and help equalize sarcomere length," and that the galvanic stimulation may be utilized effectively to interrupt the pain/contraction cycle (1992, 10).

Whatever the exact mechanism, ultrasound with stimulation can be used as a noninvasive way to break up TrPs. Either low-voltage AC muscle stimulation (sine wave) with pulsed ultrasound or high-voltage DC muscle stimulation is effective for reducing TrPs and the resultant spasticity.

In cases of TrPs in localized muscle groups, the treatment regimen is relatively straightforward. Muscle stimulation should be set to patient tolerance. If fibromyalgia pain amplification is present, patient tolerance may be quite low, so input from the patient is essential. The clinician must raise the setting slowly, holding the gelled probe-face *in motion* over the suspected TrP area to avoid overheating the tissue in any one site. (If you keep the probe stationary, heat will build and may burn the tissues beneath.) With a prone patient, activity will be first noticed in the indifferent pad, with applicator probe activity following.

My chiropractor, Craig Anderson, has found TrPs often respond to a setting of 1 to 1.5 watts/cm2. GMS or ultrasound with low-voltage muscle stimulation can also be used in a diagnostic "search and destroy" mode. Deep TrPs and latent TrPs will respond to this method, and can be located and broken up in this way. The patient will feel either a "pins and needles" sensation with more superficial TrPs, or something like a raw sore deep inside the tissue at the site of a deep TrP.

Myofascial Pain

Chronic myofascial pain syndrome, complicated by long-standing pain/contracture mechanisms and other perpetuating factors, poses a great challenge to the clinician. It is essential to find and eliminate or minimize TrP perpetuating factors. The muscle grouping with the most impact on the patient's quality of life should be the first treated. The primary TrP is often difficult to pinpoint, as satellite and secondary TrPs may be very active. Once the pain/contracture cycle has been broken, the TrP may shift—first to latency, and then breaking up. During the course of treatment, the pain may shift from side to side as more TrPs are revealed under the softening musculature. As the TrPs break up, they release toxins and wastes.

The patient needs time to detoxify. If too much therapy is done at one time, nausea and/or low-grade fever and flu-like symptoms may appear. Even a five-minute treatment may leave the especially toxic patient fatigued, and it is prudent to counsel patients to take it easy for the rest of the day. Basic contraindications for electrical therapies apply.

There are now patient units available in many types and forms. For example, Electronic Neuromuscular Stimulator (EMS), or microstimulation, delivers a very low electrical pulse through electrodes applied to the skin. It relaxes muscle spasms and muscle tightness, increases circulation, and increases the range of motion. Electronic devices should not be used on cancer patients, near patients with pacemakers, on patients with heart trouble or seizure disorders. All manufacturer contraindications and precautions should be followed.

If trigger points return after successful therapy, there is a perpetuating factor that has not been addressed. Guidelines for assessing and treating TrPs, as well as an overview of TrPs and their pain patterns are contained in my video (Starlanyl 1997).

References

Ferguson, L. W. 1995. Treating shoulder dysfunction and "frozen shoulders." *Chiro Tech* 7(3):73–81.

Hawk,C., C. Long and A. Azad. 1997. Chiropractic care for women with chronic pelvic pain: a prospective single-group intervention study. *J Manip Physiol Ther* 20(2):73–79.

Mock, L. E. 1997. Myofascial release treatment of specific muscles of the upper extremity (levels 3 and 4). Part I, II, III. *Clin Bulletin of Myofas Ther* 2(1):5-33), 2(2/3):5-22, 2(4):51–69.

Neoh, C-A. 1995. Subjective shortness of breath and trigger points of levator scapular muscles. *J Musculoskel Pain* 3(Suppl 1):27 (Abstract).

Nilsson, N., H. W. Christensen and J. Hartvigsen. 1997. The effect of spinal manipulation in the treatment of cervicogenic headache. *J Manipulative Physiol Ther* 20(5):326–330.

Rask, M. R. 1984. The omohyoideus myofascial pain syndrome: report of four patients. *J Craniomandib Pract* 2(3):256–262.

Saggini, R., M. A. Giamberardino, L. Gatteschi and L. Vecchiet. 1996. Myofascial pain syndrome of the peroneus longus: biomechanical approach. *Clin J Pain* 12(1):30–37.

Schneider, M. J. and J. H. Cohen. 1992. Nimmo Receptor Tonus Technique: A Chiropractic Approach to Trigger Point Therapy. Section 3, chapter 3, pp. 1–18. In *Chiropractic Family Practice Manual*. Ed J. J. Sweere. Aspen Publication.

Schneider, M. J. 1995. Tender Points/fibromyalgia vs. trigger points/myofascial pain syndrome: a need for clarity in terminology and differential diagnosis. *J Manip. Physiol Ther* 18(6):398–406.

———. 1992. Soft tissue effects of sacroiliac and lumbosacral joint manipulation. *Chiro Tech* 4(4):136–142.

Skargren, E. I. , B. E. Oberg, P. G. Carlsson and M. Gade. 1997. Cost and effectiveness analysis of chiropractic and physiotherapy treatment for low back and neck pain. Six-month follow-up. *Spine* 22(18):2167–2177.

Starlanyl, D. J. 1997. *Chronic Myofascial Pain Syndrome: A Guide to the Trigger Points*. Two-hour video. Oakland: New Harbinger. (800) 748-6273 or (510) 652-0215.

Travell, J. G. and D. G. Simons. 1992. *Myofascial Pain and Dysfunction: The Trigger Point Manual, Volume II: The Lower Body*. Baltimore: William and Wilkins.

———. 1983. *Myofascial Pain and Dysfunction: The Trigger Point Manual, Volume I: The Upper Body*. Baltimore: William and Wilkins (revision in process).

What Your Dentist Should Know

By Devin Starlanyl, M.D., and Wesley Shankland, II, D.D.S.

Please read "What Everyone on Your Health Care Team Should Know."

The dentist is a vital and integral part of the FMS/MPS health care team. With awareness of fibromyalgia (FMS) and/or Myofascial Pain Syndrome (MPS) symptomology and preventative care, much pain and trauma and, most importantly, inappropriate and invasive treatment may be avoided.

Trigger Points and Dentistry

Both FMS and MPS can have a large impact on dental care. It is essential for you to know that your patient may have various muscles constricted by MPS trigger points (TrPs) in such a manner as to change the occlusion, forcing the mandible to close unnaturally (Fricton 1995). When the TrPs have been treated, occlusal contacts will change (Abdel-Fattah 1997). This can be a disaster if you have equilibrated the occlusion to the contraction of the muscles (Shankland 1996; Abdel-Fattah 1997). Trigger points can be caused by malocclusion, and the reverse is also true.

Equilibration and TrP treatment must take place together. Otherwise, they may both be ineffective. Some clinicians and researchers (Abdel-Fattah 1998) believe that degrading of the articular discs and the bony structures of the temporomandibular joint can result. Patients with FMS and/or MPS may react in unusual ways to bite splints. Sometimes splinting makes things worse for them. Patients have been known to bite right through a splint in one night. Often, processed, reinforced splints are required. In addition, a medication such as amitriptyline is also required at bedtime for the severe bruxers (Shankland 1983). For those with the combination of bruxism, muscle twitches, and cramping, clonazepam may be helpful.

Teeth clenching is a default mechanism of the brain. When it doesn't know what to do to respond to mixed or erratic signals, it may clench the jaw—a sort of twiddling of the cranial thumbs. Look for masseter TrPs and temporalis TrPs. Problems swallowing, chewing pain, jaw clicking, TMJ symptoms, soreness inside the throat, excessive saliva secretion and sinusitis-like pain, drooling during sleep, and choking on saliva can all result from an internal medial pterygoid TrP, which is often overlooked.

Trigger Points and Toothaches

Unexplained toothaches can be caused by several TrPs, chiefly in the temporalis, digastric, and masseter muscles. Each TrP has its own particular toothache pattern. Any kind of immobility can activate TrPs. Usually, a TrP-induced toothache is intermittent. During long dental procedures, take periodic rests to allow your patient to exercise and relieve the jaw muscles. Find out what symptoms go along with each TrP. For example, anterior digastric TrPs refer pain to the two front lower teeth, and the resulting tooth pain is often mistaken for pulpitis. Unfortunately, many unnecessary endodontic procedures are performed in an attempt to treat the patient's tooth pain, only to have the pain continue after the pulp of the tooth is gone. Anterior TrPs may also cause difficulty swallowing. Ask your patient about localized pain elsewhere in the body. See if you can't find a pattern. Thirty percent of all

FMS/MPS patients have TMJ problems. If there is inexplicable dental pain, dysfunction, and sensitivity, suspect trigger points. Pain can be referred to the teeth from various TrPs in the upper body.

Sternocleidomastoid (SCM) TrPs

The sternocleidomastoid TrPs are responsible for many motor coordination problems. Sternocleidomastoid TrPs can cause dizziness, imbalance, neck soreness, swollen gland feeling, runny nose, maxillary sinus congestion, "tension" headaches, eye problems (tearing, blurred or double vision, inability to raise the upper lid, and a dimming of perceived light intensity), spatial disorientation, postural dizziness, vertigo, sudden falls when bending, staggering walk, impaired sleep, nerve impingement, and disturbed weight perception.

Primary TrPs in the SCM often cause secondary TrPs that invoke dental pain. Also, with SCM TrPs, it's quite common for a trigger point to develop in the opposite lateral pterygoid muscle, producing malocculsion and perpetuating the TMJ/TrP cycle of pain and dysfunction. People with SCM TrPs often have trouble glancing downward—they can become so disoriented that nausea and vomiting result. Chronic dry cough, pain deep in the ear canal, pain to the throat and back of the tongue and to a small round area at the tip of the chin can be part of the SCM TrP package. Localized sweating and vasoconstriction can be a problem, as well as pain in a "skull cap" area of the head. These TrPs can also cause pain at the mastoid process and the deep nuchal line.

Nocturnal Sinus Syndrome

FMS/MPS nocturnal sinus syndrome is not an official name. This is a nighttime sinus stuffiness occurring on one side of the head which moves to whichever side of the head is lower. Gravity drains the congestion to the lower side. This condition accompanies postnasal drip and a constantly runny nose. Trigger points can form from this irritation, which eventually may refer teeth pain.

Vasomotor Rhinitis

Almost all FMS/MPS patients have "vasomotor rhinitis" at least some of the time. That's a runny nose with no "biological" cause. I think that with muscle tightening, normal fluid passages are constricted, and fluid backs up in the sinuses. So we get a constant postnasal drip all night, although the membranes of the nose may feel very dry and even bleed.

Facial Pain

One cause of prickling "electric" face pain over the jaw area is from compression of the buccal nerve by the two parts of the lateral pterygoid muscle in chronic bruxers. This sensation is frequently experienced upon waking in the morning or during times of intense stress. This symptom may also be caused by platysma TrPs.

Jaw pain and dysfunction are often the fault of one or more masseter TrPs, although trapezius and temporalis TrPs are often involved. Cutaneous facial TrPs can cause pain in the ears, eyes, nose, and teeth. These TrPs are shallow, and can occur in many places on the face. Jaw pain and dysfunction are often the fault of one or more masseter TrPs, although trapezius and temporalis TrPs are often involved, as well. Tell your patients to try acupressure. It may be vital to find a trained trigger point myotherapist to work with you and your patients (Heinrich 1991).

Trigger Points Caused by Prophylaxis

Because FMS is a pain amplification syndrome, even routine prophylaxis can be severely painful for FMS/MPS patients. In FMS, some of the mechanoreceptors have become pain receptors and central nervous system plasticity plays a large part in amplifying all pain. (Russell 1996; Yunus 1992; Bendtsen, Norregard, Jensen, et al. 1997; Lautenbacher and Rollman 1997). Tense muscles from the pain of cleaning may cause the jaw to hurt for more than a week. You might use infiltration of local anesthetic into the gingiva, where most of the scaling is necessary.

It's also helpful if there are frequent stops to move the jaw during cleaning and other dental work. Prescribe a muscle relaxer, such as Skelaxin, before and after cleanings, to allow for more stretching of the jaw. FMS/MPS patients can experience pain even during X-ray—those squares cut right in, especially under the tongue. Have the patient work on the masseter muscle for the next few days, using moist heat and acupressure. Note that many FMS patients cannot tolerate epinephrine in the local anesthetic.

Endodontic Therapy

Root canals can be torture. FMS/MPS patients feel pain earlier in the case of a threatened nerve. We feel extreme pain longer, often when other patients would feel none at all. Sometimes it is impossible to eliminate all of the pain. It is vitally important to get all the pulpal tissue out of the tooth as quickly as possible, again allowing the patient frequent rest periods. Several people have reported cases of "myofascial neuralgia" after a root canal—with pain that lasted a month or more. A few members of the Internet group have reported teeth cracking after this procedure.

Prothodontic Treatment

People with FMS/MPS have more than the usual difficulty adjusting to dentures, probably due to the FMS amplification of pain and the alteration in function of the muscles of mastication while chewing, especially with complete dentures. It is important that dental problems be fixed promptly. Dentures must fit, and any imbalances in the occlusion must be corrected, particularly when the patient is relaxed and his/her muscles are not painful. You may have to perform a re-mount procedure when attempting to refine the occlusion. Trigger points on both sides should be treated because of the interrelation of the musculature and jaw structures.

Preventive Procedures

For the TMJ patient after a dental appointment, applying ice followed by moist heat on the masseter and temporalis TrPs a few times a day may ease the pain. Tell your patient to avoid chewing gum and hard chewy foods, to limit mouth opening, and to chew foods as evenly as possible on both sides of the mouth. Instruct patients to brace their chin and limit mouth opening, even when yawning. Spray and Stretch with fluro-methane to inactivate TrPs is described in detail in the Travell and Simon's *Trigger Point Manual, Volume I* (1983). You might even demonstrate Spray and Stretch to the patient's spouse or companion.

Ischemic compression using acupressure techniques is also often effective. Prescribing an anti-inflammatory medication the day before, the day of, and the day after the dental appointment can be very helpful. Also, consider prescribing a mild muscle relexant like Skelaxin, as well. First discuss current medications already being taken. With FMS and MPS, medications may change frequently.

If you cannot specifically identify the cause of tooth pain or any other facial pain complaint, do no harm! Don't initiate any irreversible procedure such as endodontic therapy, oral surgery, or equilibration. Also, don't assume the diagnosis is cracked tooth syndrome just because the patient complains of tooth pain from an unknown origin.

References

Abdel-Fattah, R. A. 1998. Craniomandibular Myofascial Pain: Diagnosis and Treatment. Lecture: Travell Focus on Pain Seminar, San Antonio, TX, March 12–15.

———. 1997. An introduction to occlusal biomechanics in temporomandibular disorder. *Cranio* 15(4):349-350.

Bendtsen, L., J. Norregaard, R. Jensen and J. Olesen. 1997. Evidence of qualitatively altered nociception in patients with fibromyalgia. *Arth Rheum* 40(1):98–102.

Fricton, J. R. 1995. Management of masticatory myofascial pain. *Semin Orthod* 1(4):229–243.

Heinrich, S. 1991. The role of physical therapy in craniofacial pain disorders: an adjunct to dental pain management. *Cranio* 9(1):71–75.

Lautenbacher, S. and G. B. Rollman. 1997. Possible deficiencies of pain modulation in fibromyalgia. *Clin J Pain* 13(3):189–196.

Russell, I. J. 1996. Neurochemical pathogenesis of fibromyalgia syndrome. 1996. *J Musculoskel Pain* 4(1/2):61–92.

Shankland II, W. 1996. *TMJ: Its Many Faces*. Columbus: Anadem Publishers.

———. 1983. Craniomandibular pain: current treatment options. *Ohio Dent* 57(7):53–57.

Travell, J. G. and D. G. Simons. 1983. *Myofascial Pain and Dysfunction: The Trigger Point Manual, Volume I: The Upper Body*. Baltimore: William and Wilkins (revision in process).

Yunus, M. B. 1992. Towards a model of pathophysiology of fibromyalgia: Aberrant central pain mechanisms with peripheral modulation. *J Rheumatol* 19:6:846–850.

What Your Dermatologist Should Know

Please read "What Everyone on Your Health Care Team Should Know" and "What Your ENT/Allergist Should Know."

Many of your most mysterious cases may well fall under the umbrella of fibromyalgia (FMS) and/or Myofascial Pain Syndrome (MPS). Keep in mind that people with FMS and/or MPS are not a homogeneous lot. Different neurotransmitters are involved in the biochemical dysregulation that characterizes FMS, as well as the different trigger points(TrPs) found in MPS and FMS/MPS Complex.

Those of us with FMS and/or MPS also may respond differently to medications than what is expected. However, many of us do have high histamine levels. Many people with FMS will have a neurogenic flare response to stimuli (Helme, Littlejohn and Weinstein 1987). Talk to your patient. Find out if there is a change in the way a specific antihistamine works. Be aware that about 20 percent of those who take Benedryl are kept awake by it, and FMS/MPS patients already have sleep problems. The first trial of this medication should be made during daytime, on a day when alertness is not required.

Some of us get red, angry, photosensitive rashes. This can even take the form of a lupus-like pattern across the face. Sometimes, it is a reaction to our own "toxic" acid sweat. We can develop subcutaneous trigger points (TrPs) which appear as small lumps under the skin (Bassoe 1995). There have been recent findings of dermal IgE deposits and increased mast cells in FMS (Enestrom, Bengtsson and Frodin 1997).

Many people with FMS have allergies (Tuncer, Buntun, Arman, et al. 1997; Koenig, Powers and Johnson 1977; Smart, Waylonis and Hackshaw 1997), and some of us develop multiple chemical sensitivities (Slotkoff, Radulovic and Clauw 1997). Sensitivity to chemicals can further increase our allergic response system (Schedle, Samorapoompichit, Fureder, et al. 1998). In addition, TrP symptoms will often send us running to a dermatologist. Study the following trigger point referral zone patterns.

Trigger Points and Dermatology

Trapezius TrP3, about two-thirds of the way down along the inner edge of the shoulder blade and a little toward the spine, causes spillover pain to the upper neck region of the muscles along the spinal cord, as well as a deep ache and soreness over the area above the shoulder blade. This can feel like sunburn. The clue here is that this TrP also refers pain to the mastoid area behind the ear, and to the top of the shoulder. Nothing you can do topically will stop the "sunburn," but attention to the TrP will stop the pain.

Trapezius TrP5 located in the muscle close to the upper-inner corner of the shoulder blade, causes a burning feeling between the shoulder blades. TrP7 is an oval area along the spine above TrP5. It sends an unpleasant shivery feeling and goose bumps on the outside of the upper arm, and sometimes also to the thigh. This feeling is similar to shivers that may run up and down your spine when fingernails are scraped over a blackboard.

Other TrPs can cause autonomic concomittants, especially the sternocleidomastoid trigger points (Travell and Simons 1992; 1983).

The most important aspect of treatment is to believe your patient's account of her/his symptoms. Check out Travell and Simons' *Myofascial Pain and Dysfunction: The Trigger Point*

Manual, Volume I: The Upper Body (1983) to see what these TrPs look like. Ask patients who present with any of the symptoms described above if they experience generalized or regional pain, muscle weakness, or decreased range of motion. You may be able to pick up on FMS or Chronic Myofascial Pain Syndrome that other physicians have missed.

References

Bassoe, C. F. 1995. The skinache syndrome. *J Royal Acad Med* 88:565–569.

Enestrom, S., A. Bengtsson and T. Frodin 1997. Dermal IgG deposits and increase of mast cells in patients with fibromyalgia—relevant findings for epiphenomena. *Scand J Rheumatol* 26(4):308–313.

Helme, R. D., G. O. Littlejohn and C. Weinstein. 1987. Neurogenic flare responses in chronic rheumatic pain syndromes. *Clin Exp Neurol* 23:91–94

Koenig, Jr., W. C., J. J. Powers and E. W. Johnson. 1977. Does allergy play a role in fibrositis? *Arch Phys Med* Rehab 58(2):80–83.

Schedle, A., P. Samorapoompichit, W. Fureder, X. H. Rausch-Fan, A. Franz, W. R. Sperr, et al. 1998. Metal ion-induced toxic histamine release from human basophils and mast cells. *J. Biomed Mater Res* 39(4)560–567.

Slotkoff, A. T., D. A. Radulovic and D. J. Clauw. 1997. The relationship between fibromyalgia and the multiple chemical sensitivity syndrome. *Scand J Rheumatol* 26(5):364–367.

Smart, P. A., G. W. Waylonis and K. V. Hackshaw. 1997. Immunologic profile of patients with fibromyalgia. *Am J Phys Med Rehabil* 76(3):231–234.

Travell, J. G. and D. G. Simons. 1983. *Myofascial Pain and Dysfunction: The Trigger Point Manual, Volume I: The Upper Body.* Baltimore: William and Wilkins (revision in process).

Tuncer, T., B. Buntun, M. Arman, A. Akyokus and A. Doseyen. 1997. Primary fibromyalgia and allergy. *Clin Rheumatol* 16(1):9–12.

What Your FMS/MPS Emergency Room Staff Should Know

If time allows, read "What Everyone on Your Health Care Team Should Know." If time does not allow the first ER team to read it, have someone else read it and tell you what may be pertinent to your patient. Life will be a lot simpler for you and your future patients if you read it all when you are not pressed for time.

Fibromyalgia (FMS) patients experience enhanced pain and other sensory stimuli may be also be amplified (Bendsten, Norregaard, Jensen, et al. 1997; Elam, Johansson and Wallin 1992). Expect CNS neuroplasticity (Morley 1993). The patient may have multiple chemical sensitivities and drug allergies or unusual reactions (Slotkoff, Radulovic and Clauw 1997). Get a detailed history if possible. Check out Travell and Simons' *Myofascial Pain and Dysfunction: The Trigger Point Manuals* (1992; 1983) when you have time. All good medical libraries will have them.

Myofascial Pain Syndrome (MPS) is a chronic pain condition with autonomic concomitants. Fibromyalgia is a neuroendocrine dysfunction, and will amplify other symptoms, including pain. Expect hyperalgesia (amplified pain from painful stimuli) and allodynia (pain from nonpainful stimuli such as light, noise, odors, and touch) (Kosek and Hansson 1997). *Flare*, a time when symptoms are intensified and new symptoms often appear, may be the reason why your patient has appeared in the ER, in such great need. The symptoms are *not* psychological, but very real, and stress will further amplify them (Caidahl, Lurie, Bake, et al. 1989; Simms and Goldenberg 1988; Riera, Vilardell, Vaque, et al. 1994; Simons 1987; Triadafilopoulos, Simms and Goldenberg 1991).

Symptoms of FMS/MPS Complex may mimic many urgent ER conditions. Those urgent conditions may, in fact, be present as well, and may be further complicating an already complex case. In the best of all possible worlds, the ER staff would be trained in a thorough understanding of both FMS and chronic myofascial trigger points (TrPs). In the real world, if the normal tests show nothing, but your patient is in severe distress, here are some clues that may help you help that patient.

Rapid/Fluttery/Irregular Heartbeat/ Heart-Attack-Like-Pain

Pectoralis major trigger points (TrPs) cause pain beneath the center of the chest, under the sternum. They can also transmit pain to the front of the chest and breast, extending down to the little finger side of the arm to the fourth and fifth fingers. Trigger points on the right side can produce irregular heartbeats. Trigger points on the left side can mimic heart attack pain. In the sternum area, TrPs are likely to broadcast intermittent, intense pain to the front of the chest and down the inner aspect of the arm. This can include a feeling of chest tightness, often mistaken for angina. This may be accompanied by ectopic heart rhythms (Travell and Simons 1983, 585). Spraying the area with Fluori-Methane in the pattern described by Travell and Simons may relieve the immediate symptoms if they are due to simple TrPs (Travell and Simons 1983, 662), but repeated ischemic compression or local anesthesic injection to the trigger points may be required (Travell and Simons 1983, 589). The initiating factor may indeed be a myocardial problem, so a complete workup is necessary.

These pectoralis major TrPs can also radiate pain to the inside top of the forearm, as well as to the little finger side of the hand, including the last two or more fingers. If there are irregular heartbeats and no other sign of heart problems, check for TrPs. Look especially for an active TrP in the right pectoralis major muscle between the fifth and sixth ribs. Chest pain that persists after a heart attack is often caused by these TrPs.

The subclavius TrPs send pain across the front of the collarbone and shoulder. The pain travels down the inner part of the upper arm on the same side as the TrP. The pain skips the elbow, continuing down the top part of the forearm. It skips the wrist, but can include the front and back of the thumb and first two fingers. When coronary artery disease and TrPs coexist, myofascial constriction from the TrPs can cause further narrowing of the arteries.

Pectoralis minor TrPs on the left side can mimic angina. TrPs in this muscle can entrap the axillary artery as well as the brachial plexus nerve. Numbness and odd sensations of the fourth and fifth fingers are common. The pulse at the wrist can disappear as the arm is moved into different positions. Check for paradoxical breathing which perpetuates this and other TrPs.

Sternalis TrPs produce a deep ache under the sternum, extending over the entire region of the bone and below. This referral zone can cover the upper chest and front of the shoulder on the same side. It may spread to the underarm and to the upper arm on the little finger side to the elbow. This produces an ache like a heart attack or angina, and is totally independent of body movement. Trigger points can occur anywhere within the sternalis muscle, but most often reside in the upper two-thirds and to the left of center at mid-breastbone level. A TrP located where the pectorals, sternocleidomastoid, and sternalis come together can be the source of a dry, hacking cough.

Iliocostalis thoracis TrPs at mid-chest level send pain upward toward the shoulder as well as sideways toward the chest wall. Those on the left side in this area cause pain that is often mistaken for angina. Trigger points on either side of this area are often misdiagnosed as pleurisy. Low chest iliocostalis TrPs can refer pain upwards across the shoulder blade.

Shortness of Breath

The Serratus anterior TrP is responsible for a "side stitch" and shortness of breath. There is referred pain to the side and to the back of the chest. This includes the lower interior border of the shoulder blade, sometimes running down the inner area of the arm, hand, and the last two fingers. There may be air hunger, with panting or mouth breathing. In severe cases, there may be chest pain even at rest. Trigger points cause a reduced tidal volume because of reduced chest expansion. Also, the nerve supply to the serratus anterior muscle may be entrapped due to scalene muscle TrPs.

Stiff Neck

Levator scapulae TrPs cause a stiff neck. They produce pain in the area of the neck and along the inside border of the shoulder blade. This pain can also project to the rear of the shoulder joint. If they appear in conjunction with other upper body TrPs, the presentation may mimic meningitis.

Dizziness, Headache, Visual Disturbances

Sternocleidomastoid (SCM) TrPs in the sternal portion can refer pain to the top or back of the head, over the eye, across the cheek, or to the throat and the breastbone, depending on location of the TrP. Upper sternal SCM TrPs cause pain behind but not close to the ear, and to the back of the head. Other symptoms affect the eye and the sinuses, including tearing, reddening, or drooping of the eye, inability to raise the upper eyelid, and visual disturbances, such as blurred vision. Surroundings may appear dimmer than they actually are. Strongly contrasting parallel lines, such as in the play of light and shadow from trees on a road, window blinds, or escalator treads may cause a mild seizure-like effect. Stripes, polka dots, and checked patterns can cause dizziness. Sometimes a runny nose and sinus congestion develop on the involved side. Ringing in the ear and even deafness have been reported. Headaches/migraines can also be caused by TrPs in the trapezius, temporalis, splenii, suboccipital, semispinalis capitis, frontalis, zygomaticus major, cutaneous facial, and posterior cervical muscles, as well as by coexisting *reactive* hypoglycemia.

Trigger points in the clavicular portion can cause frontal headache and earache. The mid-clavicular TrPs refer pain to the front of the head. Symptoms include dizziness caused by movement, and disturbed balance. Spatial disorientation is common. Vertigo is not unusual, with possible syncope. Episodes of dizziness can last for seconds or hours. Ataxia occurs unexpectedly. Postural responses are exaggerated. This leads to a feeling of loss of control. Nausea is common, although vomiting is infrequent, due to proprioceptor disturbances. Double/blurry/changing vision can be caused by TrPs in the internal eye muscles, temporalis, SCM, trapezius, cutaneous facial, and splenius cervicis.

Abdominal and/or Pelvic Pain

Multifidi TrPs in the low-back multifidi also transmit pain to the abdomen, and perpetuate Irritable Bowel Syndrome (IBS). All multifidi TrPs can cause nerve entrapment symptoms including supersensitivity, numbness, or lessened sensitivity of the skin on the back. All paraspinal muscles can refer pain to the upper buttock, the kidney area, or produce pain in the groin and scrotum, causing retraction of the testicle.

Abdominal muscle TrPs can influence the organs, and the organ systems can perpetuate TrPs. Trigger points usually refer pain in the same quadrant, but may transmit symptoms into any other quadrant of the abdomen, as well as to the back. These TrPs can produce projectile vomiting, anorexia, nausea, urinary bladder and sphincter spasms, and painful menstrual periods, as well as IBS symptoms such as burning, fullness, bloating, swelling, and diarrhea

Abdominal oblique TrPs cause pain reaching into the chest, across the belly, and downward. Heartburn is common, as well as reflux. Superficial TrPs in the outer abdominal wall can produce diarrhea. What Travell and Simons (1983, 662) call the "Belch button" exists at the back rim of some side abdominal wall muscles, such as the external oblique, or in the membrane covering the deep muscles of the trunk and back. These TrPs cause "stomach problems" with belching and gas. This TrP can cause spontaneous burping and even projectile vomiting.

The rectus abdominus TrPs in the upper area refer pain to the mid-back on both sides. They can produce heartburn, uncomfortable abdominal fullness, indigestion, nausea, and vomiting. The vomiting is usually due to TrPs at the very bottom of the breastbone, especially on the left side. These TrPs can also refer pain across the upper abdomen between the rib margins. A TrP in the upper-left rectus abdominus can also cause superficial pain in the area of the heart. Trigger points in other parts of the rectus abdominus can cause symptoms of gall bladder disease, gynecological disease, and/or peptic ulcer. Active abdominal TrPs, especially the rectus abdominus, can cause a lax, distended abdomen with excessive gas. Contraction of the abdominal muscles is inhibited by the TrPs. Trigger points in the rectus abdominus around the sides of the umbilicus can create sensations of abdominal cramping or colic, especially in infants. These symptoms can be relieved by vapocoolant spray. These TrPs can also cause diffuse abdominal pain, which is accentuated by movement. Lower rectus abdominus TrPs, about halfway between the navel and pubis, are often responsible for dysmenorrhea.

McBurney's Point, a TrP on the right rectus abdominus, simulates acute appendicitis. This TrP can also refer pain throughout the quadrant, a sharp pain to the penis and inner hollow of the hip and to the iliacus muscle there, as well as simulating kidney trouble. Active TrPs in the lower rectus abdominus can mimic diverticulosis and pelvic disease.

The adductor magnus has a TrP high up that can refer severe pain deep within the pelvis. The pain referral zone can include the pubic bone, vagina, rectum, and bladder. It may mimic Pelvic Inflammatory Disease (PID) or prostate trouble. Adductor magnus TrPs can also compress the femoral blood vessels. Look for this TrP at the mid-inner thigh, about an inch from the groin. You may be able to feel a taut ropy band of TrPs there. Electrical stimulation and groin stretches help ease the pain of this troublesome TrP.

Iliopsoas TrP pain is transmitted in a distinctive vertical pattern along the lumbar spine on the same side as the TrP, and can extend as high as the region between the shoulder blades. There is also a referral zone on the front of the thigh, and a tight, painful area along the sides of the navel, with belly pain that is often mistaken for appendicitis. These TrPs can make it difficult to get up from a deep chair. Mobility may be reduced to crawling on hands and knees.

Iliopsoas TrP pain is relieved by reclining, especially with the hip flexed and the leg out to the side. These TrPs cause severe appendicitis-like pain that radiates down the thigh, and also refers pain to the low- and mid-back along the spine. These TrPs can occur from prolonged sitting with the hips acutely flexed, such as on long trips. People with active or latent iliopsoas TrPs tend to walk with a stooped posture, have a forward tilt of the pelvis, and excessive curvature of the lumbar spine. Back pain caused by iliopsoas TrPs is very common in pregnancy.

Iliopsoas TrPs rarely occur alone. Check the gluteus maximus and the hamstrings. Tightness of the hamstrings contributes to most low-back pain. Functional shortening of the hamstrings causes a backward tilt to the pelvis. This overloads the iliopsoas muscle and causes TrPs. Call a physical therapist to do a bilateral release of the hamstrings before the iliopsoas can be released.

Severe Low-Back Pain/Sciatica

Quadratus lumborum TrPs cause pain in the sacroiliac joint and lower buttock. This pain can spread forward along the crest of the hip to the adjacent lower belly, groin, and the top of the thigh bone. Even at rest, these TrPs can create a persistent deep aching pain, which is severe at all times, and becomes even worse with upright sitting or standing. It becomes difficult to turn or lean to the side. When first getting up, the patient may have to crawl to the bathroom. This intense pain can extend to the groin, testes, or scrotum, or radiate in a sciatic distribution. These TrPs can also refer pain to the outer part of the upper thigh. Deep quadratus lumborum TrPs can create lightning-like jolts of pain in the front of the thigh. The patient may be unable to roll over in bed, or unable to bear the pain of standing or walking. Coughing or sneezing becomes horribly painful.

Gluteus minimus TrPs occur on the side of the hip, radiating pain down the side of the leg, including the top of the foot. Trigger points beneath the crest of the hip radiate pain down the back of the leg through the calf. This pain throbs and pulses. It is intolerably persistent and excruciatingly severe. Your patient may not be able to find a sitting or reclining position that is comfortable. S/he may stagger or limp. There can be altered sensations of pain, unusual feelings, or numbness in the reference zone.

Trigger points in the piriformis and other short lateral rotator muscles can cause Piriformis Syndrome, which includes nerve entrapment as well as TrP pain. This pain hits the sacroiliac region, spreads sideways across the back of the buttock, over the hip, and to the upper two-thirds of the back of the thigh. There can be entrapment of many different nerves, blood and lymph vessels. Pain is usually increased by sitting, standing, and walking. These TrPs are often part of a matrix of TrPs in the hip and pelvis. The sciatic radiation of pain due to nerve entrapment can extend down the back of the leg to the sole of the foot. Piriformis Syndrome can include pain and unusual sensations in the lower back, groin, perineum, buttock, hip, the back of the leg, foot, and in the rectum during bowel movements. Symptoms are aggravated by sitting or by activity. There can be swelling in the affected leg, and sexual dysfunction or painful intercourse for both sexes. The foot can feel numb, with loss of awareness of the position of the foot. This produces a broad-based, staggering gait.

Severe Leg Pain

Vastus intermedius TrPs feel like three fingers of pain, stretched like claws across the middle front of the thigh from the outside to the inside in a diagonal pattern. There is difficulty with fully straightening the knee. If TrPs are present both in the rectus femoris muscle and high in the vastus intermedius muscle, the hip can buckle.

The vastus lateralis harbors many TrP sites along the outside of the thigh from the pelvis to the knee. These can cause the knee to buckle. The knee cap may lock in place, refusing to bend.

Buckling Ankle

Peroneus longus and peroneus brevis Trps have referral zones over the outside of the ankle, above, behind, and below it. Trigger Points in the peroneus tertius refer pain behind the ankle and to the side of the heel, as well as in the local area of the TrPs and the upper-outside of the foot. These TrPs cause ankle pain and weakness. The ankles turn out and sprain easily.

Fibromyalgia Flare

Compounding the above symptoms, there may be "flaring" or worsening of the all-over flu-like achiness of FMS, and aggravation of these common symptoms: difficulty getting out known words, directional disorientation, visual perception problems, short-term memory impairment, panic attacks, confusional states, and "fugue" type states (staring into space before the brain can function again). In addition, because your patient looks healthy, s/he may have met with disbelief and been refused support normally given to others who are ill. In all likelihood, you are dealing with this patient because the normal medical support structure has broken down or has never existed for this person.

When FMS and chronic MPS occur together, FMS often initiates a symptom and TrPs perpetuate it. The TrPs are difficult to break up because the FMS perpetuates them. The FMS/MPS Complex is more than just the sum of the two syndromes. Check for and deal with TrP perpetuators such as sleep deprivation, pain, FMS and other chronic illnesses, paradoxical breathing, metabolic problems, vitamin and mineral insufficiency, adhesions, previous surgeries, previous traumas, allergies, reactive hypoglycemia, "good sport" syndrome, poor posture, poor body mechanics, poor nutrition, poor coping behaviors, smoking, alcohol consumption, chronic infection (including yeasts/fungi/parasites), Morton's foot, FMS/MPS foot, short upper arms, short lower legs, unequal leg length, hypothyroid (Total T4, Free T4, Total T3, and TSH needed), psychological stress, ill-fitting shoes, ill-fitting furniture and car seats, hypermobility, repetitious exercise and work, overwork, immobility, and inappropriate physical therapy.

The TrPs described above are some of the most common that can cause ER appearances. Before such an emergency confronts you, become familiar with TrPs by studying the medical texts *Myofascial Pain and Dysfunction: The Trigger Point Manuals, Volume I* and *Volume II* by Janet G. Travell, M.D., and David G. Simons, M.D. (1983; 1992), and my video "Chronic Myofascial Pain Syndrome: Guide to the Trigger Points."

If these or any TrPs keep recurring, in spite of proper treatment, there is a hidden perpetuating factor, such as a metabolic problem, cancer, or structural stress. Relieving the TrPs may relieve the symptoms for a short period of time, but the underlying problem will still be there. For every FMS/MPS patient who shows up in the ER with these data sheets, there will be at least a hundred who don't have this information. There will be even more who will come in undiagnosed. You may be able to supply such patients with a missing piece of the puzzle that will put them on the road to better health.

References

Bendtsen, L., J. Norregaard, R. Jensen and J. Olesen. 1997. Evidence of qualitatively altered nociception in patients with fibromyalgia. *Arth Rheum* 40(1):98–102.

Caidahl, K., M. Lurie, B. Bake, G. Johansson and H. Wetterqvist. 1989. Dyspnoea in chronic primary fibromyalgia. *J Intern Med* 226(4):265–270.

Elam, M., G. Johansson and B. G. Wallin. 1992. Do patients with primary fibromyalgia have an altered sympathetic nerve activity? *Pain* 48(3):371–375.

Kosek, E. and P. Hansson 1997. Modulatory influence on somatosensory perception from vibration and heterotopic noxious conditioning stimulation (HNCS) in fibromyalgia patients and healthy subjects. *Pain* 70:41–51

Morley, J. S. 1993. Central neuroplasticity. *Pain* 54(3):363–365.

Riera, G., M. Vilardell, J. Vaque and C. Alonso. 1994. Fibromyalgia and abdominal pain. *Surgery* 116(1):117–118.

Simms, R. W. and D. I. Goldenberg. 1988. Symptoms mimicking neurologic disorders in fibromyalgia syndrome. *J Rheumatol* 15(8):1271–1273.

Simons, D. G. 1987. Myofascial pain syndrome due to trigger points. *Internat Rehab Med Assn Monograph Series 1*. Available from Gebauer (800) 321-9348.

Slotkoff, A. T., D. A. Radulovic and D. J. Clauw. 1997. The relationship between fibromyalgia and the multiple chemical sensitivity syndrome. *Scand J Rheumatol* 26(5):364–367.

Travell, J. G. and D. G. Simons. 1992. *Myofascial Pain and Dysfunction: The Trigger Point Manual, Volume II: The Lower Body*. Baltimore: William and Wilkins.

———. 1983. *Myofascial Pain and Dysfunction: The Trigger Point Manual, Volume I: The Upper Body*. Baltimore: William and Wilkins (revision in process).

Triadafilopoulos, G. R., W. Simms and D. I. Goldenberg. 1991. Bowel dysfunction in fibromyalgia syndrome. *Digest Dis Sci* 36(1):1237–1248.

What Your ENT/Allergist Should Know

Please read "What Everyone on Your Health Care Team Should Know."

You will probably find the fibromyalgia (FMS)/Myofascial Pain Syndrome (MPS) patient to be a Gordian knot you must unravel. Many of us have allergies (Tuncer, Buntun, Arman, et al. 1997; Koenig, Powers and Johnson 1977), asthma, food intolerance and disrupted immune systems, multiple chemical sensitivities, vasomotor rhinitis (Cleveland, Fisher and Brestel 1992), postnasal drip, chronic sore throat, dizziness, and a whole constellation of other symptoms that lead us right to your office (Travell and Simons 1992; 1983). To treat FMS and MPS properly, you must become familiar with the causes behind each of them, as well as with the trigger point (TrP) referred pain patterns. Myofascial TrPs can entrap nerves and blood vessels. They can also cause proprioceptor disturbances. This often makes diagnosis a challenge.

Effects of Trigger Points

Referred autonomic TrP phenomena can include vasoconstriction and subsequent blanching, coldness, sweating, pilomotor response, salivation, vasodilation, lacrimation, coryza, and hypersecretion, in addition to weakness, tenderness, spasms (increased motor unit activity), and pain. Proprioceptive disturbances caused by TrPs include imbalance, dizziness, tinnitus, and distorted perception of the weight of objects held in the hands.

Effects of FMS

People with FMS have a hypersensitized nervous system (Bendtsen, Norregaard, Jensen, et al. 1997). Histamine is a neurotransmitter that is regulated during delta sleep. People with FMS often have disrupted delta sleep due to alpha wave intrusion. Multiple chemical sensitivities (leaky gut syndrome), sensitivity to odors, light, noise, and weather changes are also common with FMS. We are often hypersensitive to molds and yeasts. We don't always react normally to allergy skin tests (Helme, Littlejohn and Weinstein 1987). There may be in an increase in dermal IgG deposits and an increase in mast cells (Enestrom, Bengtsson and Frodin 1997). Hearing and vestibular abnormalities are not unusual (Gerster and Hadj-Djilani 1984; Rosenhall, Johannson and Omdahl 1996). Dyspnea is common (Weiss, Kreck and Albert 1998). Once you become familiar with FMS and MPS, when you take a good medical history, you can see the pattern. You may find you need a combination of therapeutic strategies to do battle with FMS/MPS Complex.

Skin Problems with FMS

Skin discoloration can be part of the HPA-axis dysregulation or due to acidic "toxic" sweat patterns. Photoreaction with the sweat can produce brown or red mottling on the skin, which can appear in the form of the lupus "butterfly" rash. The pituitary is responsible for secreting melanocyte-stimulating hormone. Light triggers the hypothalamus, which triggers the pituitary. A heavy sunblock is often necessary. Detoxification programs, such as experimental guaifenesin therapy, often can prevent mottling. This has the added benefit of helping thin the thickened mucus, which is so common in FMS.

Prickling "electric" face is most often due to a trigger point (TrP) in the platysma muscle. This TrP refers the prickling pain to the skin area over the jaw. Jaw pain and dysfunction is usually a function of the masseter TrP, although the trapezius and temporalis TrPs are often involved.

FMS and Itching

When we itch, we often look for an allergic cause. We forget about sensory itch. There are, however, pressure-plate receptors in our outer skin layer called Merkel's discs. They translate the tactile messages received by the skin to the brain. When they don't know what message to send, they have a default mechanism. Unfamiliar sensations are translated as itch. It's my theory that due to the dysregulation of neurotransmitters in FMS and/or the mechanical constriction of fluids around the Merkel's discs, as well as a hypersensitive autonomic nervous system, we itch a lot—much more than most folks. Sometimes it is so bad that it disrupts our meager amounts of sleep.

Itching can also be a sign of low-level TrPs. Cold helps to numb the itch because it numbs the pressure-plate receptors. Dryness makes the itch worse because it creates an enhanced pressure reception by the discs. Some of the itches follow TrP referral patterns, in which case the TrP must be broken up. There is a maddening, inner ear itch which is often on the masseter TrP. It can be helped by acupressure in the depression that forms in front of the ear when the jaw is opened.

Livido Reticularis

Livido reticularis is a network of fine veins and capillaries that is extremely painful. It usually forms on the legs, but it can also occur on the arms. If it occurs in a referral zone, treat the TrP.

Welts

Red welts can occur with any kind of TrP therapy as part of the histamine (neurotransmitter) and mast cell liberation at the trigger points and other traumatic sites. Neurogenic pain can occur in response to even mild touch, heat, or chemical contact. There can be alterations of sensations in FMS, including a profound change in the tolerance of heat and cold (Kosek and Hansson 1997). Skinfold tenderness increases, as well as "tactile defensiveness," or muscle tension in response to touch.

"Natural-Killer" T-Cells

"Natural-killer" T-cells require serotonin to activate them. Serotonin is regulated in delta sleep. People with FMS have alpha-wave intrusion into our delta level sleep, so we miss the restorative sleep and neurotransmitter regulation that healthy delta sleep provides. In someone with fibromyalgia, the natural-killer T-cells insist "It's not my job" when confronted by an "alien invader." Teach preventative maintenance, such as the use of warm saltwater for nose drops before bed, to reduce the amount of mucus irritating the throat at night.

Sternocleidomastoid TrPs

Sternocleidomastoid TrPs can cause dizziness, imbalance, swollen gland feeling, runny nose, maxillary sinus congestion, "tension" headaches, eye problems (tearing, blurred, or double vision, red eyes, inability to raise the upper lid, and a dimming of perceived light intensity), spatial disorientation, postural dizziness, vertigo, sudden falls while bending, staggering walk, impaired sleep, nerve impingement, and disturbed weight perception. People with SCM TrPs often have trouble glancing downward without falling forward. They can become so disoriented that they experience nausea and vomiting. Chronic dry cough, pain deep in the ear canal, pain in the throat and back of the tongue and in a small round area at the tip of the chin can be part of the SCM TrP package. Localized sweating and vasoconstriction can be a problem, as well as pain in the "skull cap" area of the head. What SCM TrPs don't often cause is a pain in the neck, although they figuratively become one due to their wide-ranging symptoms. They may cause neck soreness. The feeling of continued movement in a car after you've stopped, and the feeling of tilted "banking" as your car turns corners are also caused by SCM TrPs.

FMS/MPS Nocturnal Sinus Syndrome

FMS/MPS nocturnal sinus syndrome is not an official name. This is a nighttime sinus stuffiness on one side of the head that moves to whichever side of the head is lower. Gravity drains the congestion to the lower side. This moving violation goes along with postnasal drip and a constantly runny nose, and can disrupt already scarce sleep.

Vasomotor Rhinitis

Almost all FMS/MPS patients have "vasomotor rhinitis." Because of muscle tightening, normal fluid passages become constricted and fluid backs up in the sinuses. This causes constant postnasal drip all night, although the membranes of the nose may feel very dry and even bleed. It isn't unusual for a massage therapist to be working on a trapezius TrP and suddenly the sinuses will clear. This often happens in an area right behind the jaw, under the ear. I can often tell what side patients sleep on most, because that's usually the side with the worst head and neck rigidity. The side they sleep on most is subjected to more of the drip . . . drip . . . drip . . . like water torture, on the back of the throat, all night. The SCM TrPs and the scaleni become tight to "splint" the sore throat and digastric TrPs. I have found that very warm saltwater used as nose drops to clean the throat and nasopharyngeal area before bed will prevent or at least minimize this difficulty without the need to add medications to the system.

If dysfunction of the neurotransmitter histamine is an integral part of a patient's FMS, antihistamines and decongestants can be important. If the postnasal drip isn't treated, trouble with swallowing develops due to digastric TrPs. This leads to head and neck pain, and a feeling of "swollen glands." Warning: Digastric TrPs are sensitive. Sometimes it's best for the patient to "milk" the area of its excess fluid, using a gentle downward stroking motion from the chin to the base of the throat. Tell the patient to start gently and listen to the body.

Ear Problems

Deep masseter TrPs may cause ringing or a low roaring sound in the ears. The sound may vary. The medial pterygoid TrPs can cause deep ear pain and stuffiness in the ear. The sternal portion TrPs of the SCM can also cause deep ear pain.

Throat and Neck Problems

Chronic dry cough is often caused by a TrP at the lower end of the sternal division of the SCM. The sternocleidomastoid is not a muscle, but a muscle group. TrPs in different areas cause different symptoms. To complicate matters, a chronic dry cough can also be due to esophageal reflux. Bruxism, chewing gum, playing a wind instrument or a violin will often aggravate neck TrPs. Problems swallowing, chewing pain, jaw clicking, TMJ problems, soreness inside the throat, excessive saliva secretion and sinusitis-like pain, drooling during sleep, and choking on saliva can result from internal medial pterygoid TrPs.

Facial TrPs

Cutaneous facial TrPs can cause pain in ears, eyes, nose, and teeth. These TrPs are shallow, and can occur in many places on the face. Tell your patient to try some pressure-point work. This, along with moist heat followed by massage of the head, neck, and shoulders can bring great relief to the tightened, distressed muscles.

References

Bendtsen, L., J. Norregaard, R. Jensen and J. Olesen. 1997. Evidence of qualitatively altered nociception in patients with fibromyalgia. *Arth Rheum* 40(1):98–102.

Cleveland, C. H. Jr., R. H. Fisher and E. E Brestel. 1992. The association between rhinitis and fibromyalgia. *J Allergy Clin Immunol* 89(1):358.

Enestrom, S., A. Bengtsson and T. Frodin 1997. Dermal IgG deposits and increase of mast cells in patients with fibromyalgia—relevant findings for epiphenomena. *Scand J Rheumatol* 26(4):308–313.

Gerster, J. C. and A. Hadj-Djilani. 1984. Hearing and vestibular abnormalities in primary fibrositis syndrome. *J Rheumatol* 11(5):678–680.

Helme, R. D., G. O. Littlejohn and C. Weinstein. 1987. Neurogenic flare responses in chronic rheumatic pain syndromes. *Clin Exp Neurol* 23:91–94.

Koenig, Jr., W. C., J. J. Powers and E. W. Johnson. 1977. Does allergy play a role in fibrositis? *Arch Phys Med Rehab* 58(2):80–83.

Kosek, E. and P. Hansson 1997. Modulatory influence on somatosensory perception from vibration and heterotopic noxious conditioning stimulation (HNCS) in fibromyalgia patients and healthy subjects. *Pain* 70:41–51.

Rosenhall, U., G. Johannson and G. Omdahl. 1996. Otoneurologic and audiologic findings in fibromyalgia. *Scand J Rehabil Med* 28(4):225–232.

Travell, J. G. and D. G. Simons. 1992. *Myofascial Pain and Dysfunction: The Trigger Point Manual, Volume II: The Lower Body*. Baltimore: William and Wilkins.

———. 1983. *Myofascial Pain and Dysfunction: The Trigger Point Manual, Volume I: The Upper Body*. Baltimore: William and Wilkins (revision in process).

Tuncer, T., B. Buntun, M. Arman, A. Akyokus and A. Doseyen. 1997. Primary fibromyalgia and allergy. *Clin Rheumatol* 16(1):9–12.

Weiss, D. J., T. Kreck and R. K. Albert. 1998. Dyspnea resulting from fibromyalgia. *Chest* 113(1):246–249.

What Your Eye Doctor Should Know

Please read "What Everyone on Your Health Care Team Should Know."

Some people with fibromyalgia (FMS) can't go anywhere unless they wear dark glasses, due to extreme light sensitivity. Some are bothered only by fluorescent lighting. Some get a seizure-like effect when confronted by a pattern of light and dark, such as the shadows made by trees along a road. There is often a problem driving at night, due to the lights of the oncoming cars. Beta-carotene seems to help this somewhat. There is a study indicating eye motility dysfunction in FMS (Rosenhall, Johannson and Orndahl 1996).

Contact Lenses and Eyeglasses

People with FMS often have sicca syndrome. This means that all the mucous membranes feel dry. Coupled with the FMS sensitivity to and amplification of pain, this causes difficulty with contact lenses. The dryness, irritation, sensitivity, and the allergies often prove too much to handle. Yet the weight of glasses can aggravate trigger points (TrPs) in the head and neck area. After a regimen of eye exercises and medication (especially guaifenesin), some people with FMS/MPS Complex have been able to wear contact lenses for the first time.

Facial TrPs

Cutaneous facial TrPs can cause pain in the ears, eyes, nose, and teeth. These TrPs are shallow, and can occur in many places on the face. Try some pressure-point work on the face. If the TrPs are there, they will let you know. It is fairly common in fibromyalgia and Myofascial Pain Syndrome (MPS) for deposits to form in the corners of the eyes.

Clear Vision

In order for vision to be clear, both eyes must take the same picture at the same time. When this doesn't happen, double vision, blurry vision, and/or changing vision can result. Misalignment of the eyes can be caused by TrPs interfering with the muscles that hold the eyeballs in place. Trigger points can be responsible for contracting these muscles at different tensions. Muscle fatigue would make things worse.

Tell your patient to do this:

To check the inner eye muscles, stretch them. Put one hand on your head, above your forehead. Then try to look at that hand. This shouldn't hurt. If it does hurt, it's the TrPs in your muscles telling you they are there. With your eyes still looking upward at your hand, look from one upper corner of your eye to the other. If this hurts, the TrPs are there, and that's at least part of what is causing your eye problem. The eye exercises stretch out eye muscle TrPs.

Once your patient does this simple eye exercise regularly, the mysterious changing vision problem usually disappears. Splenius cervices TrPs can also cause blurring of near vision. This will also cause pain in the side of head to the eye on the same side, and in the eye orbit. It is also helpful to discuss your patient's reading habits. Incorrect lighting can give rise to trigger points (Travell and Simons 1983, 208).

Floaters

Floaters are common in FMS, and may accompany the overgrowth or dysregulation of connective tissue growth, which I have observed to be common in FMS.

Jumpy Pages

Orbicularis oculi TrPs will refer pain to the nose, cheek, above the eye, and cause "jumpy pages" when reading. Tell your patient to try putting clear plastic over the page to decrease print contrast. Acupressure around the eye will help.

Asymmetry

Asymmetry is a common perpetrator of TrPs. Check to see if your patient's ears are misaligned. Ensure that glasses fit well.

Sternocleidmastoid (SCM) Trigger Points

Sternocleidmastoid TrPs can cause dizziness, imbalance, swollen gland feeling, runny nose, maxillary sinus congestion, "tension" headaches, eye problems (tearing, ptosis, blurred or double vision, inability to raise the upper lid, and a dimming of perceived light intensity), spatial disorientation, postural dizziness, vertigo, sudden falls while bending, staggering walk, impaired sleep, nerve impingement, and disturbed weight perception. People with SCM TrPs often have trouble glancing downward without falling forward. They can become so disoriented that there is nausea and vomiting. Chronic dry cough, pain deep in the ear canal, pain to the throat and back of the tongue and to a small round area at the tip of the chin can be part of the SCM TrP package. Localized sweating and vasoconstriction can be a problem, as well as pain in a "skull cap" area of the head. What SCM TrPs don't cause is a pain in the neck, although they figuratively become one due to their wide-ranging symptoms. They may cause neck soreness, however.

These symptoms can include a feeling of continued movement in a car after stopping, and the feeling of tilted "banking" as the car turns corners. Some patterns of stripes, checks, and small print can cause dizziness if SCM TrPs are present.

Clumsiness

Ask your patient if s/he bumps into doorjambs, walls, and other stationary objects, and knocks things over often. FMS/MPS patients go tripping through life, cleaning up one mess after another. We learn to keep our sense of humor and a good supply of absorbent paper towels. The combination of SCM TrPs and extrinsic eye muscle TrPs seem to be chiefly responsible for visual perception problems. Reassure your patient that this is a mechanical problem that can be overcome. This knowledge alone may bring a great deal of relief.

References

Rosenhall, U., G. Johannson and G. Orndahl. 1996. Otoneurologic and audiologic findings in fibromyalgia. *Scand J Rehabil Med* 28(4):225–232.

Travell, J. G. and D. G. Simons. 1983. *Myofascial Pain and Dysfunction: The Trigger Point Manual, Volume I: The Upper Body.* Baltimore: William and Wilkins (revision in process).

What Your Gastroenterologist Should Know

Please read "What Everyone on Your Health Care Team Should Know." Please also read the section "Reactive Hypoglycemia" from chapter 3.

It has long been known that bowel motility is affected by neurotransmitters. Although fibromyalgia (FMS) may be causing some patients to head for your door (Sivri, Cindas, Dincer, et al. 1996; Triadafilopoulos, Simms and Goldenberg 1991), many irritable bowel and related symptoms are caused or aggravated by myofascial trigger points (TrPs).

Low-back multifidi trigger points transmit pain to the abdomen, and perpetuate Irritable Bowel Syndrome (IBS). At the base of the vertebrae they refer pain to the tailbone. All multifidi trigger points (TrPs) can cause nerve entrapment symptoms including supersensitivity, numbness, or lessened sensitivity of the skin on the back. All paraspinal muscles can refer pain to the upper buttocks, the kidney area, or produce pain in the groin and scrotum, causing retraction of the testicle.

Abdominal Muscle TrPs

Abdominal muscle TrPs can influence the organs, and the organ systems in turn can perpetuate the TrPs. This forms a mutually reinforcing pain network until you intervene. Abdominal TrPs usually refer pain in the same quadrant, but occasionally they may transmit symptoms into any other quadrant of the abdomen, as well as to the back. They are hard to diagnose, but much harder to endure. These TrPs can produce projectile vomiting, anorexia (Travell and Simons 1983, 660), nausea, urinary bladder and sphincter spasms, and painful menstrual periods, as well as IBS symptoms such as burning, fullness, bloating, swelling, and diarrhea.

Abdominal oblique TrPs can cause pain that reaches up into the chest, crosses the belly, and reaches long fingers of pain downward. Heartburn is a common symptom, as well as acid reflux. These symptoms may also indicate TrPs in the rectus abdominis.

Active TrPs in the muscles of the lower side abdominal wall can refer pain to the groin and testicles, and then project fingers of pain elsewhere. Superficial TrPs in the outer abdominal wall can produce diarrhea.

What Travell and Simons call the "Belch button" (1983, 662) exists at the back rim of some side abdominal wall muscles, such as the external oblique, or in the membrane covering the deep muscles of the trunk and back. These TrPs cause "stomach problems" with belching and gas. When active, this TrP can cause spontaneous burping and even projectile vomiting. Diseases of the internal organs can activate TrPs that will then perpetuate the pain and other symptoms long after your patient has recovered from the disease.

Trigger points in the upper area of the rectus abdominus can also produce symptoms of heartburn, uncomfortable abdominal fullness, indigestion, nausea, and even vomiting. The vomiting is usually due to TrPs at the very bottom of the breastbone, especially on the left side. These TrPs can also refer pain across the upper abdomen between the rib margins. A TrP in the upper-left rectus abdominus can cause superficial pain in the area of the heart.

Trigger points in other parts of the rectus abdominus can cause symptoms of gall bladder disease, gynecological disease, and/or peptic ulcer. Active abdominal TrPs, especially the rectus abdominus, can cause a lax, distended abdomen with excessive gas. In this case, contraction of the abdominal muscles is inhibited by the TrPs. Trigger points in the rectus abdominus around the sides of the belly button can create sensations of abdominal cramping or colic. This happens to infants. Fortunately, these symptoms can be relieved gently by vapocoolant spray. These TrPs can also cause diffuse abdominal pain, which is accentuated by movement.

A TrP at McBurney's point, on the right rectus abdominus, simulates acute appendicitis. This TrP can also refer pain throughout the quadrant, sending a sharp pain to the penis and inner hollow of the hip and the iliacus muscle there, as well as simulating kidney trouble. Active TrPs in the lower rectus abdominus can mimic diverticulosis and pelvic disease.

Lower abdominal pain, tenderness, and spasm can be referred from TrPs in the vaginal wall. A TrP high in the adductor thigh muscles can project pain to the lower lateral abdominal wall. There can also be TrPs in the diaphragm. These can cause an odd, fluttery feeling in the belly, as well as hiccups.

Causes of Abdominal Trigger Points

Abdominal TrPs develop in a muscle that is subjected to acute or chronic overload, or in muscles that are in the zone of pain referred from an organ disease. Peptic ulcer, parasites, acute trauma, chronic occupational stress, or an abdominal scar and adhesions will make your patient susceptible to abdominal TrPs. Other activating or perpetuating factors include total body fatigue, overexercise, emotional tension, exposure to cold, viral infections, yeast infections, constipation, poor posture, and body asymmetry. These stresses are additive. Referral patterns for TrPs in the abdominal muscles are less consistent from patient to patient than in the patterns for most other areas. Tennis ball acupressure, self-compression, good breathing techniques, pelvic tilt exercises, and lots of laughter can help to ease these TrPs.

Perpetuating Factors

If these or any other TrPs keep recurring in spite of proper treatment, you must find the perpetuating factor. That could be a hidden abdominal problem, or a systemic problem such as cancer or a metabolic disorder. Such organic disease can cause TrPs. Relieving the TrPs may relieve the symptoms for a short period of time, but the underlying problem will still be there.

References

Sivri, A., A. Cindas, F. Dincer and B. Sivri. 1996. Bowel dysfunction and irritable bowel syndrome in fibromyalgia patients. *Clin Rheumatol* 15(3):283–286.

Travell, J. G. and D. G. Simons. 1983. *Myofascial Pain and Dysfunction: The Trigger Point Manual, Volume I: The Upper Body.* Baltimore: William and Wilkins (revision in process).

Triadafilopoulos, G, R., W. Simms and D. I. Goldenberg. 1991. Bowel dysfunction in fibromyalgia syndrome. *Digest Dis Sci* 36(1):1237-1248.

What Your Mental Health Worker Should Know

Please read "What Everyone on Your Health Care Team Should Know." Please also read the section "Reactive Hypoglycemia" from chapter 3.

Any patient with diffuse bodywide aches of long duration (Bendtsen, Norregaard, Jensen, et al. 1997), coupled with a sleeping disorder (inability to fall asleep, inability to stay asleep, light sleep, inability to get restorative sleep, and/or waking early), should be evaluated for fibromyalgia (FMS). Patients with specific patterns of referred pain (trigger points), indication of nerve, lymph, or blood vessel entrapment, or proprioceptive disturbances should be evaluated for Myofascial Pain Syndrome (MPS) (Travell and Simons 1992; 1983). Once you understand the causes of FMS and MPS, you may be able to make a diagnosis that others have missed.

The "It's All in Your Head" Syndrome

Your patient may be confused or stressed during an office visit. S/he may have gone through years of misdiagnosis, and may have received a lot of criticism (Buskila, Neumann, Sibirski, et al. 1997). On the Internet, it's called the "It's All In Your Head" Syndrome, or IAIYH (Van Loon 1995). Visiting anyone in the medical care field often may have been very stressful (Jones 1996). Consequently, you may need to ask a family member to come with your patient. Note that it is wise to ask whether morning appointments are OK before scheduling these patients early in the morning, because their morning stiffness can be considerably debilitating.

Think about how you would feel if you were no longer able to practice your profession . . . if you lost the ability to control your muscles, and sometimes even to think clearly . . . if you couldn't function in your family role . . . if you were in severe pain, and your ankles were buckling, and you couldn't even pick up a glass of water without spilling it all over yourself, and yet your family and your friends thought you were crazy because you *looked just fine* . . . how would you feel? This is what it is like for many people with FMS and MPS.

Too little serotonin may trigger depression. Acute pain that diminishes in the course of a natural healing process is something that most of us can live with. Recurrent or persistent pain, especially when it is caused by an unrecognized or untreatable cause, can threaten our future function and well-being (Gritchnik and Ferrante 1991; Hitchcock, Ferrell and McCaffery 1994). This can lead to frustration, depression, and progressive disability. It is recognized that chronic pain states can cause depression (Hendler 1984). There is no specific personality type for Myofascial Pain Syndrome (Nelson and Novy 1996) or fibromyalgia (Johannson 1993). These studies indicate that "emotional disturbance in pain patients is more likely to be a consequence than a cause of chronic pain" (Gamsa 1990).

Important neurotransmitters are balanced and regulated during delta-level sleep, which is frequently interrupted in FMS (Branco, Atalaia and Paiva 1994). We usually need medication to help do what our bodies cannot do by themselves. Lack of restorative sleep impacts on cognitive function, which may already be disrupted by the chronic pain state (Grigsby, Rosenberg and Busenbark 1995).

The most intensively studied medications that modulate neurotransmitters are psychoactive drugs. *This does not mean that the patient's condition is psychological.* Depression is caused by the chronic pain state. Studies show that patients' lives are profoundly impacted by fibromyalgia (Burckhardt, Clark and Bennett 1993; Henriksson 1996).

Medications that affect the central nervous system are appropriate for FMS. They target the symptoms of sleep lack, muscle rigidity, pain, and fatigue (Yunus 1992). These medications don't stop the alpha-wave intrusion into delta-level sleep, but they do extend the amount of sleep, and may ease symptom "flares."

Chronic Pain

Please become as knowledgeable as you can about these conditions. You may have already seen many FMS/MPS patients, although many were undiagnosed or misdiagnosed. They all need your help to cope. Chronic pain from a nonmalignant cause is often treated less vigorously than cancer pain, although the level of pain may be equal or worse. Read the following quote. It is from *PAIN: A Clinical Manual for Nursing Practice* (1989) by McCaffrey and Beebe:

"The health team's reaction to a patient with chronic nonmalignant pain may present an impossible dilemma for the patient. If the patient expresses his depression, the health team may believe the pain is psychogenic or is largely an emotional problem. If the patient tries to hide the depression by being cheerful, the health team may not believe that pain is a significant problem. . . . Having an emotional reaction to pain does not mean that pain is caused by an emotional problem."

It's normal to be depressed with chronic pain, but that doesn't mean depression is causing the pain (Faucett 1994). Visits with your patient should be about empowerment, not invalidation. Your patient may have gone through a traumatizing period of not being believed, while being racked by chronic pain of unknown origin. You should encourage your patient to be an active manager and coordinator of the treatment team, and take responsibility for his/her own actions and consequences. Methods for accomplishing this are given in my first book (Starlanyl and Copeland 1996). Most patients had a high level of activity before FMS/MPS became full-blown. Now they must learn to understand their limits and be careful not to push beyond those limits. There are specific symptoms of FMS/MPS Complex that may cause you some confusion. They are as follows:

Muscle Twitching

Eye twitching is often the first noticeable twitch in FMS/MPS, and it's very common. It is often due to trigger points (TrPs) in the muscles around the eyes. Twitching muscles can become a serious problem. This can be a continuous twitch, or perhaps one or two muscles will fire off now and then. Fasiculations and waves of twitches can be due to low-level TrPs. This has been described as having your nerves plugged in to twinkling Christmas lights. Other people have severe twitches that disrupt their functioning. These can lead to painful cramping.

Trouble falling asleep, trouble staying asleep, light sleeping, interrupted sleep, waking up feeling tired and unrefreshed are all symptoms of the alpha-delta sleep disorder. It is not enough that your patients spend eight hours in bed. When they wake, they need to have had restorative sleep.

Difficulty getting out known words, especially nouns and pronouns, is part of the "cognitive deficits" package we get with FMS. Names and nouns become awfully hard to find.

It's frustrating. This may be compounded by coexisting reactive hypoglycemia (Hvidberg, Fanelli, Hershey, et al. 1996; Blackman, Towle, Lewis, et al. 1990; McCrimmon, Deary, Huntly, et al. 1996). Difficulty distinguishing right from left and/or difficulty finding places or following directions is also common. They say that there will never be a rally for fibromyalgia because none of us would be able to find where it was being held.

Short-term memory problems and confusional states are common. We often can't do a number of steps in sequence. I found that I was unable to deal with appointments on the half-hour while working on this book. My mind wouldn't register them as half-hours. I'd arrive a half-hour early or a half-hour late. The concept was too much for me to grasp, because of the extra work load. If your patient doesn't show up, it probably doesn't mean that the patient is noncompliant. You may want to flag that patient's visits for reminder calls.

Severe problems estimating distance and depth perception can cause driving to be extra exciting. Trigger points can cause severe dizziness when the field of vision is changing rapidly, as well as many other proprioceptor disturbances. Any pattern of light and dark, such as window blinds, escalator steps, trees along a road, or patterns in fabrics can cause dizziness or even a seizure-like feeling.

Free-floating anxiety, panic attacks, rapid mood swings, irritability with unknown cause, trouble concentrating, inability to recognize familiar surroundings—this is all part of what we term "fibrofog," and can be part of the neurotransmitter imbalance. This can be worsened by reactive hypoglycemia, which must be modified by diet.

"Sensory overload" is what I call the feeling that information and stimulation are coming at you so fast you can't deal with it. We either go into a "fugue" state—stare into space for a while until our brain catches up (this can happen mid-sentence)—or we close down some sensory input. In the latter case, we shut off car radios, leave noisy rooms, and avoid cities. We need our "space."

Sensitivity to cold, heat, humidity, barometric pressure, and approaching storms is a part of the body's "thermostat" regulating problems. One minute we're hot, and the next minute we have chills. We can also be hypersensitive to odors, sounds, light, and touch. Sometimes the whole world can seem alien and antagonistic. You can be the bridge to a healthier understanding of what is happening within. Listen to your patient, and don't be afraid to believe what s/he says to you.

References

Bendtsen, L., J. Norregaard, R. Jensen and J. Olesen. 1997. Evidence of qualitatively altered nociception in patients with fibromyalgia. *Arth Rheum* 40(1):98–102.

Blackman, J. D., V. L. Towle, G .F. Lewis, J. P. Spire and K. S. Polonsky. 1990. Hypoglycemic thresholds for cognitive dysfunction in humans. *Diabetes* 39:828–835.

Branco, J., A. Atalaia and T. Paiva. 1994. Sleep cycles and alpha-delta sleep in fibromyalgia syndrome. *J Rheumatol* 21(6):1113–1117.

Burckhardt, C. S., S. R. Clark and R. M. Bennett. 1993. Fibromyalgia and quality of life: a comparative analysis. *J Rheumatol* 20(3):475–479.

Buskila, D., L. Neumann, D. Sibirski and P. Shvartzman. 1997. Awareness of diagnostic and clinical features of fibromyalgia among family physicians. *Fam Pract* 14(3):238–241.

Faucett, J. A. 1994. Depression in painful chronic disorders: the role of pain and conflict about pain. *J Pain Symptom Manage* 9(8):520–526.

Gamsa, A. 1990. Is emotional disturbance a precipitator or a consequence of chronic pain? *Pain* 42(2):183–195.

Grigsby, J., N. L. Rosenberg and D. Busenbark. 1995. Chronic pain is associated with deficits in information processing. *Percept Mot Skills* 81(2):403–410.

Gritchnik, K. P. and F. M. Ferrante. 1991. The difference between acute and chronic pain. *Mt Sinai J Med* 58(3):217–220.

Hendler, N. 1984. Depression caused by chronic pain. *J Clin Psychiatry* 45(3 pt 2):30–38.

Henriksson, C. and C. Burckhardt. 1996. Impact of fibromyalgia on everyday life: a study of women in the USA and Sweden. *Disabil Rehabil* 18(5):241–248.

Hitchcock, L. S., B. R. Ferrell and M. McCaffery. 1994 The experience of chronic non-malignant pain. *J Pain Sympt Manage* 9(5):312–318.

Hvidberg, A., C. G. Fanelli, T. Hershey, C. Terkamp, S. Craft and P. E. Cryer. 1996. Impact of recent antecedent hypoglycemia on hypoglycemic cognitive dysfunction in nondiabetic humans. *Diabetes* 45(8):1030–1036.

Johannson, V. 1993. Does a fibromyalgia personality exist? *J Musculoskel Pain* 1(3/4):245–252.

Jones, R. C. 1996. Fibromyalgia: misdiagnosed, mistreated and misunderstood? *Am Fam Phys* 52(1):91–92.

McCaffrey, M. and A. Beebe. 1989. *PAIN: A Clinical Manual for Nursing Practice.* St Louis: C. V. Mosby Co.

McCrimmon, R. J., I. J. Deary, B. J. P. Huntly, K. J. MacLeod and B. M. Frier. 1996. Visual information processing during controlled hypoglycaemia in humans. *Brain* 119(4): 1277–1287.

Nelson, D. V. and D. M. Novy. 1996. No unique psychological profile found for patients with reflex sympathetic dystrophy or myofascial pain syndrome. *Regional Anesth* 21(3): 202–208.

Starlanyl, D. J. and M. E. Copeland. 1996. *Fibromyalgia and Chronic Myofascial Pain Syndrome: A Survival Manual.* Oakland: New Harbinger Publications.

Travell, J. G. and D. G. Simons. 1992. *Myofascial Pain and Dysfunction: The Trigger Point Manual, Volume II: The Lower Body.* Baltimore: William and Wilkins.

———. 1983. *Myofascial Pain and Dysfunction: The Trigger Point Manual, Volume I: The Upper Body.* Baltimore: William and Wilkins (revision in process).

Van Loon, E. 1995. Fibromyalgic depression: Surely it's all in her head? *J Musculoskel Pain* 3(Suppl 1):141 (Abstract).

Yunus, M. B. 1992. Towards a model of pathophysiology of fibromyalgia: Aberrant central pain mechanisms with peripheral modulation. *J Rheumatol* 19:6:846–850.

What Your Neurologist Should Know

Please read "What Everyone on Your Health Care Team Should Know." Please also read the section "Reactive Hypoglycemia" from chapter 3.

Neurotransmitters are your field. You know more than most physicians how fast the information is being updated in neurology and endocrinology. Neuroendocrine disorders are complex, and fibromyalgia (FMS) compounded with Myofascial Pain Syndrome (MPS) can leave you shaking your head in confusion. What's worse, most of the FMS/MPS Complex patients will come to you undiagnosed or misdiagnosed (Buskila, Neumann, Sibirski, et al. 1997).

Many of your patients may suffer from allodynia or hyperesthesia, but there are specific symptoms of FMS/MPS Complex besides pain in specific trigger point (TrP) patterns that should send up a red flag. Some of these symptoms mimic neurological disorders (Travell and Simons 1992, 1983; Simms and Goldenberg 1988).

Stiffness

FMS/MPS morning stiffness is primarily due to the immobility of the night, as well as to the lack of restorative sleep. It isn't so much the amount of sleep we get as the poor quality of sleep (Branco, Atalaia and Paiva 1994; Drewes, Gade, Nielsen, et al. 1995; Horne and Shackell 1991). Also, any time we stay in one position for any length of time, our bodies stiffen in that position due to inflexible myofascia. This stiffness may take hours to work out.

Twitching

Eyelid twitching is often the first noticeable symptom in FMS/MPS Complex, and it's very common. Check the periorbital TrPs, especially around the upper eye ridge. You will probably find some real screamers. Check the hollow slightly back from the outside corner of the eye. Also check the sternocleidomastoid, the temporalis, and the trapezius TrPs for possible causes of the eye twitch. You may also find other head TrPs. Other muscles twitching can become bothersome. Sometimes there can be a continuous twitch of many muscles. In other cases, one or two muscles will fire off now and then. This may be intensified by mineral insufficiency and/or neurotransmitter dysregulation.

Fasiculations and waves of twitches can be caused by low-level TrPs. This has been described as having your nerves plugged in to twinkling Christmas lights. Other people have severe twitches that disrupt their functioning. These can in time become painful cramping.

Sleep Problems

Trouble falling asleep, trouble staying asleep, light sleeping, interrupted sleep, waking up feeling tired and unrefreshed are often symptoms of the alpha-delta sleep disorder, which often occurs with FMS/MPS. The K-alpha sleep anomaly is also sometimes found in FMS.

Neurogenic Problems

Raynaud's syndrome is often present with FMS (Bennett 1991), and nerve, blood and lymph vessel entrapment by myofascial TrPs can compound the symptoms (Travell and Simons 1992; 1983). There may be increased neurogenic inflammation (Littlejohn, Weinstein and Helme 1987), sensory dysfunction (Kosek, Ekholm and Hansson 1996), qualitatively altered nociception (Bendtsen, Norregaard, Jensen, et al. 1997), and altered sympathetic nerve activity (Elam, Johansson and Wallin 1992) in FMS. There can also be orthostatic sympathetic derangement (Martinez-Lavin, Hermosillo, Mendoza, et al. 1997; Bou-Holaigah, Calkins, Flynn, et al. 1997).

Difficulty getting out known words, especially nouns and pronouns, is part of the "cognitive deficits" package we often get with FMS. Names and nouns become awfully hard to find. It's very frustrating. In addition, TrPs in speech muscles can create slow, "halted" speech pattern, or garbled sounds.

Difficulty distinguishing right from left and/or difficulty finding places or following directions is common. They say that there will never be a rally for fibromyalgia because none of us could find where it was held, and we'd all come on the wrong day anyway.

Short-term memory problems and confusional states are common. We may have difficulty multitasking, or performing a number of steps in sequence. You may have to arrange for your office to call your FMS patients an hour beforehand, to be sure that they remember. This behavior is common in chronic pain states (Gritchnik and Ferrante 1991; Grigsby, Rosenberg and Busenbark 1995). Long-term memory may disappear.

Your patient may have severe problems estimating distance and depth perception. This can lead to a feeling of unreality. Sternocleidomastoid TrPs can cause severe proprioceptor disturbances, including dizziness when the field of vision is changing rapidly, and many other proprioceptor disturbances. Any pattern on light and dark, such as window blinds, escalator steps, trees along a road, or patterns in fabrics can cause dizziness or even a seizure-like feeling.

Psychological Problems

Free-floating anxiety, panic attacks, rapid mood swings, irritability with unknown cause, trouble concentrating, inability to recognize familiar surroundings—this is all part of what we term "fibrofog," and can be part of the neurotransmitter imbalances. This can be worsened by *reactive* hypoglycemia (Hvidberg, Fanelli, Hershey et al. 1996; Christensen 1997; Lindgren, Eckert, Stenberg, et al. 1996), a common perpetuator of FMS and MPS, which must be modified by diet.

Expect severe headaches, which may be modified considerably by specific trigger point therapy if they are due to MPS (Travell and Simons 1983; Krabak, Borg-Stein, Oas, et al. 1996; Dunteman, Turner and Swarm 1996; Graff-Radford, Jaeger and Reeves 1986).

"Sensory overload" is what I call the feeling that information and stimulation are coming at you so fast you can't deal with it. We either go into a "fugue" state, and stare into space for a while until our brain catches up (this can happen mid-sentence)—or we learn to close down some sensory input. In the latter case, we shut off car radios, and avoid noisy rooms and cities. There are times we *need* our "space."

Depression is often caused by chronic pain states (Faucett 1994; Hendler 1984). Too little serotonin may trigger depression. Neurotransmitters are imbalanced in FMS (Russell 1996), and in the endocrine system as well (Pillemer, Bradley, Crofford, et al. 1997). Acute pain that diminishes in the course of a natural healing process is something that most of us can live with. Recurrent or persistent pain, especially due to an unrecognized untreatable cause, can threaten our future function and well-being, which can lead to frustration, depression, and progressive disability.

Physical Sensitivity

Sensitivity to cold, heat, humidity, barometric pressure, and approaching storms, light, noise, and odors may all be a part of body "thermostat" regulation problems. One minute we're hot, and the next minute we have chills. The hypothalamus at the base of the brain is our thermostat, so this is part of the disrupted HPA axis (Griep, Boersma and de Kloet 1994). The hypothalamus sends a message to the body to contract or dilate blood vessels, via neurotransmitters. Some of us run a low-normal temperature and some of us have chronic low-grade fevers. Check for hypothyroid and other metabolic dysfunctions.

Take a good history. We often have abnormal electromyographic results due to nerve entrapment by TrPs, and even abnormal EEGs, although these vary, like the symptoms, from hour to hour and day to day. Please use only surface EEGs. Remember that there is considerable pain amplification in FMS (Lautenbacher and Rollman 1997; Yunus 1992). Neuorplasticity plays a significant role in chronic pain states (Coderre, Katz, Vaccarino, et al. 1993). There are often white blotches in the MRIs. We don't yet understand their significance. Regional cerebral blood flow abnormalities have been documented in FMS (Mountz, Bradley, Modell 1995; Johansson, Risberg, Rosenhall, et al. 1995). Once you see this pattern of signs and symptoms and understand the concepts behind the diagnoses of FMS and MPS, they will become easier to recognize.

References

Bendtsen, L., J. Norregaard, R. Jensen and J. Olesen. 1997. Evidence of qualitatively altered nociception in patients with fibromyalgia. *Arth Rheum* 40(1):98-102.

Bennett, R. M. 1991. Symptoms of Raynaud's syndrome in patients with fibromyalgia. A study utilizing the Nielsen test, digital photopleysmography, and measurements of platelet alpha 2-adrenergic receptors. *Arth Rheum* 34(3):264–269.

Bou-Holaigah, I., H. Calkins, J. A. Flynn, C. Tunin, H. C. Chang, J. S. Kan and P. C. Rowe. 1997. Provocation of hypotension and pain during upright tilt table testing in adults with fibromyalgia. *Clin Exp Rheumatol* 15(3):239–246.

Branco, J., A. Atalaia and T. Paiva. 1994 . Sleep cycles and alpha-delta sleep in fibromyalgia syndrome. *J Rheumatol* 21(6):1113–1117.

Buskila, D., L. Neumann, D. Sibirski and P. Shvartzman. 1997. Awareness of diagnostic and clinical features of fibromyalgia among family physicians. *Fam Pract* 14(3):238–241.

Christensen, L. 1997. The effect of carbohydrates on affect. *Nutrition* 1(6):503–514.

Coderre, T. J., J. Katz, A. L. Vaccarino and R. Melzack. 1993. Contribution of central neuroplasticity to pathological pain: review of clinical and experimental evidence. *Pain* 52(3): 259–285.

Drewes, A. M., K. Gade, K. D. Nielsen, K. Bjerregard, S. J. Taagholt and L. Svendsen. 1995. Clustering of sleep electroencephalographic patterns in patients with the fibromyalgia syndrome. *Brit J Rheumatol* 34(12):1151–1156.

Dunteman, E., S. Turner and R. Swarm. 1996. Pseudo-spinal headache. *Reg Anesth* 21 (4):358–360.

Elam, M., G. Johansson and B. G. Wallin. 1992. Do patients with primary fibromyalgia have an altered sympathetic nerve activity? *Pain* 48(3):371–375.

Faucett, J. A. 1994. Depression in painful chronic disorders: The role of pain and conflict about pain. *J Pain Symptom Manage* 9(8):520–526.

Graff-Radford, S. B., B. Jaeger and J. L. Reeves. 1986. Myofascial pain may present clinically as occipital neuralgia. *Neurosurgery* 19(4):610–613.

Griep, E. N., J. W. Boersma and E. R. de Kloet. 1994. Pituitary release of growth hormone and prolactin in the primary fibromyalgia syndrome. *J Rheumatol* 21(11):2125–2130.

Grigsby, J., N. L. Rosenberg and D. Busenbark. 1995. Chronic pain is associated with deficits in information processing. *Percept Mot Skills* 81(2):403–410.

Gritchnik, K. P. and F. M. Ferrante. 1991. The difference between acute and chronic pain. *Mt Sinai J Med* 58(3):217–220.

Hendler, N. 1984. Depression caused by chronic pain. *J Clin Psychiatry* 45(3 pt 2):30–38.

Horne, J. A. and B. S. Shackell. 1991. Alpha-like EEG activity in non-REM sleep and the fibromyalgia (fibrositis) syndrome. *Electroenceph Clin Neurophysiol* 79(4):271–276.

Hvidberg, A., C. G. Fanelli, T. Hershey, C. Terkamp, S. Craft and P. E. Cryer. 1996. Impact of recent antecedent hypoglycemia on hypoglycemic cognitive dysfunction in nondiabetic humans. *Diabetes* 45(8):1030–1036.

Johansson, G., J. Risberg, U. Rosenhall, G. Orndahl, L. Svennerholm and S. Nystrom. 1995. Cerebral dysfunction in fibromyalgia: evidence from regional cerebral blood flow measurements, otoneurological tests and cerebrospinal fluid analysis. *Acta Psychiatr Scand* 91(2):86–94.

Kosek, E., J. Ekholm and P. Hansson. 1996. Sensory dysfunction in fibromyalgia patients with implications for pathogenic mechanisms. *Pain* 68(2-3):375–383.

Krabak, B. J., J. P. Borg-Stein, J. Oas, D. Dumais. 1996. Reduced dizziness and pain with treatment of cervical myofascial pain. *Arch Phys Med Rehabil* 77:940 (Abstract).

Lautenbacher, S. and G. B. Rollman. 1997. Possible deficiencies of pain modulation in fibromyalgia. *Clin J Pain* 13(3):189–196.

Lindgren, M., B. Eckert, G. Stenberg and C. D. Agardh. 1996. Restitution of neurophysiological functions, performance, and subjective symptoms after moderate insulin-induced hypoglycaemia in non-diabetic men. *Diabetic Medicine* 13:218–225.

Littlejohn, G. O., C. Weinstein and R. D. Helme. 1987. Increased neurogenic inflammation in fibrositis syndrome. *J Rheumatol* 14(5):1022–1025.

Martinez-Lavin, M., A. G. Hermosillo, C. Mendoza, R. Ortiz, J. C. Cajigas, C. Pineda, A. Nava and M. Vallejo. 1997. Orthostatic sympathetic derangement in subjects with fibromyalgia. *J Rheumatol* 24(4):714–718.

Mountz, J. M., L. A. Bradley, J. G. Modell, R. W. Alexander, M. Triana-Alexander, L. A. Aaron, K. E. Stewart, G. S. Alarcon and J. D. Mountz. 1995. Fibromyalgia in women. Abnormalities of regional cerebral blood flow in the thalamus and the caudate nucleus are associated with low pain threshold levels. *Arthritis Rheum* 38:926–938.

Pillemer, S. R., L. A. Bradley, L. J. Crofford, H. Moldofsky and G. P. Chrousos. 1997. The neuroscience and endocrinolgy of fibromyalgia. *Arth Rheum* 40(11):1928–1939.

Russell, I. J. 1996. Neurochemical pathogenesis of fibromyalgia syndrome. 1996. *J Musculoskel Pain* 4(1/2):61–92.

Simms, R. W. and D. I. Goldenberg. 1988. Symptoms mimicking neurologic disorders in fibromyalgia syndrome. *J Rheumatol* 15(8):1271–1273.

Travell, J. G. G. and D. G. Simons. 1992. *Myofascial Pain and Dysfunction: The Trigger Point Manual, Volume II: The Lower Body*. Baltimore: Williams and Wilkins.

———. 1983. *Myofascial Pain and Dysfunction: The Trigger Point Manual, Volume I: The Upper Body*. Baltimore: Williams and Wilkins (revision in process).

Yunus, M. B. 1992. Towards a model of pathophysiology of fibromyalgia: Aberrant central pain mechanisms with peripheral modulation. *J Rheumatol* 19:6:846–850.

What Your Nutritionist Should Know

Please read "What Everyone on Your Health Care Team Should Know." Please also read the section on "Reactive Hypoglycemia" from chapter 3. You may also want to review the medical articles in the References and Bibliography sections that specifically deal with nutrition and reactive hypoglycemia.

People with FMS and/or MPS are not homogenous, they have different sets of symptoms. The biochemistry of your clients with fibromyalgia (FMS) and/or Myofascial Pain Syndrome (MPS) may be considerably out of balance. Many neurotransmitters are involved with energy metabolism. There is also a great deal about the FMS/MPS combination that we don't know.

Metabolism

Metabolic abnormalities such as reactive hypoglycemia and hypothyroid states are common coexisting conditions with FMS. They are frequent perpetuating factors of both FMS and MPS. To gain some measure of control over FMS and/or MPS, the client must identify and deal with as many perpetuating factors as possible. The medical history you take must be thorough and complete, for that is where you will find the clues you need to help unravel these symptoms for your client. You are a vital part of the healing process. For example, growth hormone is often low in FMS (Griep, Boersma and de Kloet 1994). Growth hormone plays an important part in glucose counterregulation (Cryer 1996). Glucose counterregulation is essential in the prevention and control of hypoglycemia (Cryer 1993).

Carbohydrates

In the study of nutrition, many of us have learned the importance of stressing healthy carbohydrates. A great many clients with FMS/MPS Complex are intolerant of grains, especially whole grains. They often require a more balanced diet than the traditional "food pyramid," which is bottom-heavy with carbohydrates. They are carbohydrate intolerant, insulin-resistant (Reaven, Brand, Chen, et al. 1993), and have reactive hypoglycemia or postprandial hypoglycemia (Eisinger, Plantamura and Ayavou 1994). Whatever reactive hypoglycemia is called, and it has many other names, it is slowly being recognized as an important fact of modern-day life, often leading to the destructive duo of obesity and type II diabetes. I hope that there will be more studies on this. I have seen it so frequently that the connection has become obvious to me. Reactive hypoglycemia will not show up on the normal glucose tolerance test (Genter and Ipp 1994), but the symptoms are well known and the resolution of the problem is usually the restoration of a healthy, balanced diet.

I have observed a subset of reactive hypoglycemics who are very thin. Often they have trigger points (TrPs) and metabolic concomitants that cause nausea and intolerance to most foods. They are put on high carbohydrate diets which then cause further worsening of their illness. Often these clients have no desire to eat protein-rich foods. This can set up a spiral wherein the FMS symptoms worsen the MPS symptoms, and the reverse is also true. The reactive hypoglycemia may cause cognitive deficits, which lessen the client's ability to recognize the problem (Blackman, Towle, Lewis, et al. 1990; Christensen 1997; Hvidberg, Fanelli, Hershey, et al. 1996; McCrimmon, Deary, Huntly, et al. 1996).

I have talked to more than one person who was totally disabled and bedridden because of a few TrPs and reactive hypoglycemia, and sometimes with developing FMS. With the proper diet and care, however, they were walking within a week, and were relatively healthy within a month. You can make this kind of difference in your clients' lives, too.

It is essential that you find a diet regimen that works for your client. Often, the diet found in Barry Sears' books (1995; 1997a) are a good place to start. There is even a Zone recipe book, *Zone Perfect Meals in Minutes* (Sears 1997b). You may find, however, that your client requires more protein than these books indicate is needed.

Start by questioning your client about diet. Frequently there are two types—the open "carbo-junky" diet, which means feasting on cookies, chocolate, and potato chips, and the "healthy" carbo-hidden diet. People on the latter diet often mistakenly believe they have good nutrition. They eat hot or cold cereal or fruit and toast for breakfast, a salad and vegetable for lunch, and a pasta dish for dinner. Get them started on alternatives, like cottage cheese, meat and fish, and even tofu if necessary. Make sure every meal is balanced with protein, carbohydrate, and a little fat.

There may be a short period of intense headaches as your client's body adjusts to a new, healthier balance, but encourage the client to be firm. Once the headaches pass, the amount of energy and vitality the client will have will be surprising and well worth the effort. The client need not be a slave to measuring and weighing food, and once a healthy pattern is established, cheating once in a while is allowed. Your client may remark that when s/he cheats, however, there is a backlash of symptoms.

You may find that supplements such as chromium (McCarty 1996; Anderson, Polansky, Bryden, et al. 1987), magnesium and malic acid (Abraham and Flechas 1992), and carnitine (Bengtson, Cederblad and Larsson 1990) are helpful to your client. Bowel dysfunction may be part of FMS (Triadafilopoulos, Simms and Goldenberg 1991), but much of your client's discomfort may stem from myofascial trigger points.

Trigger Points

It is important that you be aware of some of the trigger points (TrPs) that may aggravate gastric symptoms, so that you will be alert for their presence. Check your medical library for *Myofascial Pain and Dysfunction: The Trigger Point Guide* by Travell and Simons (1983), or my video "Chronic Myofascial Pain Syndrome: A Guide to the Trigger Points."

The serratus anterior TrP is responsible for the "side stitch," as well as shortness of breath. This is the TrP that frequently develops if there has been repetitive vomiting. There is referred pain to the side and to the back of the chest. This includes the lower interior border of the shoulder blade, and sometimes runs down the inner area of the arm, hand, and the last two fingers. There may be air hunger, with panting or mouth breathing, as well as air swallowing and resultant gas. In severe cases, there will be chest pain, even at rest. A reduced volume of air goes in and out of the lungs due to reduced chest expansion. Also, the nerve supply to the serratus anterior muscle may be entrapped because of scalene muscle TrPs. There may also be a dry cough, because of low sternocleidomastoid muscle TrPs.

Iliocostalis thoracis TrPs at mid-chest level send pain upward toward the shoulder, as well as sideways toward the chest wall. Trigger points on the left side in this area cause pain that is often mistaken for angina. Trigger points on either side on this area are often misdiagnosed as pleurisy. Low chest iliocostalis TrPs can refer pain upwards across the shoulder blade. This pain can extend around to the belly, and down over the lumbar area.

Multifidi muscle TrPs along the spine refer pain to corners of the vertebrae. Low-back multifidi also transmit pain to the abdomen, and perpetuate Irritable Bowel Syndrome (IBS). At the base of the vertebrae they refer pain to the tailbone. All multifidi muscle TrPs can cause nerve entrapment symptoms including supersensitivity, numbness, or lessened sensitivity of the skin on the back. All paraspinal muscles can refer pain to the upper buttock, the kidney area, or produce pain in the groin and scrotum, causing retraction of the testicle.

Abdominal muscle TrPs can influence the organs, and the organ systems can perpetuate the TrPs. This forms a feedback spiral that worsens the symptoms.

In medicine, the abdominal area is separated into four parts, called quadrants. Trigger points usually refer pain in the same quadrant where they reside, but occasionally they may transmit symptoms into any other quadrant of the abdomen, as well as to the back. They are hard to diagnose, but much harder to endure. These TrPs can produce projectile vomiting, anorexia, nausea, urinary bladder and sphincter spasms, and painful menstrual periods, as well as IBS symptoms such as burning, fullness, bloating, swelling, and diarrhea (Travell and Simons 1983, chapter 49).

Abdominal oblique muscle TrPs cause pain that reaches up into the chest, crosses the belly, and reaches long fingers of pain downward. Heartburn is a common symptom, as well as acid reflux. Reflux occurs when the contents of the stomach—gases, liquids, or solids—return to the esophagus. It gives a new meaning to the term "gut reaction."

Active TrPs in the muscles of the lower side abdominal wall can refer pain to the groin and testicles, and then project fingers of pain elsewhere. Trigger points in the upper rim of the pubis and the inguinal ligament region close to the side can cause urinary frequency, retention of urine, and groin pain. In older children, they can also be the cause of bed-wetting. Superficial TrPs in the outer abdominal wall can produce diarrhea.

The "Belch button" is what Travell and Simons (1983) call the TrP that exists either at the back rim of some side abdominal wall muscles, such as the external oblique, or in the membrane covering the deep muscles of the trunk and back. These TrPs cause "stomach problems" with belching and gas. When active, this TrP can cause spontaneous burping and even projectile vomiting. Several TrPs can refer pain to the abdomen and produce effects that, together, can make you think that your patient has a diseased abdomen. Diseases of the internal organs can activate TrPs that will then perpetuate the pain and other symptoms long after the patient has recovered from the disease.

The rectus abdominus is a long, flat muscle in the front center of the body. Trigger points in the upper area refer pain to the mid-back on both sides. They can also produce symptoms of heartburn, uncomfortable abdominal fullness, indigestion, nausea, and even vomiting. The vomiting is usually caused by TrPs at the very bottom of the breastbone, especially on the left side. These TrPs can also refer pain across the upper abdomen between the rib margins. Active abdominal TrPs, especially the rectus abdominus, can cause a lax, distended abdomen with excessive gas. In this case, contraction of the abdominal muscles is inhibited by the TrPs. Trigger points in the rectus abdominus around the sides of the belly button can create sensations of abdominal cramping or colic. These TrPs can also cause diffuse abdominal pain, which is accentuated by movement.

These trigger points may be secondary or satellite trigger points from a primary TrP higher or lower in the body. If you suspect TrPs, discuss the possibility with the patient's primary care physician and physical therapist. If these or any TrPs keep recurring, in spite of proper treatment, there is a hidden perpetuating factor. That could be an unsuspected heart or abdomen problem, for example. Although, at first your patient may seem like a person with a bizarre collection of unrelated symptoms, listen carefully. Once you begin to grasp the concepts behind the facts of FMS and MPS, the symptoms often come together to give you the clues you need to help your patient.

References

Abraham, G. E. and J. D. Flechas. 1992. Management of fibromyalgia: rationale for the use of magnesium and malic acid. J *Nutritional Res* 3:39–59.

Anderson, R. A., M. M. Polansky, N. A. Bryden, S. J. Bhathena and J. J. Canary. 1987. Effects of supplemental chromium on patients with symptoms of reactive hypoglycemia. *Metabolism* 36(4):351–355.

Bengtson, A., G. Cederblad and J. Larsson. 1990. Carnitine levels in painful muscles of patients with fibromyalgia. *Clin Exper Rheum* 8(2):197–198.

Blackman, J. D., V. L. Towle, G. F. Lewis, J. P. Spire and K. S. Polonsky. 1990. Hypoglycemic thresholds for cognitive dysfunction in humans. *Diabetes* 39:828–835.

Christensen, L. 1997. The effect of carbohydrates on affect. *Nutrition* 13(6):503–514.

Cryer, P. E. 1996. Role of growth hormone in glucose counterregulation. *Horm Res* 46(4–5): 192–194.

———. 1993. Glucose counterregulation: prevention and correction of hypoglycemia in humans. *Am J Physiol* 264 (2 pt 1):E149–E155.

Eisinger, J., A. Plantamura and T. Ayavou. 1994. Glycolysis abnormalities in fibromyalgia. *J Am Col Nutri* 13(2):144–148.

Genter, P. M. and E. Ipp. 1994. Accuracy of plasma glucose measurements in the hypoglycemic range. *Diabetes Care* 17(6):595–598.

Griep, E. N., J. W. Boersma and E. R. de Kloet. 1994. Pituitary release of growth hormone and prolactin in the primary fibromyalgia syndrome. *J Rheumatol* 21(11):2125–2130.

Hvidberg, A., C. G. Fanelli, T. Hershey, C. Terkamp, S. Craft and P. E. Cryer. 1996. Impact of recent antecedent hypoglycemia on hypoglycemic cognitive dysfunction in nondiabetic humans. *Diabetes* 45(8):1030–1036.

McCarty, M. F. 1996. Chromium and other insulin sensitizers may enhance glucagon secretion: implications for hypoglycemia and weight control." *Med Hypo* 46(2):77–80.

McCrimmon, R. J., I. J. Deary, B. J. P. Huntly, K. J. MacLeod and B. M. Frier. 1996. Visual information processing during controlled hypoglycaemia in humans. *Brain* 119(4):1277–1287.

Reaven, G. M., R. J. Brand, Y. D. Chen, A. K. Mathur and I. Goldfine. 1993. Insulin Resistance and insulin secretion are determinants of oral glucose tolerance in normal individuals. *Diabetes* 42(9):1324–1332.

Sears, B. 1997b. *Zone Perfect Meals in Minutes.* NY: ReganBooks, HarperCollins.

———. 1997a. *Mastering the Zone.* NY: HarperCollins.

Sears, Barry and B. Lawren. 1995. *Enter the Zone.* NY: HarperCollins

Travell, J. G. and D. G. Simons. 1983. *Myofascial Pain and Dysfunction: The Trigger Point Manual, Volume I: The Upper Body.* Baltimore: William and Wilkins (revision in process) .

Triadafilopoulos, G. R., W. Simms and D. I. Goldenberg. 1991. Bowel dysfunction in fibromyalgia syndrome. *Digest Dis Sci* 36(1):1237–1248.

What Your OB/GYN Should Know

Please read "What Everyone on Your Health Care Team Should Know."

It is vitally important that every OB/GYN specialist understands the concepts that lie behind the facts of fibromyalgia (FMS) and Myofascial Pain Syndrome (MPS), because they will have an impact on every aspect of your dealings with your FMS/MPS patient. Often it is you who will make the diagnosis, due to the nature of your interactions with your patient, and an understanding of trigger points (TrPs) is essential in this task. To learn about TrPs see *The Trigger Point Manuals* by Travell and Simons (1992; 1983).

For example, piriformis TrP nerve entrapment can be the cause of sharp pain during pelvic exams. Other TrPs in that area can cause pain and muscle spasms during vaginal and rectal exams. Because the experience of pain is amplified by FMS, that may require you to modify some of your procedures. Also, people with FMS often have sicca syndrome. This means that all the mucous membranes can dry, including the lining of the vagina, and the GI tract. Fibromyalgia has a direct effect on the HPA axis, which in turn affects the gonadal axes (Torpy and Chrousus 1996). Fibromyalgia can interact with and be affected by the sex hormones (Carett, Dessureault and Belanger 1992) and reproductive events (Ostensen, Rugelsjoen and Wigers 1997).

Pregnancy and Health Issues

Stretches and other physical therapy to promote myofascial elasticity are important for the FMS/MPS patient during pregnancy, as well as extra vitamins and minerals. Benedryl is a remedy for sleep suitable in pregnancy. Unfortunately, for some FMS/MPS patients, it causes insomnia. Many of us have the alpha-delta sleep anomaly and get little restorative sleep. Disruption of delta sleep may be tied to hormone dysregulation. Many of us also have nutritional problems, because of a malabsorption condition in the GI tract. I have observed that some women with FMS have had prolonged gestational periods, perhaps due to the unbalanced adrenaline serotonin axis. This may be the result of lowered serotonin. Nontraditional symptom management methods may be useful during pregnancy if there are complications of FMS and/or MPS (Schneider 1992; de Aloysio and Penacchioni 1992).

I have observed that people with FMS/MPS have a tendency to form cysts, fibroids, heavy scarring, and adhesions. Even our cuticles and pierced earring holes overgrow. This is something to keep in mind when surgery is contemplated.

Hysterectomy

Many FMS/MPS patients have had hysterectomies to relieve pain. Often just the uterus is removed, but in many cases the ovaries are taken out later to balance hormonal swings and ovarian pain, which can refer pain to the groin and legs.

The Menses

FMS is a pain amplification syndrome (Sorensen, Graven-Nielsen, Henriksson, et al. 1998). and our autonomic nervous system is hypersensitized. Both central and peripheral mechanisms seem to be involved (Yunus 1992). Your patient really hurts. During menses, it is not unusual for the patient to be able to feel what area of the uterus is sloughing off. Some have said that it is like being skinned alive on the inside, every month. Menstrual problems such as severe cramping, irregular periods, long periods with a great deal of bleeding, membranous flow, late periods, missed periods, and periods with blood clots are common in FMS/MPS. Irregular periods and long flows are also common, due to neuroendocrine and gonadal imbalances mentioned earlier. There seems to be an increased incidence of female urethral syndrome, as well (Wallace 1990).

Trigger Points

Some part of these menstrual problems can be caused by coccygeus, iliocostalis, rectus abdominis, pyramidalis, and other pelvic and low-back TrPs. There is also a TrP high in the adductor magnus which refers a diffuse pain and soreness throughout the pelvic area, and can mimic pelvic inflammatory disease (PID). Even some multifidi muscle TrPs refer pain to the abdominal area. It's not unusual for pregnancy or even dysmenorrhea to activate TrPs. Find a good TrP-savvy physical therapist to work with your FMS/MPS patients.

Active TrPs in the abdominal muscles, especially in the rectus abdominus, may cause a lax, pendulous abdomen with gas problems. Your patient can't pull in the gut because the TrPs inhibit contraction. A fat pad forms over the abdomen. That fat pad is hard to get rid of, due to the TrPs. The first thing to do is to find and eliminate the back muscle TrPs that refer pain to the abdomen. These can cause burning, fullness, bloating, and swelling. Only then can you hope to eliminate the belly TrPs.

Genetics

Because studies show that 50 percent of the children of people with FMS/MPS may have an inherited tendency to develop the condition, female children of parents with FMS/MPS should be monitored carefully during their first menses (Pellegrino, Waylonis and Sommer 1989). If severe dysmenorrhea occurs, the patient should be checked out for signs of FMS/MPS.

Therapies

I have found that if patients use tennis-ball acupressure before their period, (it hurts, but it flushes out the TrPs), there will be less constriction in the abdominal area, and less bloating. It is especially important to work the line where the leg joins the trunk. Patients can do this by lying on the floor and placing the tennis ball between their bodies and the floor. If the area is extremely sore, there is a TrP there. Nerve entrapment by TrPs may be present as well, leading to neuropraxia. If there is nerve involvement, often ice will help ease the pain. If the pain is muscular alone, the patient will find heat more comforting.

Vaginal Discharge

Vaginal discharge, sometimes with an itch, is common. So is mittelschmerz. This pain, as in menstrual pain, often triggers the adductor longus and iliopsoas TrPs. These TrPs can respond to galvanic muscle stimulation, sine-wave ultrasound with electrostimulation, Spray and Stretch, and Cranio-Sacral Release.

Yeast Infections

Frequent yeast infections, an itch on the roof of the mouth after eating tangy cheese, and bloating after drinking beer may be signs that your patient has a yeast problem. This is usually a sign of increased acidity and toxicity. Many people with FMS/MPS have reactive hypoglycemia which sets up conditions favorable for rapid yeast growth. The "Zone" diet works well for this (Sears 1997b). I also find that allergy shots for molds are very helpful, as well as guaifenesin therapy.

Breast Pain

Hypersensitive nipples and/or breast pain are commonly due to pectoralis TrPs. Many of us have latent pectorals and sternalis trigger points. "Doorway stretches" help these TrPs. Fibrocystic breasts are also common in FMS/MPS Complex. This may be due to ductal entrapment by myofascial TrPs.

Medication Effects

Many FMS/MPS patients have unusual reactions to medications due to their altered metabolism. Sometimes, just a small portion of a normal dose of a medication will have very strong effects. At other times, we can take whopping doses of a medication and feel no effects at all.

Secretions

A lot of us have thick secretions. Guaifenesin ends this problem, and the way it thins secretions may be part of why it is so effective in "reversing" the effects of FMS. I've heard that it has been used to help promote conception (Check, Adelson and Wu 1982). It seems to help us get rid of accumulated toxins and acids.

Sexual Intercourse and Pain

Pain with intercourse is often due to vaginal TrPs and pelvic floor TrPs. For aching discomfort and cramps during coitus, check for abdominal and low back TrPs. For sharp pain, check for a piriformis muscle TrP with pudendal nerve entrapment. Vulvar vestibulitis, vulvodynia, hyperesthesia, and general pelvic muscle aches are also common. Progesterone will affect the levels of serotonin, and serotonin levels may vary from day to day as the amount of delta sleep varies. Expect mood swings and difficulties with neurotransmitter fluctuation, and hormonal irregularities.

References

Carrett S., M. Dessureault and A. Belanger. 1992. Fibromyalgia and sex hormones. *J Rheumatol* 19(5):831.

Check, J. H., H. G. Adelson and C. H. Wu. 1982. Improvement of cervical factor with guaifenesin. *Fertil Steril* 37(5):707–708.

de Aloysio, D. and P. Penacchioni. 1992. Morning sickness control in early pregnancy by neuguan point acupressure. *Obstet Gyn* 80 (5):852–854.

Ostensen, M., A. Rugelsjoen and S. H. Wigers. 1997. The effect of reproductive events and alterations of sex hormone levels on the symptoms of fibromyalgia. *Scand J Rheumatol* 26(5):355–360.

Pellegrino, M., G. W. Waylonis and A. Sommer. 1989. Familial occurrence of primary fibromyalgia. *Arch Phys Med Rehab* 70(1):61–63.

Schneider, M. J. 1992. Soft tissue effects of sacroiliac and lumbosacral joint manipulation. *Chiro Tech* 4(4):136–142.

Sears, B. 1997. *Mastering the Zone.* NY: HarperCollins.

Sorensen, J. T., K. Graven-Nielsen, G. Henriksson, M. Bengtsson and L. Arendt-Nielsen. 1998. Hyperexcitability in fibromyalgia. *J Rheumatol* 25(1):152–155.

Torpy, D. J. and G. P. Chrousos. 1996. The three-way interactions between the hypothalamic-pituitary-adrenal and gonadal axes and the immune system. *Baillieres Clin Rheumatol* 10(2):18–198.

Travell, J. G. and D. G. Simons. 1992. *Myofascial Pain and Dysfunction: The Trigger Point Manual, Volume II: The Lower Body.* Baltimore: William and Wilkins.

———. 1983. *Myofascial Pain and Dysfunction: The Trigger Point Manual, Volume I: The Upper Body.* Baltimore: William and Wilkins (revision in process).

Wallace, D. J. 1990. Genitourinary manifestations of fibrositis, and increased association with female urethral syndrome. *J Rheumatol* 17(2):238–239.

Yunus, M. B. 1992. Towards a model of pathophysiology of fibromyalgia: Aberrant central pain mechanisms with peripheral modulation. *J Rheumatol* 19:6:846–850.

What Your Pharmacist Should Know

Please read "What Everyone on Your Health Care Team Should Know."

Each of us with fibromyalgia (FMS), Myofascial Pain Syndrome (MPS), or FMS/MPS Complex needs a trustworthy pharmacist to coordinate our medications and keep us informed. New medications are coming out so rapidly that it is impossible for physicians to keep up with them all. Our health care team often comprises many specialists, and they don't always communicate with each other. Most of us are on many medications of different kinds, and people with FMS tend to react unusually to medications. Some of our medications can interact unpleasantly. For example, Soma (carisoprodol) can react with niacin if taken at the same time, producing nausea and a painfully hot flush and rash.

FMS/MPS Complex and Medication

Often, people with FMS/MPS Complex have to try many medications before they find the best ones. We react differently to each medication, and there is no "cookbook recipe" for FMS or MPS. What works well for one of us can be ineffective for another. A medication that puts one person to sleep may keep another awake. There is a whole subset of FMS/MPS Complex patients who find medications such as Benedryl, Ultram, Pamelor, and Paxil stimulating. Some of these people may look healthy, but their suffering can be great. We all have our own unique combination of neurotransmitter disruption and connective tissue disturbance. We need doctors who are willing to stick with us until an acceptable symptom relief level is reached. We also need a compassionate and understanding pharmacist to work with us.

The most-studied medications that modulate neurotransmitters are psychoactive drugs. *This does not mean that the patient's condition is psychological.* Fibromyalgia patients have enhanced nociception (Bendtsen, Norregaard, Jensen et al. 1997) and are often in great pain. Medications that affect the central nervous system are appropriate for FMS. The target symptoms are sleep lack, muscle rigidity, pain, and fatigue. These medications don't stop the alpha-wave intrusion into delta-level sleep, but they do extend the amount of sleep, and may ease symptom "flares."

It is the rule rather than the exception that an FMS/MPS client will save strong pain medications from a surgery or an injury for when they are *really* needed—for an FMS/MPS "flare." This behavior indicates that their prescription needs are not being met. FMS is often misunderstood (Jones 1996) by the medical profession, and your clients may turn to you for guidance and understanding.

Medications and Narcotics

It's normal to be depressed by chronic pain, but that doesn't mean depression is causing the pain. FMS is a sensory amplification syndrome (Kosek, Ekholm and Hannson 1996). Maintenance with mild narcotics (Darvocet, Tylenol #3, Vicodin-Lorcet-Lortab) for nonmalignant (noncancerous) chronic pain conditions is a logical, humane alternative if other reasonable attempts at pain control have failed. The main problem with raised dosages of these medications is not with the narcotic components per se, but with the aspirin or acetaminophen that is often compounded with them. There can be serious side effects with NSAID usage (Gardner and Simpkin 1991). Please keep an eye on the level of your client's medications.

Clients with FMS/MPS Complex need adequate pain control to break the pain/contraction/pain/contraction spiral. It does not serve them well if you treat them like addicts. They get no pleasure from their medications, just some symptom relief. However, the level of medication should not be rising steadily. That is a sign that the perpetuating factors are not being treated properly, and/or that the level of pain relief is not adequately treated with the current medication. During a symptom flare, these clients often need more medications, but the level should decrease again after flare has subsided.

Narcotic analgesics are sometimes more easily tolerated than NSAIDs (Reidenberg and Portenoy 1994). Neither FMS nor MPS is inflammatory, and anti-inflammatory medications often contribute to malabsorption in the gut. NSAIDs may disrupt stage 4 sleep, and delta sleep is already interrupted in FMS. Prolonged use of narcotics may result in physiological changes affecting tolerance or physical dependence (withdrawal), but these are not the same as psychological dependence (addiction).

Be sure to ask your FMS/MPS clients about multiple chemical sensitivities. Many of us are lactose intolerant, and can't deal with even the small amounts of lactose used as fillers in many medications. Be patient. Many of us will appear confused at times, due to "fibrofog." We need your help to cope with the difficulties of living with an invisible chronic illness.

References

Bendtsen, L., J. Norregaard, R. Jensen and J. Olesen. 1997. Evidence of qualitatively altered nociception in patients with fibromyalgia. *Arth Rheum* 40(1):98–102.

Gardner, G. C. and P. A. Simpkin. 1991. Adverse Effects of NSAIDs. *Pharm Ther* 16:750–754.

Jones, R. C. 1996. Fibromyalgia: misdiagnosed, mistreated and misunderstood? *Am Fam Phys* 52(1):91–92.

Kosek, E., J. Ekholm and P. Hansson. 1996. Sensory dysfunction in fibromyalgia patients with implications for pathogenic mechanisms. *Pain* 68(2-3):375–383.

Reidenberg, M. M. and R. K. Portenoy. 1994. The need for an open mind about the treatment of chronic nonmalignant pain. *Clin Pharmacol* 55(4):367–369.

What Your Physical Therapist Should Know

Please read "What Everyone on Your Health Care Team Should Know" and "Perpetuating Factors."

Fibromyalgia (FMS) is *not* a "wastebasket diagnosis." It does not simply mean "achy muscles," and it is *not* the same as trigger points (TrPs), or chronic Myofascial Pain Syndrome (MPS), or FMS/MPS Complex. Each of these conditions requires different types of physical therapy. Your client may get much worse if you treat TrPs as you would FMS. Single or multiple TrPs are much less complicated than bodywide chronic MPS, and if there are no perpetuating factors, can be eradicated.

Fibromyalgia is not just a form of muscular rheumatism. It is a systemic, nondegenerative, noninflammatory, nonprogressive dysfunction of the neurotransmitters. Chronic MPS is bodywide and neuromuscular. There can be nerve and vascular entrapments. With FMS/MPS Complex, you have both a severe pain condition in MPS, and the pain amplification condition that is a characteristic of FMS. Keep this in mind. Everything you do to these clients will amplify their discomfort/pain, and sometimes the pain will be delayed. Urge your clients to give you constant feedback.

FMS/MPS clients need to learn good coping behaviors. Their struggles are intense and yet they constantly hear, "You look 'just fine.'" This adds another psychological stress to their lives, and makes things worse. One result of invisible chronic pain is the disbelief with which it is often met.

Fibrofog

With FMS and FMS/MPS Complex, there can come an inability to concentrate, think clearly, or remember things. This goes beyond frustration and can become frightening. "Fibrofog" can be aggravated by weather changes, cold, humidity, excessive physical activity, physical inactivity, hormonal fluctuations, sleeplessness, anxiety, stress, depression, or mental or physical fatigue. It is a great stressor. Write out your instructions for clients, no matter how clear your verbal explanations may be.

Trigger Points

Palpating TrPs can severely exacerbate clients' referred pain activity for a day or two. Warn them before you do an initial TrP mapping. A lump at a TrP site could be caused by the damming of blood and other fluids by obstructed blood flow. Trigger point acupressure must be applied to a *relaxed muscle.* It won't work if the client is tense. If the muscles are taut due to spasticity, you may need to work with galvanic electrical stimulation or other methods to reduce spasticity before attempting acupressure. Hot, moist packs will sometimes help to relax the muscle.

During TrP acupressure, the TrP is pressed with sustained pressure to what Travell and Simons (1983, 87) call a "tolerably painful" level. As the discomfort eases, pressure is increased. If the discomfort does not ease, try hot, moist packs and passive range of motion.

"Vigorous massage of hyperirritable TrPs can cause an adverse reaction with a marked increase in pain" (Travell and Simons 1983, 87). When the client is experiencing pain while at rest for a considerable part of the time, the TrPs are very active and rarely respond favorably to anything more than gentle, passive stretches and hot packs. Myofascial release and Cranio-Sacral Release can be very useful physical therapies, and they can often be tolerated at these times. Stripping massage and lymphatic drainage may have to wait until the TrPs calm down.

Mechanical stresses, such as body asymmetry, poor body mechanics, short upper arms and/or short lower legs, head-forward posture, and paradoxical breathing perpetuate TrPs in most clients with persistent MPS. When the client has pain without even moving the affected area, gentle stretching in a hot bath may help. Tell your client not to overdo movement.

Ask your client to keep an ongoing list of symptoms that occur between treatments. Symptoms that your client might not recognize as being related to TrPs include the following: cold or hot spots on the body, sweating, teary eyes, a constantly runny nose, goose bumps, balancing problems, dizziness, ringing in the ear, and burning, blanching, or reddening of the skin. Many more symptoms are described in my video and in Travell and Simon's *Trigger Point Manuals* (1992; 1983).

Your client will come in with complaints caused by the most recently activated TrP. Don't become discouraged if, once that is deactivated, the pain shifts to another TrP. This happens. Also, expect the pain to switch sides as secondary TrPs that have developed in muscles used to compensate for those weakened by primary TrPs start screaming for attention. Be sure to check both sides of the body.

As a rule, treat the muscle group first that is causing or adding to sleep disruption. Then deal with the one causing greatest pain, or restriction of movement. Ask the client which TrP is most troublesome. Find out what the client does for a living, or for a hobby, and plan your therapy accordingly. First restore flexion, then side bending, rotation, and then, finally, extension.

Fatigue

The client may have fatigue and nausea after a physical therapy session, no matter how gentle. If therapy is effective, toxins trapped in the myofascia and/or intracellular space may be released into the bloodstream. Make sure that the client has recovered from one session before you begin work again. This may mean that beginning work is slow. This may be the reverse of many of your usual practices; but at first the client may be able to tolerate only a half-hour of physical therapy, once a week. This may be increased as the first flush of toxins are dealt with. Be sure to monitor the client's fatigue carefully.

Exercise

If there are active trigger points, according to Travell and Simons (1983, 97), "... at that stage, active exercise that loads a contracting muscle is not indicated." Be cautious in recommending exercise, as FMS clients have reduced growth hormone secretion, which plays an important role in muscle tissue repair. In MPS or with simple TrPs, repetitive exercise can be destructive. Trigger points *must* be inactivated before muscles can be strengthened.

Exercise should be regarded as a prescription. You must ensure that the client gets the proper kind, dose, and timing. Specify rate, number of repetitions, how often in one day and conditions (not when client is overstressed, ill, cold, etc.). Specify relaxation and breathing between each cycle of exercise. If mild muscle soreness results, but is gone by the next day, that's a sign that the exercise may continue. If soreness continues, postpone the exercise. If the soreness is there after the third day, change the exercise plan to a lighter one. Use rest and moist heat to help postexercise soreness.

Increased referred TrP pain during or after exercise is an indication that the exercise should be stopped. Delayed-onset muscle soreness, which appears a day or two following overdoing it, is a function of FMS and not of TrPs.

Forget the famous line, "No pain, no gain." *It does not apply in fibromyalgia or Myofascial Pain Syndrome, or even in simple TrPs.* There is good evidence that continuing to exercise in spite of the pain will simply aggravate the abnormal pain filter present in FMS. (Bennett 1997). In FMS clients, exercise causes a reduction in temperature and cerebral blood flow. They often can't think clearly enough during exercise to set limits. Tell them to set a timer, or to exercise with a friend who can keep track of the time.

Therapies

Any pool with a temperature outside the 88- to 94-degree range can cause long-range worsening of symptoms in MPS or TrPs. Cramps can also result from cooler temperatures, sometimes immediately. Hotter temperatures may bring nausea and extreme fatigue, if toxins flood the system. Hot tubs and hot baths should be limited to fifteen minutes or less, at least at first. Watch for chlorine sensitivity. Many of these clients will have multiple chemical sensitivities.

You can use galvanic electrical stimulation or ultrasound with electrostim as a "search and destroy" method, as both modalities cause pain in the immediate area of the TrP until it's broken up. When setting the controls, listen to your client's responses. Keep the sound head moving as you increase the power slowly, and gently move over a suspected TrP area. Ask the client to let you know when his or her tolerance level is reached. Some clients may not be able to tolerate the lowest setting, and so you may need other modalities to begin treatment of the TrPs. Inquire if the client is on guaifenesin therapy. If so, be sure the gel used contains no salicylate or aloe.

If using Spray and Stretch, be very careful to use the *exact* treatment strategy taught in the Travell trigger point tapes, which are often available at your local hospital physical therapy department. For this therapy to be effective, the client must be positioned properly for each TrP, and the spray must be applied in a specific pattern, in a specific direction, at a specific distance, interspersed with a stretch. The TrPs must be released in a specific order. Then, you run through a passive range of motion for the muscle group, and then reward the client. All these steps are necessary for effective treatment.

Specific trigger point myotherapy training is available through the following sources:

- The Academy for Myofascial Trigger Point Therapy, 1312 East Carson Street, Pittsburgh, PA 15203. (412) 481-2553

- Robert Gerwin, M.D., Travell Seminars, Pain and Rehabilitation Medicine, 7830 Old Georgetown Road, Suite C-15, Bethesda, MD 20814-2432. (301) 656-0220; and

- Mary Maloney, PT, Naugatuck Physical Therapy, 175 Church Street, Naugatuck, CT 06770. (203) 723-0533

Cold will relieve nerve entrapment pain. Warm, moist heat will relieve muscle pain. If TrPs recur after effective treatments, there are hidden perpetuating factors, or perpetuating factors that have not been treated. If the pain recurs but the TrP is gone, notify the doctor immediately. It is time to look for another cause, including cancer and other systemic diseases.

It is important to be familiar with *Myofascial Pain and Dysfunction: The Trigger Point Manual, Volume I* and *Volume II* by Travell and Simons (1983; 1992). You are an educator. As your client learns more self-physical therapy techniques—tennis ball acupressure, stretching, good body mechanics and posture—he or she will become responsible for more of the physical therapy required. Healing can begin only when the cycle of pain/contracture is broken.. With perseverance, guiding FMS/MPS clients on the healing path can be an exceedingly fulfilling task.

References

Bennett, R. 1997. *Fibromyalgia Network Newsletter*, July, p. 5.

Travell, J. G. and D. G. Simons. 1992. *Myofascial Pain and Dysfunction: The Trigger Point Manual, Volume II: The Lower Body*. Baltimore: William and Wilkins.

———. 1983. *Myofascial Pain and Dysfunction: The Trigger Point Manual, Volume I: The Upper Body*. Baltimore: William and Wilkins (revision in process).

What Your Podiatrist Should Know

Please read "What Everyone on Your Health Care Team Should Know."

It is important that you remember that people with fibromyalgia (FMS) have a hypersensitive autonomic nervous system. This means that pain sensations are amplified. Often you can do quite a bit to relieve your patient's pain because many perpetuating factors of Myofascial Pain Syndrome (MPS) occur in your realm of expertise. Trigger points (TrPs) in the leg often refer pain to the feet, and hip conditions, such as piriformis syndrome, often cause symptoms that will drive patients to your door (Vecchiet, Giamberardino and Saggini 1991; Saggini, Giamberardino, Gatteschi, et al. 1996).

If your patient has a foot that falls outward when s/he is lying on a treatment table, consider piriformis syndrome on the leg with the pronated foot. Often both feet will be pronated, which indicates bilateral piriformis syndrome.

Trigger Points (TrPs)

Tibialis anterior TrPs send pain and tenderness to the front of the ankle. This can spill over to the top surface of the great toe. The ankle hurts when walking, and feels worse climbing stairs. The toes drag, and are responsible for many unexpected trips and frequent falls. The inability of the foot to clear the ground during stride greatly increases "balance problems." Walking over rough ground can cause these TrPs to develop, as can tightness in the calf muscle or Morton's foot. Tell your patient to brace the feet at night with a pillow or a rolled blanket at the bottom of the bed under the covers. This will keep the feet in a neutral position, and may prevent activation of these TrPs.

Peroneus longus and **peroneus brevis** TrPs have referral zones over the outside of the ankle, above, behind, and below it. This pain pattern may also extend a short distance along the outer part of the foot. Sometimes you will see a spillover pattern over the outer side of the middle third of the lower leg. Trigger points in the peroneus tertius refer pain behind the ankle and to the side of the heel, as well as in the local area of the TrPs and in the upper outside of the foot.

Ankle pain and weak ankles are prime symptoms of these TrPs. The ankles turn out and sprain easily. Unusual sensations and sensitivities may develop on the ankle and the top of the foot. Peroneus TrPs can result from prolonged immobilization of the leg and foot in a cast. Other instigating and perpetuating factors are wearing high heels, tight elastic around the calf (check for an indented red line on the leg after wearing socks), flat feet, Morton's foot, and the FMS/MPS foot (wide in front and narrow in back). This latter condition can begin with an arch that is very high. If perpetuating factors are not adequately dealt with, however, the arches may fall. Entrapment of the common peroneal nerve can occur with TrPs in the peroneus longus. This results in numbness and tingling on the top of the foot in a triangle between the first and second toes.

Soleus TrPs refer pain to the lower back part of the leg and the bottom surface of the heel. Pain may also be projected to the sacroiliac joint on the same side of the body as the TrPs. Trigger points in the upper part of the soleus muscle usually refer pain and tenderness over the back of the calf. In the soleus, TrPs may cause walking uphill or up and down stairs to be difficult or impossible. Entrapments of blood vessels and the tibial nerve can be aggravated by high soleus TrPs. Upper soleus TrPs are more likely to interfere with the venous pump, and can cause ankle and foot swelling.

The soleus TrP at the base of the calf may cause unbearable pain in the heel. In fact, soleus TrPs often may be the true cause of heel spur pain. If there are spurs on both heels, but only one causes pain, look for TrPs. There is an unusual pain referral pattern from the TrP at the base of the calf muscle—it initiates jaw pain. This TrP seems to be more common in people with FMS/MPS Complex.

Tibialis posterior TrPs refer pain over the Achilles tendon above the heel. A spillover pattern extends from the TrP down over the calf, covering the entire heel, the sole of the foot, and the bottom of the toes. Pain can be severe in the arch of the foot and the Achilles tendon. Running or jogging, especially on a slanted, uneven, or irregular surface, or wearing badly worn shoes may activate or perpetuate these TrPs. Wearing corrective orthotics is often terribly painful, because they press on the region of referred pain.

The feet are exquisitely tender to pressure. Janet Travell and David Simons, in their medical text, *Myofascial Pain and Dysfunction: The Trigger Point Manual: Volume II* (1992), explain that patients with TrPs will not tolerate hard orthotics. They suggest using the modified Travell insert shown on page 389 of their text, and on page 61 of the book I wrote with Mary Ellen Copeland, *Fibromyalgia & Chronic Myofascial Pain Syndrome: A Survival Manual* (1996). Teach your patients to avoid high heels, and make sure their shoes have sensible soles.

TrPs in the long extensors of the toes cause pain primarily on the top of the foot. Extensor digitorum longus TrP pain may extend nearly to the tips of the middle three toes. Extensor hallucis longus TrPs cause pain in the region behind the great toe, which may extend nearly to the tip of the great toe. These TrPs can cause night cramps in the long extensors of the toes, and growing pains in children. They can cause entrapment of the deep branch of the peroneal nerve. This may cause weakness, and is still another cause of your patients falling over their own feet.

Flexor digitorum longus TrPs transmit pain primarily to the middle of the sole of the foot just before the four lesser toes, with spillover pain to the toes themselves. There also may be spillover pain from the TrP to the ankle and the front of the heel area.

TrPs in the flexor hallucis longus refer strong pain to the bottom surface of the great toe and to the pad behind it. The chief symptom of these TrPs is painful feet, especially when standing or walking. This is most obvious after the patients have been off their feet for a while. Toe flexor cramping is usually caused by TrPs in the intrinsic flexors of the toes.

TrPs in the extensor digitorum brevis or extensor hallucis brevis create local pain over the top of the foot. Pain and tenderness from the abductor hallucis TrP center along the inner side of the heel, with spillover pain to the instep and to the back of the heel.

The **abductor digit** TrP causes pain and tenderness along the bottom of the pad behind the toes, and may spill over onto the nearby sole and onto the side of the foot near the toe. Pain and tenderness from the flexor digitorum brevis TrPs center over the ball of the foot behind the second to fourth toes.

These TrPs cause sore feet and pain on walking. If the TrPs are severe, there will also be deep, aching pain when at rest. They can cause a staggering walk, a painfully restricted range of motion, and a diffuse deep tenderness on the bottom of the foot. These TrPs can entrap the posterior tibial nerve. Your patient may feel as though the ankle is sprained, but the ankle itself does not hurt.

The pain from these TrPs is most obvious in the morning. *The first steps are severely painful until the plantar fascia and the muscles have been stretched.* These TrPs are often misdiagnosed as plantar fasciitis. For relief, I recommend golf-ball or rolling-pin foot exercisers. Unless there a structural deformity, orthotics are usually unnecessary after the TrPs have been inactivated.

Quadratus plantae TrPs refer pain and tenderness to the bottom surface of the heel. The adductor hallucis TrPs send pain to the ball of the foot, as well as hurting locally. Trigger points in the transverse head of this muscle can cause a strange "fluffy" feeling of numbness, and a sense that the skin over the ball of the foot is swollen.

Referred pain from the flexor hallucis brevis covers the bunion pad area of the first toe, and may spill over to include all of the first toe and much of the second toe. Trigger points of the interossei muscles cause pain and tenderness along the side of the toe, and to the ball of the foot behind each toe. First dorsal interosseous TrPs can cause tingling in the great toe.

These TrPs cause impaired walking because of pain. There might also be numbness of the foot, or a swollen feeling. Orthotics can cause intolerable pain. Common aggravators of these TrPs are excessive turning in or out of the foot; restricted range of motion; or hypermobility of the toes, forefoot, and hindfoot; weakness of the toes, Morton's foot; calluses; and improperly designed and fitted shoes.

References

Saggini, R., M. A. Giamberardino, L. Gatteschi and L. Vecchiet. 1996. Myofascial pain syndrome of the peroneus longus: biomechanical approach. *Clin J Pain* 12(1):30–37.

Starlanyl D. J. and M. E. Copeland. 1996. *Fibromyalgia & Chronic Myofascial Pain Syndrome: A Survival Manual.* Oakland: New Harbinger Publications.

Travell, J. G. and D. G. Simons. 1992. *Myofascial Pain and Dysfunction: The Trigger Point Manual: Volume II: The Lower Body.* Baltimore: William and Wilkins.

Vecchiet, L., M. A. Giamberardino and R. Saggini. 1991. Myofascial pain syndrome, clinical and pathological aspects. *Clin J Pain* 7(Supp1):S16–S22.

What Your Pulmonary Specialist Should Know

Please read "What Everyone on Your Health Care Team Should Know."

Research studies have shown that chronic dyspnea is common in people with chronic primary fibromyalgia (FMS), but is not due to cardiac or pulmonary causes (Caidahl, Lurie, Bake, Johansson, et al. 1989). Respiratory pressures are low, but spirometric values have been reported as normal (Lurie, Caidahl, Johansson, et al. 1990). Sleep apnea is not an uncommon coexisting condition in FMS, especially in males (May, West, Baker, et al. 1993).

There has also been a study noting overnight fall in arterial oxygen saturation (Alvarez Lario, Alonso Valdivieso, Alegre Lopez, et al. 1996). Some of this problem may be traced to constricted bronchi due to neurotransmitter dysregulation. This can also contribute to excess mucus, which is often thicker than normal. These problems may be aggravated by coexisting allergies/asthma. Patients are often short of breath due to paradoxical respiration and mouth breathing. Some of this can be traced to myofascial trigger points (TrPs).

Trigger Points

Sternocleidomastoid (SCM) TrPs sometimes contribute to a runny nose and sinus congestion on the involved side. Paradoxical breathing can also overload the SCM, which is an accessory muscle to the process of respiration.

Lateral (external) pterygoid TrPs cause pain in front of the ear, as well as chewing difficulties. There is pain deep into the TMJ and maxillary sinuses. Usually, there is a chronic drip from the maxillary sinuses, and clicking noises from the TMJ, as TrP-tightened muscles pull the bones slightly out of alignment.

Scalene muscle TrPs can also cause nerve, blood vessel, or lymph entrapment. All three major scalene muscles can refer pain to the front and back of the body in a widespread pattern. In the front, they cause a persistent aching pain over the chest and down the front and back of the arm to the forearm. The chest feels "tight." This pattern skips the elbow and extends to the thumb and index finger. On the left side, this pain may be mistaken for angina. Shallow pain can also be referred to the inner-upper boarder of the shoulder blade. There can be signs of obstruction of veins and arteries and compression of the motor and sensory nerves of the arm. Sleep is often disturbed by pain from these TrPs. Your patient may have to sleep sitting up or propped up on pillows. There may be numbness, tingling, and odd sensations in the fourth and fifth fingers and the little finger side of the hand and forearm. Paradoxical respiration often causes these TrPs.

Pectoralis major TrPs cause pain under the sternum. They can also transmit pain to the front of the chest and breast, extending down to the little finger side of the arm to the fourth and fifth fingers. Trigger points on the right side can produce irregular heart beats. Trigger points on the left side often mimic heart attack pain.

Trigger points of the pectoralis can occur in any of the muscle layers, in any place, but they are most common in certain areas. In the area of the collarbone, TrPs cause local pain. They also refer pain over the front of the shoulder muscle. In the breastbone area, TrPs are likely to broadcast intermittent, intense pain to the front of the chest and down the inner aspect of the arm. This can include a feeling of chest tightness, often mistaken for angina.

These TrPs also can radiate pain to the inside top of the forearm, as well as to the little finger side of the hand, including the last two or more fingers. If you find arrhythmias and no other sign of heart problems, check for TrPs, especially in the right pectoralis major muscle between the fifth and sixth ribs. Chest pain that persists after a heart attack is often due to these TrPs. Trigger points in the side border of this muscle cause breast tenderness and hypersensitive nipples. They may also cause breast pain.

Pectoralis minor TrPs send pain over the front of the chest and shoulder. Pain may run down the inner side of the arm, and include the last three fingers. Pain from a left side pectoralis minor TrP can mimic angina. These TrPs can entrap the axillary artery as well as the brachial plexus nerve. The radial pulse can disappear as you move the arm to different positions. Numbness and odd sensations of the fourth and fifth fingers are common. There may be peculiar sensations over some parts of the forearm and over the palm side of the first three fingers.

Paradoxical breathing may again be the perpetrator. Check standing and sitting movements. Ask the patient if s/he is sleeping curled up on the side with the lower shoulder forced strongly forward.

Sternalis TrPs produce a deep ache under the breastbone, which extends over the entire region of the breastbone and below. This can cover the upper chest and front of the shoulder on the same side. It may spread to the axillary area and upper arm on the little finger side to the elbow. This produces an ache like a heart attack or angina, and is totally independent of body movement. Trigger points can occur anywhere within the sternalis muscle, but are more common in the upper two-thirds and to the left of center at mid-sternal level. A TrP located where the pectorals, SCM, and sternalis insert can be the source of a dry, hacking cough.

Serratus posterior superior TrPs can be the source of a hard-to-locate, deep upper back pain. Often, there is shoulder blade pain as well, radiating to the upper area. There can also be pain in the back of the shoulder and back of the upper arm. This may spread to the elbow point, down the forearm to the hand and little finger. In the front, it may include the chest and part of the palm on the little finger side.

The serratus anterior TrPs are responsible for the "side stitch," as well as shortness of breath. There is referred pain to the side and to the back of the chest. This includes the lower interior border of the shoulder blade, and sometimes runs down the inner area of the arm, hand, and the last two fingers. Expect air hunger, with panting or mouth breathing. This can be frightening, especially to people who also have asthma or other respiratory problems. In severe cases, there may be chest pain, even at rest. Your patients may get out of breath simply by talking, because they have a reduced volume of air going in and out of the lungs due to reduced chest expansion. Also, the nerve supply to the serratus anterior muscle may be entrapped due to scalene muscle TrPs.

Thoracolumbar paraspinal TrPs can produce the low-back pain known as lumbago.

Iliocostalis thoracis TrPs at mid-chest level send pain upward toward the shoulder, as well as sideways toward the chest wall. Those TrPs on the left side in this area cause pain often mistaken for angina. Trigger points on either side of this area are often misdiagnosed as pleurisy. Low chest iliocostalis TrPs can refer pain upwards across the shoulder blade. This pain can extend around to the belly, and down over the lumbar area.

Multifidi TrPs in the thorax refer pain to corners of the vertebrae. Low-back multifidi also transmit pain to the abdomen, and perpetuate Irritable Bowel Syndrome (IBS). At the base of the vertebrae they refer pain to the tailbone. All multifidi TrPs can cause nerve entrapment symptoms including hyperesthesia, numbness, or lessened sensitivity of the skin on the back. All paraspinal muscles can refer pain to the upper buttock, the kidney area, or produce pain in the groin and scrotum, causing retraction of the testicle.

The diaphragm can also develop TrPs. These can cause an odd, fluttery feeling in the belly, as well as hiccups. The diaphragm may lose flexibility when riddled with TrPs. More about diaphragmatic TrPs will be forthcoming in the revision of *Myofascial Pain and Dysfunction: The Trigger Point Manual, Volune I* by Travell and Simons, publication due in late 1998.

References

Alvarez Lario B., J. I. Alonso Valdivieso, L. J. Alegre Lopez, S. C Martel Soteres, J. L. Viejo Banuelos and A. Maranon Cabello. 1996. Fall in hemoglobin oxygenation in the arterial blood of fibromyalgia patients during sleep. *Am J Med* 101:54–60.

Caidahl, K., M. Lurie, B. Bake, C. Johansson, et al. 1989. Dyspnoe in chronic primary fibromyalgia. *J Intern Med* 226(4):265–270.

Lurie, M., K. Caidahl, C. Johansson and B. Bake. 1990. Respiratory function in chronic primary fibromyalgia. *Scand J Rehabil Med* 22(3):151–155.

May, K. P., S. G. West, M. R. Baker and D. W. Everett. 1993. Sleep apnea in male patients with the fibromyalgia syndrome. *Am J Med* 94(5):505–508.

What Your Surgeon Should Know

Please read "What Everyone on Your Health Care Team Should Know."

Patients with fibromyalgia (FMS) and/or Myofascial Pain Syndrome (MPS) may react unusually to surgery and its associated care. Fibromyalgia is a pain amplification syndrome. Be prepared for more intense postsurgical pain, as well as longer healing time due to low growth hormone and associated healing factors. Immobility will usually cause MPS symptoms to worsen, and muscles to contract. Sometimes, patients will not be able to endure the hard hospital beds. Some of us with FMS/MPS Complex find even water beds too hard, and need additional padding. Darkness and quiet may be necessary for restorative sleep.

It is of utmost importance that the reasons for surgical intervention are clear. Myofascial trigger points may mimic surgical conditions (Flax 1995). There are many "carpal tunnel" conditions and "thoracic outlet syndromes" that are from myofascial trigger points. A list of some of these can be found in the article, "Myofascial Pain Syndrome Due to Trigger Points" (Simons 1987), along with the specific TrP muscular origins, references, and common diagnoses.

Patients with FMS and/or MPS are more prone to develop adhesions, fibroids, cysts, overgrowths, and abnormal scarring. It's common for trigger points (TrPs) to form along incisions. This can be prevented by using procaine to inject the surgical area immediately before incision.

Positioning of the patient during surgery is critical. It is important to place no undue stress on the body. Myofascial Pain Syndrome, itself, has been considered a postoperative complication (Prasanna 1993), possibly due to overstretch of muscles and lack of adequate support for muscle groups during the surgical procedures.

During surgical repair, take extra care to approximate myofascia, and repair it whenever possible. Keep in mind that patients with FMS, MPS, or FMS/MPS Complex tend to form thickening myofascial tissue in the form of ropy bands or lumps. This leads to contractured, shortened muscles, which, in turn, lead to more TrPs.

Surgery and Medications

People with FMS/MPS often have atypical reactions to medications. The normal medication regimen for your patient may have to be "beefed up" during the recovery time to prevent flare. Flare is a condition when symptoms worsen and intensify. Surgery, or any change, may be a flare trigger. It is best to minimize the impact of surgery as much as possible.

Anesthesia and FMS/MPS

It is not unknown for FMS or MPS symptoms to go into remission after general anesthesia. It may be due to the total relaxation of the muscles and subsequent removal of myofascial "splinting," and to a change in the nature of ground substance. Clearly, more research is needed to study this phenomenon. As more physicians become familiar with the difference between single muscle group TrPs, bodywide chronic MPS, FMS, and the FMS/MPS Complex, patterns will become clearer.

Failed Procedures

There are several common "failed surgical procedures" caused by pain from TrPs. You should be familiar with these TrPs and their pain patterns. Trigger point pain is very specific. If you suspect TrPs, ask the patient about bodywide achiness and the sleep disruption of FMS, as well as inquiring about the presence of other TrPs. Patients may have undiagnosed chronic MPS.

Trigger Points

The quadratus lumborum TrP causes pain when walking, when turning in bed, when getting up from a chair, or when coughing or sneezing. It is often the cause of "failed surgical back syndrome." Patients get a deep "lightning bolt" pain from the quadratus lumborum to the front of the thigh. Pain may extend to the groin, testes, scrotum, or down the leg like sciatica. The quadratus lumborum TrP can cause a heaviness in the hips, a cramping of the calves, and burning sensations in the legs and feet. This can cause satellite TrPs to develop in those areas.

Subscapularis, infraspinatus, supraspinatus, upper trapezius, and **levator scapulae** TrPs often cause pain when the arms are raised overhead. The subscapularis TrP not only causes a "toothache pain in the shoulder," it also refers pain to the wrists. Check candidates for carpal tunnel surgery for TrPs. It isn't unusual to see someone who has had failed carpal tunnel surgery on both wrists. In every case so far, treatment of the subscapularis and related TrPs has resulted in remission of wrist pain.

Myofascial trigger points cannot be removed surgically. This may seem self-evident, but I have seen patients who had been treated by doctors who tried. Sometimes, repeatedly. So much TrP preventative work can be in the hands of the surgeon. Once s/he is aware of the possible complications of FMS/MPS, necessary surgical procedures should cause no undue trauma, and unnecessary ones can be avoided. Cutaneous TrPs, however, can be removed surgically with minimal problems and sometimes the procedure provides considerable relief.

Trigger points can mimic atypical facial neuralgia, arthritis, subdeltoid bursitis, collateral ligament damage, thoracic outlet syndrome, appendicitis, heel spurs, trochanteric bursitis, and carpal tunnel syndrome. They can cause sciatica, contractures, back pain, and meralgia paresthetica. Checking for TrPs can save a lot of unneeded aggravation, time, pain, and cost.

References

Flax, H. J. 1995. Myofascial pain syndrome—the great mimicker. *Bol Assoc Med PR* 87 (10-12):167–170.

Prasanna, A. 1993. Myofascial pain as postoperative complication. *J Pain Sympt Manage* 8(&):450–451.

Simons, D. G. 1987. Myofascial pain syndrome due to trigger points. *Internat Rehab Med Assn Monograph Series 1.* Available from Gebauer (800) 321-9348

Travell, J. G. and D. G. Simons. 1992. *Myofascial Pain and Dysfunction: The Trigger Point Manual, Volume II: The Lower Body.* Baltimore: William and Wilkins.

———. 1983. *Myofascial Pain and Dysfunction: The Trigger Point Manual, Volume I: The Upper Body.* Baltimore: William and Wilkins (revision in process).

What Your Urologist Should Know

Please read "What Everyone on Your Health Care Team Should Know" and "What Your OB/GYN Should Know."

There are many aspects of fibromyalgia (FMS) and Myofascial Pain Syndrome(MPS) that directly concern the urologist. Female urethral syndrome frequently coexists with FMS (Paira 1994). Also, there is a type of insomnia called Compulsive Urination Insomnia that I've found to be very common in FMS/MPS Complex. Most people urinate before they go to bed. There is usually a small amount of urine left in the bladder. People with FMS/MPS Complex have hypersensitive nerve endings, and can feel the pressure, so we get up and go again. We are conscious of how hard it is for us to get some sleep, and we don't want to take a chance on being awakened in the night by having to go again, so whenever we wake (sometimes with every alpha intrusion), we take a trip to the bathroom. This can happen more than thirty times a night. Lidocaine ointment on the urinary opening will stop some of the sensitivity, but the patient should first be checked for a possible yeast or low-grade bacterial infection. Any infection can be a perpetuating factor either for FMS or MPS. There are many medications that help FMS/MPS, and there are physical therapy modalities that are effective in defusing the trigger points (TrPs) of MPS.

Irritable bladder or bowel: This can be caused by the pyramidalis, multifidi, and abdominal TrPs, as well as by yeast overgrowth in the GI tract. Neurotransmitter dysfunction may have an impact on the body's sphincters, causing loss of control.

Trigger Points

I have found that TrPs in the upper rim of the pubis add to the irritability and spasms of the genital-urinary (GU) tract. This is at least part of the reason why so many of us have urinary frequency. Not only is the bladder hypersensitive, it won't hold much. In addition, we can't empty the bladder totally. There is also a TrP that can form high on the adductor magnus muscle, in the center inner thigh, about an inch from the join of the leg to the trunk. Often you will be able to feel a taut, ropy band of TrPs. These TrPs refer soreness into the pelvic region. This can mimic Pelvic Inflammatory Disorder (PID), prostate trouble, or other visceral conditions.

I have a theory that we also lose bladder elasticity, as the myofascia in that area tightens and "splints" the stressed muscles. This is also a common occurrence as we age. It just seems to happen earlier for those of us with FMS/MPS. Fortunately, there are ways to reverse this process. Often, in cases of irritable bladder and bowel, TrPs in the lower internal oblique muscle and possibly lower rectus abdominus are involved.

Burning or foul-smelling urine is fairly common, and also occurs as a result of guaifenesin treatment. It can mimic a urinary infection. I don't know why, although I suspect the body is trying to rid itself of wastes and toxins.

Impotence Occurring Secondary to Myofascial Trigger Points

The following information is taken directly from *Myofascial Pain and Dysfunction: The Trigger Point Manual, Volume II* by Janet G. Travell and David G. Simons (1992) and references are to that volume. I include page references because so many patients have said to me that their doctors "don't believe" this is in the *Trigger Point Manuals*. It is.

To understand how impotence can occur secondary to myofascial TrPs, it is necessary to understand the basic anatomy of the region. Both the bulbospongiosus and ischiocavernosus muscles enhance erection of the penis. These muscles can develop TrPs. The bulbospongiosus essentially wraps around the corpus spongiosum of the penis, which is the central erectile structure through which the urethra passes. The anterior and middle fibers of the bulbospongiosus and ischiocavernosus muscles contribute to erection by reflex and voluntary contraction that compresses the erectile tissue of the bulb of the penis and also its dorsal vein. Contraction of the ischiocavernosus muscle maintains and enhances penile erection by retarding the return of blood through the penis. Trigger points in the bulbospongiosus muscle can cause impotence (1992, 118). Trigger points in scar tissue produced by surgical incision are well known (1992, 121). Trigger points in the pelvic floor muscles are sometimes activated by surgery in the pelvic region (1992 121).

The piriformis is a major intrapelvic muscle which is a frequent site of TrPs. Entrapments are numerous. The nerves and blood vessels that pass through the greater sciatic foramen along with the piriformis are subject to entrapment (1992, 187). Exiting the pelvis along the lower border of the piriformis are the pudendal nerve and blood vessels. The pudendal nerve innervates the bulbocavernosus, ischiocavernosus, and sphincter urethrae membranacea muscles and the skin and corpus cavernosus of the penis. Innervation of these structures is essential to normal sexual function (1992, 191). "Patients may complain of . . . sexual dysfunction . . . impotence in the male" (1992, 192). "Pudendal nerve entrapment may cause impotence in men" (1992, 194). The piriformis TrP is most commonly found with a complex of other TrPs (1992, 203). This is a complex area with multiple layered muscles and opportunities for entrapment. After a surgical procedure, such as a hernia repair, a regimen of stretches can often help prevent adhesions and TrPs.

References

Paira, S. O. 1994. Fibromyalgia associated with female urethral syndrome. *Clin Rheumatol* 13(1):88–89.

Travell, J. G. and D. G. Simons. 1992. *Myofascial Pain and Dysfunction: The Trigger Point Manual, Volume II: The Lower Body*. Baltimore: William and Wilkins.

8

Medications:
Perceptions and Realities

Man stands in his own shadow and wonders why it is dark.

—Zen saying

Generic Drugs

Generic and brand-name drugs are not always exact equivalents. Some fibromyalgia (FMS) and Myofascial Pain Syndrome (MPS) patients may be sensitive to the differences. It is important that your doctor be on the alert for this. It is also important that s/he believe you if you require the brand name, so that your pharmacist can be advised. In recent years, because of all the highly publicized attempts to rein in drug prices, doctors have been under a lot of pressure to substitute generics for brand-name drugs. If a company wants to market a generic as being exactly the same as a brand-name drug (this is legal after the drug patent expires), it must pass the Food and Drug Administration (FDA) bioequivalency program.

This means that it isn't sufficient for the generic to be made of the same chemical components in exactly the same strengths as the brand name. The company manufacturing the generic must prove that when someone takes the drug, *the amount of the active substance released by the generic is the same as would be obtained with the brand-name drug.* Doctors, and patients, are led to believe that this means the generics are the same as the brand names, except perhaps for packaging. This is not true. "The FDA considers two formulations as bioequivalent when the rate of adsorption varies no more than –20% or +25%" (Banahan and Kolassa 1997). Only 17 percent of the physicians responding to a survey knew this. This means that there can be 20 percent less usable medication in a dose, or 25 percent more.

People with FMS and/or MPS are usually what the industry calls "polydrug" users. We have so many symptoms that we often require a variety of medications. Medications for other conditions (often perpetuating factors) can interact with FMS and MPS medications. For example, Zocor, a drug for high cholesterol, can interact with niacin, erythromycin, and azole antifungals such as ketoconazole. It is important to use one pharmacy for all your medications because that enables the pharmacist to help you keep track of possible drug-drug interactions.

It is also important to know which drugs you can take at the same time as other medications, and which ones you can't. For example, I have observed that some medications taken with Soma (carisoprodol) seem to dissolve faster in the stomach. For some medications this is not important. For timed-release medications, it is. Your pharmacist can teach you a lot about the ways your medications work. It is wise to learn as much as you can, especially about the medication(s) you take to control the symptom that might otherwise dictate the course of your life—pain.

Obtaining Pain Relief

People with MPS have a chronic pain syndrome with individual trigger points (TrPs) they routinely describe as "intolerable" and "torture." People with FMS have a nearly constant, generalized achy flu-like feeling, and they may also experience the amplification of the muscular pain of MPS. In addition, we are often subject to pain from other causes. To advocate for pain relief most effectively, it is essential for you to understand the concepts that underlie the diagnoses and treatments for FMS and MPS.

Pain itself is one of the prime perpetuating factors of both FMS and MPS. Inadequate pain control leads to problems like muscle contraction and sleep loss, and these problems, in turn, push patients further down the symptom spiral. Health insurance officials will cover thousands of dollars in surgery charges without blinking an eye, but they continue to fail to provide coverage for medications for pain management.

There are many possible pain therapies and medications. It can be a long and winding road to find what works best for you. The reward at the end of the road should be adequate pain relief. For some patients, even when all known perpetuating factors have been dealt with, an unacceptable level of pain remains. When treating chronic pain patients, most physicians require "an attitude adjustment" of "challenging proportions" (Sees and Clark 1993). Physicians must be made to understand that you are trying to obtain relief from pain so that you can get on with your life, not to get "high."

Some doctors refuse to even consider prescribing *standard* FMS and MPS medications that have been tested and documented as efficacious, such as amitriptyline (Brenne, Van der Hagen, Machlum, et al. 1997), tramadol (Aronson 1997), specific serotonin reuptake inhibitors (SSRIs) (Jung, Staiger and Sullivan 1997), or carisoprodol (Vaeroy, Abrahamson, Forre, et al. 1989) for chronic pain. There can be no acceptable justification for this attitude. There is a subset of chronic pain patients who require special consideration, especially those who have been in unremitting pain for a long time, and those who have pushed themselves (or have been pushed), beyond their capacity. These are patients who have pain that is inadequately relieved by these medications or who do not tolerate them. If you are in this subset of patients, it is important to understand that there are often new medications, such as Zanaflex (tizanidine), which may help, but you need a doctor who is willing to prescribe them. There are also other older paths to take to obtain pain relief, but they are roads strewn with potholes and roadblocks. There are many people working to change this, but the change is not easy.

Insurance, Medical Providers, and the DEA

A powerful triangle has formed, with insurance companies situated at one point, the Drug Enforcement Agency (DEA) at the second, and medical care providers at the third. The formation of this triangle has been well documented. These three factions are, at present, locked in a battle of perceptions.

The insurance company must be perceived to be cutting costs, since its prime responsibility is to its stockholders, and the bottom line, of course, is profitability. The DEA must be perceived to be keeping illegal drugs out of the hands of addicts. That is its job. Their administrators have no responsibility to the chronic pain patient. They carefully monitor doctors and pharmacists, who, in turn, must be perceived as being exceedingly cautious when prescribing and dispensing controlled substances.

Medical care providers are responsible to the DEA. The "war on drugs" has generated such fear that some providers refuse to write *any* prescriptions for *any* scheduled substances. Furthermore, many providers are increasingly dependent on the insurance companies for their wages and increasingly aware that any suggestion of impropriety will bring the other two factions crashing down on them. Where is the chronic pain patient in all of this? Right in the middle! The right to prescribe pain medication has become a battle over turf, and the patient has become the battleground. And, as in any battle, those on the battleground *always* suffer.

Television shows and movies glorify the patient who bears pain heroically in silence. We rarely see a depiction of death without adequate pain control, although that is more common than the medical establishment would have us believe. We pump millions of dollars into a misdirected, and increasingly ineffectual, "war on drugs," and we fail to draw the connections between that "war" and the stories we read about physician-assisted suicide. Would the "Kevorkian option" be necessary if we had adequate pain control? I think not. Those of us in "the trenches" know that raw pain is undignified, messy, and dehumanizing. Most of us know, too, that in most cases, there is no valid reason for it not to be treated adequately.

Perceptions of Pain

Studies show that the drug regulatory agencies have dictated the prescribing of opioid drugs, or rather the lack of it, to the medical provider (Hill 1996), to the point where "patients who have a legitimate need for the relief that these drugs can provide have become the unintended victims of the drug control systems" (Angarola 1990). In addition, "controlled substances laws appear to create financial disincentives for pharmacies and hospices to use them" (Joranson 1994).

Today we know (or should know) that unrelieved pain can cause increased stress, raised metabolic rate, blood clotting dysfunction, water retention, delayed healing, hormonal imbalances, an impaired immune system, impaired gastrointestinal functioning, decreased mobility, feelings of powerlessness, hopelessness, low self-esteem and depression, as well as increased muscle contraction. *Pain is a major perpetuating factor in both FMS and MPS.*

People with FMS and or MPS are often given expensive and unnecessary tests and surgeries in an attempt to find a pain mechanism *understandable to the doctor*. But the undertreatment of pain sometimes results in suicide. Since my last book was published, at least three of the "alleged Kevorkian suicides" were young patients with fibromyalgia.

Why Pain Relief Management Is Inadequate

Why, with all our scientific and medical advancement, don't we provide adequate pain relief? You might think this a simple question, but there are deeply entrenched roadblocks on the way to an answer, and they are formidable.

Lack of Training

One big hurdle is that medical students and doctors do not receive training in the concepts that underlie the proper diagnoses of FMS and MPS. Thus, they can have no understanding of the magnitude of pain that we endure. Generally, there is also a lack of training in chronic pain management. Often, chronic pain patients are placed in the same category as terminal patients. The customary paradigm of medical practice, at least in the United States is, "Meet the patient. Treat the patient. Cure the patient." When this doesn't happen, medical personnel often feel guilty, as though they had failed.

This may be an unconscious response, but it can surface at the most inopportune times. When doctors don't know what to do, they often do nothing. Frequently, they mistakenly believe that nothing *can* be done. We must demand that our doctors be trained to treat chronic pain. Medical schools must begin to make this a required part of the basic curriculum. We must refuse to give our money to people who know less than we do about our condition and how to treat it.

Law Enforcement Issues

Even when the doctor is adequately trained, there are other roadblocks. Doctors have a great well-warranted fear of the law enforcement agents and agencies who don't know the difference between use and abuse. Drug enforcement agencies monitor all narcotic prescriptions. Triplicate prescriptions are required for a number of drugs. One copy is retained by your doctor, one sent to the pharmacist, and one to the DEA.

More than two hundred pharmacists and doctors a year are arrested on charges of prescribing narcotics too freely. Many doctors are afraid of making an honest mistake, so they refuse to prescribe refills. Some refuse to prescribe narcotics at all for any reason. Most of them are concerned with the fear of societal perceptions or law enforcement regulators. Consider these two statements: "Medical practice with respect to the use of opioids for the treatment of pain has been heavily influenced by societal perceptions of problems of addiction and by laws governing the use of opioids" (Savage 1996). "The available data suggests that medical decision-making regarding the use of opioids continues to be unduly influenced by regulatory policies or fear of regulators"(Portenoy 1996).

Doctors and pharmacists have a just fear of enforcement agencies, even when pain medications are appropriately used. These organizations have been so focused on the war on drugs, they roll right over those of us struggling to obtain legitimate pain relief. They make no distinctions between use and abuse, or between the emotionally impaired addict trying to get high and the chronic pain sufferer trying to get relief from pain.

Faith and the "Just Fine" Appearance

People with chronic pain may look "just fine." Our doctors have no "objective" proof that we are in pain, or how badly we are hurting. That's why they have to listen carefully when they take our histories and believe us when we describe that pain with which we live. In the final analysis, adequate pain relief, like many other important things in life, comes down to faith. Faith is not something the doctor and pharmacist can fill out in triplicate and send to DEA. Neither is our pain, although many of us would like to be able to package it and send it to some of the folks who have denied us adequate pain relief.

There are doctors who do not believe what their chronic pain patients say about their pain and their need for proper medication. Such doctors are condescending, and even cruel, to these patients. It's not uncommon for a well-meaning doctor to dismiss chronic pain patients' complaints and send them to mental health specialists, or to substance abuse programs. This is like the doctors who all too recently performed major surgery on unanesthetized babies. It's the old "Well, it doesn't hurt me. I can't feel a thing" approach. There was no regard for the lasting trauma done to the infants (Wellington and Rieder 1993). The emotional, and we now know physical, damage done to chronic pain patients by callous doctors is comparable.

Some doctors will not consider using narcotics to treat patients with chronic pain, but will prescribe them for cancer patients (read patients with "real" pain), although, in truth, the cancer patient may be in less pain than the chronic pain patient who has been refused effective medication. Here, again, the patient pays for the doctor's ignorance. This is neither fair nor just. We must create a new era of fairness and justice.

The Difference Between Drug Dependence and Drug Addiction

Many doctors don't understand the difference between dependence and addiction. People taking narcotics to control and alleviate pain will develop a physiological dependence and will experience physiological withdrawal if the drug is abruptly stopped, but that is not the same as addiction. "Physical dependency does not, in and of itself, imply addiction" (see Appendix B: "Public Policy Statement on Definitions Related to the Use of Opioids in Pain Treatment").

Addiction is a pathological psychological state. The American Society of Addiction Medicine defines addiction *as the abuse of any psychoactive substance with compulsion and loss of control despite adverse consequences.* One study found not a single case of addiction in one hundred chronic pain patients who were taking opioid medications over a four-year period (Zenz, Strumpf and Tryba, 1992).

Opioids

No one should think that opioids are to be taken lightly. Only when other therapies fail should you and your doctor consider them, and they should not be used alone. The healing regimens of diet, bodywork, mindwork, lifestyle modifications, and so forth must be continued, and hidden perpetuating factors must be identified and treated. If the central nervous system (CNS) has been sensitized to a great degree (see chapter 5, "Chronic Pain"), and other medications and therapies either don't work or aren't tolerated, then narcotics should be considered a legitimate option for pain control.

The public perception of opioid use is changing, but it's often hard to separate the myth from the reality. In 1997, the American Academy of Pain Management and the American Pain Society issued a "Public Policy Statement Related to The Use of Opioids for the Treatment of Chronic Pain," a joint policy statement. The statement in its entirety can be found in Appendix B. It states:

> Misunderstanding of addiction and mislabeling of patients as addicts result in unnecessary withholding of opioid medications. Addiction is a compulsive disorder in which an individual becomes preoccupied with obtaining and using a substance, the continuing use of which results in a decreased quality of life.

Here are some additional pertinent statements from other researchers on opioids and chronic pain management:

> Disciplining practitioners using standards based on myths, prejudices, etc., reinforces physicians' fears of prescribing opioids for nonmalignant pain. Patients with nonmalignant pain who are not relieved if opioids are not provided will continue to suffer until regulatory boards/drug enforcement agencies define the standards of practice for opioid use for nonmalignant pain in clear and unequivocal terms (Hill 1996).

> Certain diseases and drugs, like chronic nonmalignant back pain (CNMBP) and opioids, are maligned by society, resulting in sufferers and users experiencing discrimination within the health care system which has the effect of increasing, rather than alleviating their pain and suffering. Many patients with severe CNMBP suffer not because their pain is untreatable but because their pain and personhood have not been validated by doctors and nurses who are opiophobic (Gardner and Sandhu 1997).

> From a purely pharmacologic point of view, opioids have perhaps the best side effect profile (for chronic pain) in our armamentarium (Horning 1997).

> Many patients with opioid sensitive pain are being undermedicated.... The most important reason for this undertreatment is the fear of addiction engendered by opioids, a fear that is greatly out of proportion to the real risk (Friedman 1990).

Many states' controlled substance laws hinder appropriate opioid prescribing through (a) the use of ill-defined terms, (b) restriction of pain prescriptions to a specific number of dosage units; and/or (c) utilization of multiple-copy prescription programs (Shapiro 1994).

Natural Opioids

Naturally occurring opioids such as the endorphins, the enkephalin/interneurons, and the dynorphins are the body's own pain defenses. Opiate receptors are common in nature, and have a function in the evolutionary scheme. Neurotransmitters such as serotonin and norepinephrine are involved in pain modulation, but not enough is known yet about the interactions of these biochemicals. It may be that people with FMS need replacements for deficiencies, just as a diabetic needs to replace missing insulin.

Kappa Opioid

Women may respond better to a specific class of opioids called kappa opioids, rather than the normally prescribed mu opioids. That is, they respond without side effects (Gear, Miaskowski, Heller, et al. 1997). Kappa opioids such as pentazocine, nalbuphine, and butorphanol may be more effective for women than the more commonly given morphine, codeine, oxycodone, and methadone (Gear, Miaskowski, Gordon, et al. 1996).

Two kappa opioids, nalbuphone and butorphanol, were tested as pain relievers. It seems that men and women biologically process pain relief in different ways. Other researchers have found that, in mice, morphine is much more available to the male brain than to the female brain (Candido, Lutfy, Billings, et al. 1992). Perhaps such research provides hope for more specific pain relief for women.

Chocolate and Marijuana

Another study recently found that chocolate contains cannabinoids that create a CNS modulation, which may be why so many of us crave it when we hurt (di Tomaso, Beltramo and Piomelli 1996). Chocolate, however, contains lots of fat and sugar which create serious side effects, such as reactive hypoglycemia and obesity. Marijuana *abuse* has been studied but not its *use*, not in FMS or MPS. It is illegal. Marinol is the legal form of the active ingredients, and some doctors say that their FMS and/or MPS patients do well on it.

Morphine and Codeine

People who take opioids for chronic pain need the medication to return as close to a normal life as is possible. They take opioids to be able to resume family life and other commitments, such as work. Such people tend to take as little as possible of the medication because it would interfere with their other life goals. People who take opioids to get high do so to get out of their lives, to avoid family and other commitments, and to escape from their normal existence.

The patient should understand that pain management is an important function of the health care team. The biggest problems arise with patients who are undermedicated and have "learned helplessness" in regard to pain control. Just as diabetics who require insulin injections are not addicts, chronic pain patients who use opioids to reestablish normal functioning are not addicts either.

Before prescribing opioids, your doctor should first determine your use of over-the-counter or other previously prescribed medications. The doctor will need the following information: Does the medication work? Does the pain go away in twenty to thirty minutes after you take it? How long does the pain relief last? This information should let the doctor know whether it is appropriate to consider narcotic use. At the initial evaluation, someone in the patient's family or support system may be needed because some patients may describe having no pain at all due to the fact that they severely limit their activities to avoid pain.

Patients struggling for pain relief can get caught in another kind of turf war. The primary care physician may feel uncomfortable prescribing narcotics, and send the patient to a psychiatrist for medication. The psychiatrist may feel that pain control isn't his/her responsibility, and send the patient to a rheumatologist. The rheumatologist may not be aware of the severity of FMS and/or MPS, and will either undermedicate the patient or otherwise prescribe inappropriately. The patient gets frustrated, and receives inadequate care. Pain management belongs to everyone on the health care team. They must communicate and choose appropriate and effective strategies. If they feel uncomfortable with the situation, a pain management specialist who understands both FMS and MPS may be needed to stabilize the patient's medications, and to establish a regimen that meets the patient's needs adequately and optimizes her/his functionality and quality of life.

Drug-Drug Interactions

It is important that doctors prescribing opioids be familiar with the actions of the drugs. For instance, many people with FMS and MPS are on a benzodiazepine medication (Klonopin, Tranxene, Xanax, Halcion, Restoril), and yet it is known that benzodiazepines enhance GABA (see chapter 2, "The Neurotransmitters"), which blocks opioid analgesia (Gear, Miaskowski, Heller, et al. 1997). These medications should not be given with opioids. Conversely, there are medications such as promethazine, often used as an antihistamine, which enhance the action of opioids. This type of medication may minimize the amount of opioid needed to effect pain control. Research on NMDA receptor antagonists is underway (Dickenson 1997). These medications show promise not only for potentiating the action of opioids, but also for blocking central nervous system hypersensitivity on their own.

The oral form of morphine can be titrated to precise pain requirements, so that there is pain relief without side effects, often at a very small dosage. "Titrated" means that the medication can be adjusted by exact amounts to give maximum pain relief with the fewest side effects. This can vary from day to day as needs change. There are also oral medications, such as Vicodin Tuss™ , which contains hydrocodone and guaifenesin. This has the benefit of the hydrocodone without the common NSAID accompaniment. It can be titrated so that you can take the lowest dosage possible to get the pain relief you need at a given time. Opioid medication doesn't have to be a long-term, full-time treatment. For some of us it's needed only for major flares.

Opiate Side Effects

Once a patient is on a stable dose of an opiate, new side effects will almost always signal another nonanalgesic problem. But constipation is common with this medication, so if necessary, begin a bowel regimen the first day of opiate use. Here's a rule of thumb—for each 30 mg of morphine or the equivalent—take one senna tablet. Note that it is common for patients to sleep a great deal during the first days of effective pain control. You have a lot of catching up to do. This is normal. You should then be able to work toward resuming function. Remember, improving or restoring function requires *control of pain.*

Methadone

Methadone, like many opioids, is surrounded by negative myths. Medical personnel associate it with addicts who are withdrawing from heroin. Presently, it is still the only effective medical treatment for heroin addiction. Unfortunately, this often links methadone with addiction in the minds of physicians and public alike.

Methadone is a good medication that has a built-in timed-release function. After it's taken, it is stored in the liver and then slowly released. Because of this, your doctor must make sure that your liver is metabolizing correctly, so that you can get the benefit of the methadone. The effects of one dose of methadone can last for twenty-four hours or more. It is slowly passed to the brain as needed to fill opiate receptors. Oral forms are available to titrate the needed dose precisely.

For pain relief, the medications, used in conjunction with adequate treatment of perpetuating factors, are in place. All we have to do is change the system.

Advocating for Pain Control

There are doctors who just *won't* understand that pain is one of the most frequent perpetuating factors for both FMS and MPS. Although pain is a logical side effect of perpetual muscle contraction and insufficient, inadequate sleep, these doctors refuse to acknowledge that logic. They just don't want to know.

If you are seeing a physician who is skeptical about the pain you experience, refer that doctor to this chapter. Be prepared to be met with disbelief. All the documentation in the world won't help you with doctors who won't read it, or don't believe in FMS or MPS. Furthermore, all the references in the world won't help you with the physicians who don't believe in giving *any* pain medications for chronic conditions. In such cases, vote with your feet. Walk away from such negativity generators and find a compassionate doctor who will listen to you and will prescribe medication suited to your specific needs.

9

Treatment Options
and Alternatives

*"One doesn't discover new lands without consenting
to lose sight of the shore for a very long time."*

—André Gide

Complementary Medicine

Perceptions in the field of health care are changing. They are changing at different speeds in different parts of the country. Many of these changes are positive. The phrase "alternative medicine" has begun to metamorphose into "complementary medicine." One study concluded, "Alternative medicine practices were currently being used by almost all FMS patients" (Pioro-Boisset, Esdaile and Fitzcharles 1996). This may be because complementary medicine frequently is more open to understanding "bizarre" symptoms.

Los Angeles now has two hospitals offering courses in complementary medicine (Cedars-Sinai Medical Center and Daniel Freeman Marina Hospital). An Office of Alternative Health was established in 1992 as part of the National Institutes of Health. A state-funded clinic for alternative health practices now exists in King County in Washington. A residency program at Mercy College in Dobbs Ferry, New York now allows interns in Western medicine and traditional Asian medicine to study each other's respective disciplines. There is a Department of Complementary Medicine at the Postgraduate Medical School at the University of Exeter, in the United Kingdom. This is just a beginning. Eighty percent of the world uses what we still call "alternative medicine." Of course, we haven't accepted the metric system yet either.

I know M.D.s who are studying homeopathy, hypnosis, acupuncture, meditation, and other forms of healing. Not only have some patients become more accepting and willing to try diverse healing therapies, but we have begun to question more of the tenets of Western medicine, and we will no longer accept the answer "Because the doctor says so." We are learning to explore the mind/body connection. A great deal has been written in the popular press about this, and change results from education and exposure. We have begun to stretch the time-hardened envelope, but change comes slowly.

Tough Choices

We all face tough choices dealing with perpetuating factors. I know I face some rather formidable ones. Just like everyone else, I have limited time and energy. I also have severe and long-standing FMS/MPS Complex. The biggest perpetuating factors in my case are overwork and travel, and I know I must drastically cut my work hours and do it *now*. I'm just one person, and can't possibly deal with each FMS and/or MPS person who contacts me individually. I do hope that people reading this book will realize this, and not try to contact me personally. My focus must be on teaching as many people as possible how to help themselves, without endangering my own health.

Your Right to Alternate Care

Try to decrease your pain and other symptoms in as many non-medicinal ways as is possible. Each of us reacts differently to specific medications. Some of us can't tolerate any medication at all. As of this writing, there is no medication that is universally effective for fibromyalgia (FMS) or Myofascial Pain Syndrome (MPS). You will probably have to teach your medical team— and your insurance carrier—that perpetuating factors are the key to your well-being.

Some perpetuating factors, such as reactive hypoglycemia (RHG), require nonmedicinal means to treat them (for RHG, a balanced diet works best; see chapter 3). This often means a change of lifestyle. There is no "quick fix." You may have to convince your insurance company/HMO that alternative methods are legitimate ways to ease the symptoms of your FMS and/or MPS.

Teaching Your Doctor

It is important to present new information to your primary care physician in the most positive and specific manner possible. For example, if you say, "I hear electrotherapy is helpful for pain. Would you write me a prescription for a unit?" you may not get very far. Use the References and Bibliography sections in the back of this book to reinforce your case. Rather than copying the sections and handing them to your doctor, read through them carefully looking for articles that sound relevant to your needs. Then, make a list of the references about the specific therapy you wish to try. In the case of electrotherapy cited above, you could present your doctor with a short list of articles specifically relating to electrotherapy, such as the sample list of references below. (You can read about electromagnetic sensitivity in the section called "The FMS and/or MPS X-Files" later in this chapter.)

Sample Reference List

This list of ten references is provided as a sample of what a short list of articles relating to a single specific topic should look like.

Airaksinen, O. and P. J. Pontinen. 1992. Effects of the electrical stimulation of myofascial trigger points with tension headache. *Acupunct Electrother Res* 17 (4):285–290.

Allegrante, J. P. 1996. The role of adjunctive therapy in the management of chronic nonmalignant pain. *Am J Med* 101(1A):33S–39S.

Deluze, C., L. Bosia, A. Zirbs, A. Chantraine and T. L. Vischer. 1992. Electroacupuncture in fibromyalgia: results of a controlled trial. *BMJ* 305(6864)1249–1252.

Hainaut, K. and J. Duchateau. 1992. Neuromuscular electrical stimulation and voluntary exercise. *Sports Med* 14(2):100–113.

Kaziyama, H. N. S., M. Miyazaki, M. Imamura, S. T. Imamura, L. R. Battistella, L. T. Yeng, et al. 1995. Fibromyalgia: continuous physical therapy program with or without long-term medical supervision. *J Musculoskel Pain* 3(Suppl 1):126 (Abstract).

Lewis, P. J. 1993. Electroacupuncture in fibromyalgia. *Brit Med J* 306:393.

Mercola, J. M. and D. L. Kirsch. 1995. The basis for microcurrent electrical therapy in conventional medical practice. *J Advan Med* 8(2):107–120.

————. 1993. The usefulness of cranial electrotherapy in the treatment of headache in fibromyalgia patients. *Am J Pain Manag* 3(1):15–19.

Ward, A. A. 1996. Spontaneous electrical activity at combined acupuncture and myofascial trigger point sites. *Acupunct Med* 14(2):75–79.

White, A. 1995. The fibromyalgia syndrome: electroacupuncture is a potentially valuable treatment. *Brit Med J* 310(6991):1406.

A doctor receiving such a list won't have to wade through a lot of irrelevant data, and will be much likelier to check the specific references. Using an abbreviated reference list could help you gain access to chiropractic care, physical therapy, or adequate pain medication. You can even use such a list to prove the existence of reactive hypoglycemia, or of FMS or MPS. It is a sorry state when patients must be responsible for the education of their doctors, but, sadly, in many cases that is where we are. I have tried to make your task, and the task of your doctors, as easy as possible.

After you hand your reference list to your doctor, add some relevant comments gleaned from my work and others, such as "TENS units are not the best electrical unit for breaking up trigger points, because they don't create the necessary muscle contraction. Microstimulation, neuromuscular electrical stimulation, and galvanic stimulation work well. A personal unit can be obtained with a prescription from the doctor. Devin Starlanyl finds that ultrasound is more useful in trigger point therapy when it is coupled with galvanic stimulation."

The Rule of "P to the Third Power"

Medical research is governed by the rule of "P to the 3rd power" (proof of performance by pounds of paper). Research and documentation take time. As a rule, it takes about ten years for a medication or therapy to be properly documented. (For Myofascial Pain Syndrome, the theories have been discussed for more than fifty years, it has been well

(Continued on next page.)

Canaries and Sentinels

In my last book, I said that I believe those of us with FMS and MPS are like the "canaries used in the mines in the nineteenth century." We are the sentinels, the sensitives. The stresses the planet is enduring are affecting us greatly, forcing us to become creative problem solvers. We have had to develop diagnostic skills to ferret out our perpetuating factors. Then, we have had to find ways to mitigate them, if possible. Studies are now showing that oil spills and other toxic exposures can account for FMS (Godfrey 1997; Alonzo-Ruiz, de la Hoz-Martinez and Zea-Mendoza 1985), and pollutants contribute to perpetuating factors of MPS such as allergic rhinitis, nutritional inadequacies, and breathing difficulties. I believe

documented, and still the majority of medical workers remain ignorant of it!) Today, there is considerable research being conducted on the use of myotherapy, acupuncture, chiropractic, electrical stimulation, and other healing methods for MPS, and more information is constantly being published. Ongoing research is also being conducted on FMS.

Nonmedicinal Symptom Relievers

The following list is not a comprehensive one. It does, however, list some of the methods frequently used by patients with FMS and MPS to decrease their reliance on traditional American medicines. Some practitioners, such as many osteopaths, combine these methods with traditional medications to ease their patients' symptoms.

Acupuncture: Care and effectiveness depend on which medical conditions you have, your perpetuating factors, on the skill of the practitioner, and his/her experience with FMS/MPS Complex and the life-force called "chi," as well as on your particular body's responses to the treatment. Acupuncture is proving useful in both fibromyalgia (Zborovskii and Babaeva 1996) and Myofascial Pain Syndrome (Travell and Simons 1983, 20).

Chiropractic manipulation: The use of blocking or an activator is recommended, and gentle manipulation. Many MDs are reluctant to refer patients to chiropractors, yet there may be a chiropractor near you treating FMS and/or MPS patients with some success. Chiropractic helps muscles ease back into their proper alignment after TrP work. Chiropractic manipulation is based on the interplay of structure and function, and with MPS it is precisely this interplay that is out of whack.

Present your primary care physician with a list of relevant journal articles from the References and Bibliography sections, along with a request that s/he consider referring you to a chiropractor. Even if you are in an HMO, your doctor may read the medical references. If the HMO won't refer you, you will be better able to appeal that decision. Sooner or later, they'll become educated.

Cold: Reduces blood and lymph flow and inflammation. It reduces spasticity or muscle tightness. It diminishes the pain caused by the tightness by reducing nerve conduction velocity, so that it takes the pain signals longer to reach your brain. That gives you a greater chance to sidetrack the pain signals with mind- and bodywork. Unfortunately, many of us are cold intolerant. If your pain eases in response to cold, that's often a sign that a nerve is entrapped. When medicines fail, ice or heat may work as pain relievers.

Exercise: Exercise should be considered as carefully as a prescription. Be *very* cautious with aerobic exercise. You need the right dose, the right timing, and the right kind. Repetition "loads" the muscles electrically. Exercise should never be done when your muscles are tired or cold. Muscle physiology works best when muscles are warm. As trigger points are inactivated, you should begin carefully graded exercises to increase strength and endurance. A physical therapist will be your best guide in this.

Stretch each muscle periodically. Take it slowly—your muscles may have grown shorter over time due to TrP contraction. Don't try to rush it. Overstimulation will trigger more contraction. Once the TrPs are treated, you can slowly start aerobic exercise. Find what works for you, and what you enjoy doing.

If mild exercise soreness disappears after the first day, you can repeat it on the second day. If it persists to the second day, postpone any more exercise until the third day. If soreness persists on the third day, your exercise routine must be changed. This rule of thumb is true for any treatment, such as massage or electrical stimulation. Note that stretching which involves rolling the head around in all directions is hazardous, and is likely to activate trigger points. Nonrepetitious exercise is best.

Galvanic electrical stimulation: Galvanic stimulation is a direct, continuous, and unidirectional flow of current between a positive to negative source. It can cause a contraction in denervated or rigid muscle tissue, causing an increase in circulatory flow. This leads to an increase in tissue metabolism and to reduced pain. Alternating current changes constantly, and doesn't seem to work as effectively on trigger points. There is a difference between direct (galvanic) and alternating (faradic) currents. TENS units use alternating current. No one with artificial cardiac pacemakers, defibrillators, insulin pumps, or a history of cancer should consider using these alternatives. Studies are showing that different types of electrical simulation are helpful in different types of pain (Hsueh, Cheng, Kuan, et al. 1997).

Heat: Heat increases blood flow and elasticity of connective tissue. It also increases swelling and inflammation. Trigger points are areas with long-term insufficiency of blood flow. Trigger points that are causing muscle pain generally respond to moist heat.

Homeopathy: There are different types of homeopathy. Classical homeopathy is very complex, and works by stimulating the body to help itself. It uses minute amounts of the vital force of medications to act upon the vital force of the patient. The medication is tailored to the biochemistry of the specific patient, rather than to the medical condition the patient has. It is used more extensively in other countries, as are acupressure and other forms of healing.

Massage: Proceed carefully and slowly. The right kind of massage can help; however, too vigorous a massage can cause rebound tenderness and make things worse. Cranio-Sacral

that the answers *we* find for our problems may someday help *everyone* to survive the changes the earth is experiencing. Mankind has changed the planet drastically. As we destroy more forests, spill more pollutants in the oceans, and endanger the ozone layer, many species are being threatened. We are crowding other species off the map, unwilling to recognize that we are dependent on the intertwining of biodiverse life for our own survival. The changes we have wrought are now impacting more obviously upon our own lives, and the canaries—those of us with FMS and/or MPS—are sounding the alarm.

Release or myofascial release are often effective. Avoid deep tissue work at first. Acupressure massage may fail if the trigger point is too tender, if you have perpetuating factors, or if the therapist uses improper trigger point technique, for example, if the therapist presses too hard at first, causing involuntary tensing.

There are also nonelectrical acupressure devices such as the Back Knobber and the Acu-Masseur which are sold through health and fitness catalogues and many physical therapy departments.

I use a tennis or lacrosse ball to aid in self-acupressure. I also use two balls tied tightly in a knee sock. Lie on your back on the floor. Place the sock at the base of your skull, arch your back, and slowly roll it down your spine. You can also press on your TrPs by leaning against a wall or a chair, with the filled knee sock against your head or back.

Pool therapy: If you have trigger points, avoid the repetitive motion of some water aerobics. It is also important to avoid exercises that include lifting a water jug overhead. Be sure that the water in the pool is at the proper temperature for you. A cool pool means an initial increase in heart rate and vasoconstriction, although the antigravity effects of the water may help. Water that is *too* cool can have disastrous effects on trigger points, causing cramping and severe pain. Fortunately, with the onset of the Arthritis Foundation's Aquatic Program, warm pools are becoming more common. Warm water is beneficial for many medical conditions. Muscles were designed to operate better in a warm state. The Arthritis Foundation's aquatic therapy brochure states that water therapy is best done in a pool of 83 to 88 degrees. This is a little cool by MPS standards, but it is better than many. *A pool temperature of 88 to 94 degrees F seems optimal.* Unfortunately, it may take a few incidents of severe cramping and subsequent legal action before something is done. Various types of hydrotherapy have proved valuable in the treatment of FMS, but we have yet to educate many doctors and insurance companies about this. One study clearly states, a "continuous program of hydrotherapy, exercises and permanent medical supervision is essential to improve the clinical performance of patients with fibromyalgia" (Kaziyama, Miyazaki, Imamura, et al. 1995).

Spray and Stretch: Practitioners need to be thoroughly familiar with the methods taught by Travell and Simons (1983; 1992). Each specific TrP technique is described in detail in their book and videos. Each muscle must be positioned properly, and the spraying must be done in the proper direction, interspersed with stretching, and then more spraying at the proper distance from the muscle. Then rewarming and passive range of motion exercises must be performed.

Stress reduction and Cognitive Behavioral Therapy (CBT): These complementary therapies carry with them the danger that doctors and others may assume "It's All In Your Head." It is important that your mental health professional, and the rest of your medical team, be aware that stress is but *one* perpetuating factor of FMS and MPS. All perpetuating factors need to be addressed, including nonrestorative sleep, pain, diet, and others that can contribute to your overall stress and symptom load. Easing your stress through therapy is helpful, but it is just one part in any program.

Your body is striving for balance and harmony, which is the natural state of any healthy living organism. You are trying to find as many ways to help it achieve that balance as possible. Reducing your stress levels and your perception of stress can be very helpful.

Trigger point injection: If you find a physician who knows and understands TrP injection therapy as well as perpetuating factors, and is educated enough to treat your whole body and not "just do trigger point injections," you are fortunate indeed. By all means, have them done. In the right hands, they can work magic. Specific methods are covered in Travell and Simons' *Trigger Point Manuals* (1983; 1992), although the technique has advanced considerably since the publication of those books.

You must prepare for this therapy, such as ensuring adequate amounts of vitamin C before the injections. Too many doctors just look at the pictures in the Travell and Simons' manuals, and then begin sticking needles into patients. These patients receive only temporary relief. Note that patients with both FMS and MPS may not find TrP injections as effective as patients who have only MPS do. The injections may hurt more, and their effects last for shorter periods of time. This will also depend on the expertise of the injector

I recently had six days of therapy with Hal Blatman, M.D., a former student of Dr. Travell. He has taken TrP injection to a higher plane. Using a variety of needles and injection techniques, coupled with myotherapy, spray and stretch, acupressure, lacrosse ball stretching, and nutrition counseling he was able to dramatically increase my range of motion. The injections are fast but painful, and they can release long-standing ropy bands of TrPs. Stretched and injected muscles are likely to be sore for two to three days following treatment.

Janet Travell wrote: "The gastrocnemius is very prone to soreness. . . . This muscle may remain sore for as long as five or six days following TrP injection and, for the first day or two, the patient may experience marked discomfort while walking and standing. For this reason, one should avoid injecting TrPs in both the right and left gastrocnemius muscle at the same visit; doing so might immobilize the patient" (Travell and Simons 1992, 416).

I not only had both gastrocnemius muscles injected in one day, I had many other muscles injected. I saw patients with Dr. Blatman and worked on this book, and then went from his office to speak to a Cincinnati support group. I was on my feet speaking for over two hours, and I did not have one moment of soreness in the gastrocnemius muscles. His technique is marvelous.

Some insurance carriers will not pay for TrP injections, in spite of the documentation done by Travell and Simons. Much of the ignorance in the medical world is due to one fact—the inability of most medical personnel to differentiate between FMS and MPS. Some insurance companies will pay, but only for a few injections. For some of us with head-to-toe TrPs, there is no logic to this policy.

It is important that TrP injections not be done with Marcaine (bupivacaine). It is toxic to muscles (Ishiura, Nonaka and Sugita 1986). The use of steroids is to be condemned in TrP injection. For example ". . . the addition of steroid to bupivacaine increases the initial tissue damage and prolongs the healing phase" (Guttu, Page and Laskin 1990).

Studies I have read since my visit with Dr. Blatman lead me to believe that in the genetically susceptible, the use of Marcaine for TrP injection might begin the neurotransmitter cascade that initiates FMS. ". . . [B]upivacaine interacts with cellular energy metabolism and leads to a depletion of high-energy phosphates" (Sztark, Tueux, Erny, et al. 1994).

Strenuous activities should be avoided for the period of muscle soreness, including shopping, gardening, and traveling. If TrP injections are unsuccessful, you may have had inadequate treatment of all the trigger point areas. Latent as well as active TrPs must be treated. It could be that your muscles were too tense, or that there are untreated perpetuating factors.

Myotherapy

I find myotherapy to be the most efficient form of massage, coupled with stretching and ball work, to maintain the health of my muscles. This requires the services of a trained trigger point myotherapist. Fortunately, trigger point myotherapists now have a national registry (see "Agencies and Organizations" in the Resources section).

Water Massage

My husband came upon on a relatively new type of muscle relaxation therapy while attending a seminar in Atlanta. It is called dry water massage therapy, and is done with the patient fully clothed—sort of a warm, massaging waterbed. The treatments can be localized. I recently experienced this first-hand in an AquaMed massage bed in Cincinnati—very soothing after trigger point injections.

After specific therapy trigger point therapy such as acupressure, trigger point injection, or electrical stimulation, the physical therapist should follow the therapy with hot packs or neutral warmth. The warmth can be achieved by wrapping your body in a warm blanket or even by the therapist's hand pressure. This should be followed by a passive full-range-of-motion exercise for the muscle or muscle group treated.

After any kind of TrP treatment, you can usually expect some soreness as your muscles adjust to a healthier mode of function. This involves tissue movement and change. Change is not easy to accomplish.

Some Over-the-Counter Alternatives

As electronic communication becomes more rapid, more people will have greater access to overseas studies. It is not yet obvious to the insurance companies that it is in their financial interests to pay for more research. They *must learn* that providing preventative medicine is in their best interest. Presently, preventative medicine is a foreign notion to "the system," which is why so many of us are in such bad shape. We wouldn't have to work so hard to dig ourselves out of the "hole" if "the system" hadn't failed us so deeply. Many of us must pay for myotherapy, physical therapy, and chiropractic treatments out of our own pocket, or do without. This can become very costly. And, for some of us, it is so prohibitive as to be inaccessible.

The following list of comments and observations regarding over-the-counter medications is not meant to be a list of recommendations. They are by nature brief, due to the scope and focus of this book. We are all different; what works for one of us may not work for another. We must each try to find what helps our own unique bodies most effectively. Often, there is no prescription medication that will remove all of the pain. There may, however, be nontraditional remedies that will remove or alleviate some of the perpetuating factors. A note of caution: Be very careful with the use of herbs and other natural treatments. They are not simple. Many have multiple effects. Don't take over-the-counter medications lightly.

Breathing: You don't need a prescription for this one! The need for clean oxygen to reach all of our tissues, and to have our circulatory and respiratory systems working at optimum efficiency is too often taken for granted. Bodywork, mindwork, and breathing exercises help (see *Fibromyalgia & Myofascial Pain Syndrome: A Survival Manual* [Starlanyl and Copeland 1996] for relevant exercises).

Bromelain: This may help some of the swelling and pain caused by inflammation.

Capsaicin: Used topically capsaicin helps some of us with pain control. It helps others with skin itch control, if they are able to tolerate the initial burning sensation. Use this very cautiously at first. Test it on a very small, relatively insensitive area. Capsaicin causes depletion of substance P and other peptides. People with FMS often have too much substance P in some areas of the body, but we are not sure yet about other peptides.

Caffeine: You may find that a small amount of caffeine reduces trigger point pain, but too much caffeine generally increases muscle tension and TrP irritability. Some people with fibromyalgia have no tolerance for caffeine at all. Caffeine inhibits some biochemicals, such as adenosine (and phosphodiesterase) which slow metabolism. It also increases adrenaline and noradrenaline, those neurotransmitters that can set our hearts racing.

Chromium picolinate: This seems to be helpful for curbing carbohydrate hunger.

DHEA: Not all FMS patients have low DHEA. If you are considering using DHEA, ask your doctor for a test for DHEA sulfate levels. Dr. Jorge Flechas (see "Oxytocin and Nitric Oxide Therapy" later in this chapter) recommends that the DHEA sulfate level should be around 200 mcg/dl or greater. If your level is lower, consider DHEA hormone therapy. Go cautiously and wisely, arming yourself with as much information as possible.

Ginger: This spice inhibits the formation of the inflammatory compounds prostaglandin and thromboxane. It may be very helpful for nausea, and to "warm" the body.

Herbs: Be careful with herbs. One herbal preparation may interfere with another, or with a prescription medication. Many will block guaifenesin due to their high salicylate content. Some herbal mixtures have potent ingredients and you may be very sensitive to them. Become familiar with the ingredients of any mixture before taking it. For example, licorice can affect blood pressure, as well as being very high in salicylates. It strongly activates and strengthens cortisol, and also can interact with many prescription medications. Willow bark is also natural aspirin (salicylate). Guarana is a stimulant containing a chemical similar to caffeine. However, *homeopathic* amounts of herbs may be fine, even for people taking guaifenesin.

Kombucha tea: This is not a mushroom, but a yeast. Used long-term, it can have antibiotic effects that may promote bacterial resistance to antibiotic therapy. This is not good. Grown in the home, this "tea" may be contaminated with a variety of yeasts and fungi. Some may even be carcinogenic or poisonous. Larvae have been found wriggling on top of some Kombuchas. Some people have reported nausea, vomiting, head and neck pain, and allergic reactions. Kombucha is not listed in any Eastern pharmacopoeia, ancient or modern (Srinivan, Smolinske and Greenbaum 1997).

Marijuana: It isn't exactly "over-the-counter," but it is sometimes used for sleeplessness, antitremor, antinausea, antiataxia, spasticity (muscle tightness), and pain. I have heard many reports that it is extremely helpful. Of course, it hasn't been tested on people with FMS or MPS. Marijuana itself is not uniform, and it may contain compounds damaging to your lungs or immune system. Right now it is illegal, except in two states, Arizona and California, and if you are caught, the resultant stress will be *very* damaging to your health and well-being. Marijuana seems to potentiate (activate and/or strengthen) melatonin. It can also increase appetite. Most of us don't need that, although there are, of course, some of us who do. We don't know what else marijuana might do. We don't know what kinds of pain it can control.

I know one physiatrist who prescribes Marinol (the active medicinal ingredient in marijuana) for many of his FMS patients, and he has had good results. It is interesting to note that chocolate contains marijuana-related substances (di Tomaso, Beltramo and Piomelli 1996).

Melatonin: This seems to help some of us to sleep better. Some do better with the sublingual type, and others prefer timed-release melatonin. Some of us find that it causes depression. Recent studies show that people with FMS have normal levels of melatonin (Press, Phillip, Neumann, et al. 1998).

NSAIDs: Non-steroidal anti-inflammatory drugs can cause many deleterious effects. More than 107,000 people are hospitalized every year in the United States for NSAID-related stomach bleeds and other complications, and 12–15 percent of those patients die from those bleeds (Singh, Ramey, Morfield, et al. 1996). Doctors tend to suggest their use frequently, but adequate pain control is neither easy nor simple. Here are some guidelines regarding NSAID usage:

Stomach Toxicity of NSAIDs/Aspirin by Risk

- **Lowest Risk:** nambumetone, etodolac, salsalate, sulindac

- **Medium Risk:** doclofenac, ibuprofen, ketoprofen, aspirin, naproxen, tolmetin

- **Highest Risk:** flurbiprofen, piroxicam, fenoprofen, indomethacin, meclofenamate, oxaprozin

(From Doctor's Guide, "Aspirin and Its Cousins Ranked by Stomach Risk" <http://www.pslgroup.com/dg/44876.htm> page 3 of 4)

Rhus toxicodendron: or "**Rhus tox:**" This is a homeopathic remedy some people find helpful for muscle aches, especially for the subset of FMS folks who also have MS.

St.-John's-wort: This plant extract can cause photosensitivity, in addition to affecting neurotransmitters. It affects serotonin, dopamine, and norepinephrine in nearly equal amounts. Do these neurotransmitters all need boosting in nearly equal amounts? Too many serotonin reuptake medications can lead to serotonin syndrome—sweating, agitation, confusion, and tremors. Don't take St.-John's-wort with MAO inhibitors or some diet drugs.

Turmeric: This herb is used by some healers for pain, much like an NSAID—without the stomach irritation.

Vitamins and minerals: Supplementation of vitamins, minerals, and amino acids can work wonders, but you have to be aware of your specific needs. We all differ. What works for me is a natural preparation including high B vitamins and minerals (such as Solgar Formula V

"VM-75"), *at least* 500 mg timed-release vitamin C capsules twice a day, and 400 IU (mixed tocopherols) of vitamin E.

I have deleted thymus from my daily supplements due to concerns about prion transfer. Prions are infectious protein particles that can transfer from one species to another. Raw glandular extracts carry this danger. This common vitamin regimen should be adjusted to complement *your* nutritional profile. Many of us need to boost our magnesium. A magnesium and malic acid combination seems effective for many people (Abraham and Flechas 1992). Check with your pharmacist and/or doctor to ensure that the vitamins and minerals you take do not interfere with your other medications. For example, the medication Neurontin may be blocked by magnesium. Tetracyclines are blocked by calcium. Be sure to talk to your pharmacist.

We don't have many rights when it comes to health coverage for alternative or "complementary" medicine, but this is changing, too. It's just that we have a long way to go. Western medicine has not studied many of these medicine forms extensively, especially in regard to FMS and MPS, although this is changing as well. Use the References and Bibliography sections. These sources will provide the information and documentation that will encourage change. Remember, we must *create* justice. See the Resources section for information on alternative resources.

> **Potassium Supplements**
>
> I find that in the summer, when I am working in the garden and am sweating more, I need extra potassium. Of course, I take these supplements along with medications for sleep/pain/muscle rigidity, my proper dose of guaifenesin, and many nonmedicinal therapies to attack my perpetuating factors. This enables me to work. Now I have to attack overwork, my main perpetuating factor, and avoid travel as much as possible—another TrP perpetuating factor *for me*. Find out what works for *you*.

New and Experimental Treatments

The medical establishment has taken FMS and MPS seriously for a very short time. As many of you know to your dismay, there are a lot of doctors and other health practitioners who *still* don't believe these conditions really exist. The result is that many useful therapies are still experimental. I've found none that work well in all cases of FMS and/or MPS. At least some of this lack of success is due to the lack of understanding and training on the part of the medical team members.

We are each different, and we each require individualized attention. Even when attending to those perpetuating factors that we know about, we may have others that are hidden. Some of these therapies deal with perpetuating factors with varying success. Your insurance company or HMO may try to persuade you to avoid trying these. But you must do your own risk analyses. You may also be faced with insufficient medication, and a worsening condition, in spite of all that you have been able to do.

I was roundly criticized for offering experimental treatments without medical references in my last book (Starlanyl and Copeland 1996) and will probably receive some more brickbats for this one. I believe that too many people are afraid to offer new possibilities because "hardening of the attitudes" is a very common ailment in medical circles. Some of us have to break new ground, or we'd never get anywhere. Many previously "undocumented" therapies and medications that I cited have now been more thoroughly studied, and can be found in the References and Bibliography sections in the back of this book.

Some therapies are being studied in other countries, but that makes them no less valid. The world is growing smaller, and research that is being done in other countries cannot go ignored. Some authorities tell me that I shouldn't "stick my neck out," and that I should move slowly and wait for more medical documentation. None of these authorities has FMS and/or MPS.

I am not willing to have even one person suffer needlessly. I have looked for the best and safest experimental help I could find, and I present it to you here and elsewhere in the book. There are a lot of promising new therapies out there. Check the References and Bibliography to find the scholarly documentation you need to persuade your doctor to try these therapies. Use the documentation to impress your doctor and insurance company with the amount of pain and other symptoms you are experiencing, and do your best to broaden your options. Each of us can add a voice to the chorus. Find out what works best for you. There is always hope. There is always tomorrow.

Perpetuating Factors

It's essential to explain the concept of perpetuating factors to your doctors and insurance company so that they understand it. Then, you can work together for the best possible functional outcome. It's not enough to be able to return to work, or to continue working, if you come home exhausted and crying in agony, unable to fix and eat dinner. It is also vital that you be able to participate in and enjoy your life. You need to discover where you are functioning, and where you are not. Let your doctors and insurance companies know what you can and cannot do. Let them know what your realistic expectations are, and how you would like to achieve them.

You will want to ease the overall pain burden in as many ways as possible. You may find that you need to take chromium picolinate to help you avoid excess carbohydrates, or you may need to settle into the Zone diet (Sears 1997b) before you can deal effectively with reactive hypoglycemia. Booster vitamins and minerals may help you to avoid catching a communicable illness that would send you into a flare. You may want to try light therapy for Seasonal Affective Disorder (SAD). Stay open to new possibilities. Don't resign yourself to a life of pain. Don't be afraid to try new therapies. There is too much to be gained.

Neurotransmitters

Neurotransmitter research is exciting, with a lot of new information cropping up every day, with possible applications for the future. For example, there is some interesting work being done on adenosine receptors. The theory is that caffeine and similar compounds stimulate by blocking the adenosine receptors. For those of us who chase elusive sleep, it may be a hope for the future (Radulovacki 1995; 1991). Injections of adenosine often provoke sleep.

You may have heard of the "sleepy cat" studies. Researchers deprived cats of sleep by playing with them (fair game, since cats often do the same to us!). After sleep deprivation the adenosine in the cats' brains had doubled.

Some patients are trying the serotonin precursors l-tryptophan and 5 HTP. I have a warning for those of us whose bodies utilize the alternate kynurenine pathway (see chapter 5). If these medications cause you to feel much worse, you may be making more quinolinic acid, a *neurotoxin,* instead of more serotonin. Some of us even feel bad when we eat a lot of turkey or peanuts, which usually stimulates the production of serotonin. That's a clue. Quinolinic acid has been implicated in Parkinson's disease (Miranda, Boegman, Beninger, et al. 1997) and AIDS dementia (Kerr, Armati and Brew 1995; Miranda, Boegman, Beninger, et al. 1997).

Increased quinolinic acid formation also occurs after an acute systemic immune stimulation (Heyes, Achim, Wiley, et al. 1996). It has been found that kynurenines in the hippocampus can contribute to seizure disorders, which may help to explain the subset of us that has conditions of this sort, as yet unexplained (Schwarcz 1987). These researchers aren't working with FMS or MPS, but their work shouts *clues* to me. Research is ongoing in several countries, including the United States, on NMDA antagonists. Some studies show that at least a part of chronic pain is the result of NMDA receptor hyperactivity (Siegan 1997).

Take comfort in knowing that a lot of research is being done in the field of chronic pain. The "baby boomers" are aging, and they are not content to suffer. It's revolution time. And it's about time! Furthermore, there *are* FMS- and MPS-savvy doctors out there. The number is growing, and many of them are working to make life easier for all of us.

Surface EMG/ergonomics

Kenneth Hoelscher, M.D., a physiatrist and good friend, is compiling a surface EMG/ergonomics software package that the doctors on our health care teams should find very useful. Using a surface EMG and a video cassette recorder, a simultaneous visual and kinesiology study can be recorded of the patient as s/he works. The surface EMG will record the electrical signals from eight different muscles. It will be possible to tell which muscles are firing and at what level or intensity, during the performance of any given task.

It will be able to prove the effects of lowering a chair, tilting a keyboard, and so forth. Eventually, it will be possible to calculate the chances of an injured worker being able to return to a specific job, or the chances of a worker being injured if that job is undertaken. This will help us to compute our ability to "return to work" with much more exactitude. This product came into being because a compassionate and knowledgeable doctor wanted to prevent the damage being done by work hardening and similar programs. (Contact: Kenneth Hoelscher, M.D., 600 E. Genesee Street, Suite 329, Syracuse, NY 13202.)

Darice Putterman, P.T., works with dynamic functional movement assessment with surface EMG. The Noraxon telemetry equipment she uses is able to show muscle guarding, contractures, muscle imbalances, muscle spasm, and a great many other parameters. The charts and graphs are easy to read, and provide documentation for those of us with doctors or insurance companies who believe "It's All In Your Head." For information, your doctor can contact Darice Puterman, P.T., CAAPM/Owner/Director Valley Therapy Services, 8300 North Hayden Road A 104, Scottsdale, AZ 85258.

FMS and Thyroid Supplements

John Lowe, a chiropractor and good friend, has investigated the use of thyroid supplements in FMS. He sent me the following information:

We believe that a number of factors can cause the symptoms and signs of fibromyalgia. In fact, any factor can that impedes metabolic processes of the specific tissues from which fibromyalgia symptoms and signs arise. The metabolism-impeding factors must be controlled or eliminated before a fibromyalgia patient can significantly improve.

In our protocol, we measure the patient's fibromyalgia status, graph it, and adjust the treatment based on the quantification and graphing. We use five objective measures of fibromyalgia status. The clinician's subjective judgment of the patient's status is important in making therapeutic decisions, but decisions are primarily data-driven by the scores of the objective measures.

All patients do not require thyroid hormone therapy to improve or recover. They improve or recover when nutritional deficiencies are relieved, when they become better conditioned, or more often, when a combination of metabolism-impeding factors are controlled or eliminated. Of patients who do require the use of thyroid hormone some use T4 and others T3. We start treatment with T4 if the patient has any form of hypothyroidism, and with T3 if the patient is euthyroid (has normal thyroid function test results). For many patients, particularly euthyroid patients, effective dosages are supraphysiologic. [Note: Supraphysiologic means a dose greater than is normally used for healthy individuals.] Nonetheless, extensive follow-up testing has clearly demonstrated that only rarely have such dosages induced clinically significant tissue overstimulation. It is especially noteworthy that bone mineral density in female fibromyalgia patients taking supraphysiologic dosages is typically greater than of age-matched controls.

We assume this results from the patients' significantly increased physical activity level following metabolic therapy.

Most patients' pain scores maximally improve only after they undergo effective specific treatment for a local or regional musculoskeletal problem, such as myofascial trigger points. Many fibromyalgia patients' musculoskeletal problems are resistant to local treatment before metabolic therapy. Afterward, however, most patients are normally responsive to local musculoskeletal treatment.

It is now well-established that emotional "disturbance" in fibromyalgia results from, rather than causes, fibromyalgia. We believe that relieving such disturbance is like clearing away rubble left by a hurricane or tornado. Whether trying to maintain emotional equilibrium during fibromyalgia, or "clearing away" adverse emotional sequelae after recovery, various psychological self-help methods are helpful. Some individuals, however, have been so severely scathed by their experiences as fibromyalgia patients that the assistance of a professional mental health practitioner is necessary. We urge these patients to consult only practitioners who are knowledgeable about and sympathetic to fibromyalgia patients.

For information, your doctor can contact Dr. Lowe at the Fibromyalgia Research Foundation, P.O. Box 271722, Houston, TX 77277 (713) 666-0882.

FMS and Growth Hormones

As part of the study of neurotransmitters, there is continuing research in the area of how growth hormones affect FMS. I cited a subset of tall, thin people with fibromyalgia in my first book (Starlanyl and Copeland 1996) who may not have their growth hormone affected in the same way as many of us with FMS. They often exhibit teeth grinding, restless leg syndrome, myoclonus muscle twitching, and they respond to Klonopin. I've been getting a lot of feedback from this subset. There seems to be another subset of women with FMS who also have breast cancer. It is interesting to note that one of the promising experimental drugs for breast cancer chemotherapy is Octreotide, a drug that resembles somastatin (growth hormone). Are these clues?

Studies show that at least some of the symptoms of fibromyalgia may be due to a secondary growth hormone deficiency (Bennett, Clark and Walczyk 1998; Bagge, Bengtsson, Carisson, et al. 1998) due to the dysfunctional HPA-axis (Bennett, Cook, Clark, et al. 1997). Very recent studies indicate that insulin-like growth factor (IGF-1) interacts with estrogen to moderate breast cell growth. High levels of IGF-1 may have implications both in breast cancer and the aggressiveness of breast cancer (Ng, Ji, Tan, et al. 1998; Westley, Slayton, Daws, et al. 1998). As this book goes to press, we can't be sure of the implications of these studies. They are a reminder, however, that everything in the body is connected to everything else. Adjusting the balance of the body by adding one biochemical will affect the whole body. Restoring that balance is not easy, neither is it a one-step process. Please be patient with research and researchers. We are uncovering clues, and doing the best we can to find the safest way back to health.

Nerve-Muscle Interactions

There is ongoing research in the field of nerve-muscle interactions. How cells communicate within the brain and elsewhere is being studied. The neurotransmitter acetylcholine is of prime importance in the neuromuscular junctions where nerve and muscle cells interface. This research may hold the key to some of the information we need for a cure.

Electrical Stimulation

There is also research into the effects of electrical stimulation. Electrical stimulation can even strengthen the muscles (Montes Milina, Galen Tabernero and Martin Garcia 1997). Electrical stimulation causes nerve depolarization and activation of the muscle fibers. This can help "flush out" the trigger point areas, and improve their circulation. Recently, I have heard of exciting research in the field of alpha wave brain stimulation. We need more research in this field.

Guaifenesin

I will consider changing my medications, my physical therapies, and even my exercise routines, but I will not consider going without guaifenesin, nor will I take anything that might block its effect. It's too important to my well-being. I must still practice sound nutrition, bodywork, mindwork, and the other lifestyle modifications important to the FMS/MPS

Complex patient, but I feel that guaifenesin has made a decided difference in the quality of my life, and allowed me to do much more than I could have done without it. I want others to know that this option exists.

Guaifenesin therapy was developed by Dr. R. Paul St. Amand. It is experimental. We don't know how it works. The one study done on guaifenesin and FMS was flawed, through no fault of those who ran it (St. Amand and Potter 1997). We didn't know all the variables at the time the study took place, including the importance of diet for reactive hypoglycemia, and the need for adjusting dosage for each patient.

What Is Guaifenesin and Where Do You Find It?

Guaifenesin is a common over-the-counter expectorant. It has been around for about seventy years, first as guaiacum and then as guaiacolate, and for about twenty years as guaifenesin. Guaifenesin is not a cure for FMS. It does seems to allow the kidneys to eliminate something harmful that has been stored in the body. Dr. St. Amand feels that at least part of what is eliminated is phosphates, and I agree. Oxalates may also be part of this package of unwanted stored matter that is released by guaifenesin. Excess oxalates seem to be responsible for some of the vulvitis and vulvodynia experienced by female FMS patients.

St. Amand found that with guaifenesin therapy, there was an increased excretion of 60 percent phosphates, 30 percent oxalates, and 30 percent calcium. Although excess calcium is lost, none of St. Amand's patients has exhibited any sign of osteoporosis or calcium loss. Emphysema patients on guaifenesin often take 2400 mg a day for many years without experiencing any side effects.

Guaifenesin is safe and even available in pediatric dosages. It is also sold as a prescription medication available in 600 mg caplets or capsules. It is important to ensure that there are no other medications mixed in with the guaifenesin, as there often are in cough and cold formulations. You can buy guaifenesin from Hyrex Pharmaceuticals as 200 mg pills by phone at (800) 238-5282, or from Star Pharmaceuticals at (800) 274-6400.

How Do You Know It's Working?

St. Amand believes that FMS develops in a cyclical process. At first, there are times when we experience symptoms interspersed with periods when we feel fine. Sometimes we are unaware of what is happening at this stage. Then, the periods without symptoms get shorter, the symptomatic episodes become more frequent and the symptoms worsen. This is what St. Amand calls "cycling." He believes that guaifenesin therapy reverses this process.

As guaifenesin takes effect, your urine and sweat may become dark and odorous. I think that this indicates a release of wastes, excess acids and, I believe, toxins, as well as substances such as quinolinic acid, the nerve toxin produced by the kynurenine pathway of tryptophan metabolism (see "The Alternative Tryptophan Pathway" in chapter 5). This release into the bloodstream is accompanied by muscle aches, headaches, and often overwhelming fatigue. These responses include physical problems as well as psychological ones, including feeling depressed at times during the cycle.

With the release of the wastes into the bloodstream, your body can begin to process these unwanted substances, and get rid of them through urine, feces, and sweat. Your feces may become irritating, and you may experience anal itch or soreness. This can be eased by

Bag Balm, anesthetic ointment, or cortisone ointment. You may also experience burning on urination, caused by the excess acid (see Starlanyl and Copeland 1996).

After the initial flush of wastes, you will begin to go through a reverse of the cyclical process. Every once in a while you will have a period where your symptoms ease. You may then begin to experience whole days where you feel well. It is important not to overdo on these days. Your body is struggling to regain balance. Don't overtax it.

When you get to the point where there are clusters of good days, the contrast can be remarkable. Knowing what is happening helps you to deal with the reversal symptoms. The bad days are still bad, but you know why, and you know you are on a path to better health.

Guaifenesin Therapy

Before you begin guaifenesin therapy, use the "Symptom Mapping Creature Chart" in chapter 5 to map your areas of pain. This will allow you to record any progress. The typical regimen is to start with 300 mg twice a day. However, I have seen some people start gentle guaifenesin therapy on 200 mg a day. It is important to find the dosage that works for you. This varies from patient to patient. If, after one week, no obvious change occurs, increase the dose to 600 mg twice a day for about a month. Check your "Symptom Mapping Creature Chart." The breakup of pain areas in spite of an increase in symptoms means that the stored waste matter is leaving your body.

Guaifenesin and Diet

There is no "guaifenesin" or "fibromyalgia" diet. It is important that those of you with coexisting reactive hypoglycemia follow a low carbohydrate diet if you want to feel better during guaifenesin therapy. I have found the Zone diet helpful (Sears 1997b). A strict low carbohydrate diet is a must for those who are overweight as well as hypoglycemic.

The Salicylate Blocking Effect

The effect of guaifenesin therapy may be blocked by salicylates. Dr. St. Amand explains what happens in this way:

All cells have little garages called "receptors." They are each unique for certain chemicals and hormones. To work, any medication must have the ability to enter and park in the garage in order to signal the cell to do a certain job.

Guaifenesin parks in receptors to get the kidney cells to do the work you need done. Unfortunately, salicylates are a much better fit for that garage and the valet will

---

The Decision to Take Guaifenesin

I have sat with many patients, agonizing over their decision as the guaifenesin takes effect. I have held hands, rubbed backs, soothed heads, and encouraged those going through the first cycles toward healing, as the wastes and toxins (another area in which the good doctor and I disagree) came out of their hiding places and flooded the body, producing the aggravation of symptoms. I have also rejoiced with many who were able to return to their lives and, often, their jobs. I have seen the magic of guaifenesin work, both in my life and in the lives of others. I respect and love Dr. St. Amand, who has given so much to so many, receiving nothing in return but the knowledge that he has been able to help people.

park salicylates in preference to anything else. When guaifenesin arrives in the parking lot, there are no available garage spaces. Thus no signal is given for our desired effect.

The effects of a guaifenesin blocking agent may last about twenty-four hours. Salicylates are found in some medications and topical creams, for example, some muscle rub products and sunscreens. It is also present and often hidden in a great array of cosmetics, some ultrasound gels, mouthwashes, and herbal preparations. Everyone on guaifenesin should avoid obvious sources of salicylates such as aspirin and other blatant salicylates (Diflunisal, methyl salicylate, trisalicylate), including plant extracts (aloe, licorice, pycnogenol, St.-John's--wort, ginko, quercetin, etc.).

Each person seems to have a different sensitivity to the guaifenesin blocking effect of certain salicylates. If you've found your proper dosage and suddenly the cycling stops and your symptoms worsen, check out secondary sources such as camphor, almond oil, coconut oil, lauric acid, and so forth. This has happened to me and to others, and we've always been able to track down the offending salicylate and eliminate it, with a subsequent return to improvement. These setbacks and subsequent resolutions are yet another indication to me that we are on the right track with guaifenesin.

Only phosphate is known to decrease adenosine-triphosphate (ATP) formation when it accumulates in the mitochondrial matrix. ATP is essential to almost all cellular functions. Low ATP has been found in people with FMS (Park, Phothimat, Oates, et al. 1998; Eisinger, Plantamura and Ayavou 1994). The mitochondria are the body's energy factories, and ours are polluting badly.

Both Dr. St. Amand and I suspect a lowered pH is at least part of the FMS problem. The pH is a measure of the acid/base balance of the body. Low pH indicates acid. Dr. St. Amand used his observational skills and deductive logic to theorize what is happening in our cells. Sherlock Holmes would have been proud.

At 300 mg guaifenesin twice a day, Dr. St. Amand found that about 20 percent of his patients reverse—and this reversal is often swift and strong. About 70 percent patients reverse at 600 mg twice a day. The rest of us need a stronger dosage. Once your symptoms are made distinctly worse by a given dose, that is probably the proper dose for you. Just remember, your body has a limited capacity for clearing out the debris. Give it the time it needs, and be gentle with yourself when you begin guaifenesin therapy.

If your symptoms have been relieved, it may be time to see if you can do without your other medications, one at a time. Talk to your doctor about this. Once this has been done, and if your symptoms don't return, you may want to try to drop the guaifenesin dosage. Do this gradually. According to Dr. St. Amand, some people cut back a half pill at a time and wait about three months or so before they cut back another half pill. People are reluctant to jeopardize their hard-won health. You have cut down too far when the symptoms return, so just resume the dosage you were on when you had no symptoms. That is your maintenance dose.

Internet Guaifenesin Support

To join the guaifenesin support group on the Internet, send an email to the following address:

LISTSERV@MAELSTROM.STJOHNS.EDU

with the message: SUB GUAI-SUPPORT and your full name and any changes in your protocol or condition.

Your doctor may contact Dr. St. Amand at the following address:

R. Paul St. Amand M. D.
4560 Admiralty Way, Suite 355
Marina del Rey, CA 90292
Phone: (310) 577-7510

Conclusion

Guaifenesin hasn't taken away all of my symptoms. I have an exceedingly long-standing and severe case of FMS/MPS Complex, with many perpetuating factors, and I have also been pushing my body and mind to the edge. My first book (Starlanyl and Copeland 1996) led to the video and website, which were followed immediately by work on this book. Overwork is my main perpetuating factor. My priority as soon as I finish this book is to work on all my perpetuating factors, including greatly scaling down my workload. Nevertheless, I would not have been able to accomplish these projects without guaifenesin. I strongly believe that in ten years, many doctors will be jumping on the guaifenesin bandwagon. I intend to use the next ten years undergoing guaifenesin therapy, and becoming healthier.

Oxytocin and Nitric Oxide Therapy

An intriguing alternative therapy for FMS and CFIDS has been introduced by Jorge Flechas, a physician in private practice in Hendersonville, N.C. He has developed a protocol for treatment using oxytocin (OT), a hormone often given to women to induce labor. He believes that FMS and CFIDS are neuroendocrine/metabolic disorders, and that it is a deficit in microcirculation that causes the abnormal metabolism. He has been getting good results by using a combination of OT and, when needed, DHEA (a particular thyroid hormone), and nutrients such as malic acid and magnesium.

Oxytocin stimulates nitric oxide, which restores microcirculation in the head, hands, and feet. Nitric oxide, among other things, increases the amount of serotonin and dopamine, two neurotransmitters that are often low in people with FMS. Oxytocin stimulates concentration, contributes to mental alertness and improved memory, and also stimulates the libido, diminishes pain sensitivity, relieves anxiety, and enhances sleep. It may help neurally mediated control of blood pressure, and relieve depression.

We know that oxytocin can provide pain relief for low-back pain (Yang 1994). We know it can moderate pain from the gut (Bueno, Fioramonti, Delvaux, et al. 1997). We know what an increase in serotonin and dopamine can mean to those of us who have fibromyalgia (see chapter 2). We also know that oxytocin plays a part in the effectiveness of nonpainful sensory stimuli (Uvnas-Moberg, Bruzelius, Alster, et al. 1993).

Dr. Flechas believes that there are many factors in the world today that join forces to decrease normal oxytocin levels for many people. High levels of fat in the blood decrease nitric oxide. Many of us have cholesterol problems. Stress decreases oxytocin, and many of us are in a constant "fight or flight" stress state. One study showed that children with recurrent nonorganic abdominal pain had low levels of both oxytocin and cortisol (Alfven, de la Torre and Uvnas-Moberg 1994). We often deal with varying levels of chronic abdominal pain. Oxytocin is also important in the release of glucagon, a substance in which we are often in short supply (see the section "Reactive Hypoglycemia" in chapter 3).

Inositol, a biochemical found in fruits and vegetables, is needed for oxytocin to stimulate nitric oxide production. A healthy diet containing a lot of fresh fruits and vegetables is an important part of the lifestyle changes Dr. Flechas recommends. He has found that tobacco smoking is one of the worst perpetuators of FMS. He told me that one cigarette can shut down the microcirculation of the hand by 40 percent. He tells his patients, "If you keep smoking, you are choosing to live with pain."

Some patients do not have adequate nutrients to use the oxytocin to create nitric oxide. Only 20 percent of his patients respond to an oxytocin test dose, and these patients require supplements before they can begin to use the oxytocin effectively. Dr. Flechas has developed a treatment protocol for physicians wishing to use his therapy. This includes a list of laboratory work, and tells what to do on the basis of the results of that laboratory work. It is also important to monitor the patient's response to the oxytocin.

For further information on the Flechas Protocol, your doctor can contact Jorge D. Flechas M.D., M.P.H., 724 Fifth Avenue West, Hendersonville, N.C. 28739; fax: (828) 693-4471, phone: (828) 693-3015.

Relaxin

Samuel K. Yue, a physician and director of HealthEast Pain Clinic in St. Paul, Minnesota, is currently studying the effects of relaxin, a pregnancy hormone, on fibromyalgia. Dr. Yue noticed that his female fibromyalgia patients reported an increased severity of their symptoms one week before and during menstruation on a regular basis. Some of his patients said their FMS symptoms either began, or worsened greatly, during menopause. Many FMS patients told him their symptoms went into remission during their pregnancies, only to return one to two months after delivery. He also knew that frequently Raynaud's phenomenon completely disappeared during early pregnancy.

Dr. Yue saw that his FMS patients often had tight and contracted muscles. He began to look for a natural substance in the body that would affect this tightening and contraction, and would also account for his other observations. He found a little-known hormone called relaxin, which, in most mammals, is produced in ten times higher amounts during pregnancy than at any other time. Relaxin's effects, include the production and remodeling of collagen, increasing the elasticity and relaxation of muscles, tendons, and ligaments. Relaxin has been little studied except for its more obvious effects during pregnancy.

Relaxin affects the release of several hypothalamic-pituitary hormones, as well as oxytocin and vasopressin (Geddes and Summerlee 1995). Medicinal relaxin is prepared from animal products, and was used quite extensively in the 1950s and 60s to shorten labor. It has also been used for the treatment of scleroderma, a condition of thickened collagen, and for peripheral vascular disease.

Recently, human recombinant DNA relaxin has been approved as an investigational drug in the treatment of sceleroderma (Seibold, Clements, Furst, et al. 1998). Among other functions, it also inhibits the release of histamine by mast cells (see chapter 2), and affects microcirculation (Bani 1997).

Dr. Yue believes that relaxin will release the sustained muscle contracture or spasm in many fibromyalgia patients, which would result in the resolution of their tender points and muscle originated pain, spasm, and fatigue. Because relaxin improves integrity and quality of collagen within the nervous tissues, normal conductivity and response of these nervous tissues will be restored, along with normal central nervous system function.

The FMS and/or MPS X-Files

If you are intimidated by free-ranging theories, abstract thought, and the unknown, don't read this section. If, on the other hand, you are adventurous and enjoy a voyage through the speculative and a chance to stretch your thought processes, read on! I received more responses to my mention of electromagnetic sensitivity than to any other specific topic in my first book. If the skeptics tar and feather us, we shall simply learn to fly! Most of what you find here are again simple observations or comments. There are no answers, there are only questions. That can make life exciting. There is an old Chinese curse, "May you live in exciting times!" Those of us with FMS/MPS Complex lead lives that are seldom dull. It helps to know that we're together in experiencing these odd phenomena.

Chi

Chinese "chi," ("ki" in Japan, "prana" in India, and "sila" among the Inuit peoples) has no counterpart in the Western tradition. In this culture, we demand things that we can instantly touch, see, and quantify. We do have the "Force" from the Star Wars sagas, and other attempts to explain and label this all-pervasive essence, but they remain in the realm of popular fiction. There is a saying, "In the United States, we build muscle. In China, they build chi."

However, more and more of us in the United States and elsewhere are learning to build chi as well as muscle, using many of the methodologies that were discussed in my first book (Starlanyl and Copeland 1996). This takes dedication, and much unlearning of precepts that we were taught as truths. Unlearning is much harder than learning. If, as children, we had been taught, "this is what we call a table," perhaps we would be more flexible. Instead, we are taught "this *is* a table," immediately nullifying the majority of people who call a like object something else. In my observations, people with FMS seem to have an edge when it comes to chi, due to what I call inherent electromagnetic (EM) sensitivity. I have no idea what causes this. Perhaps extra neurotransmitter traffic opens EM channels that people without FMS lack?

Microcurrent

A chiropractic physician in Portland, Oregon, Carolyn McMakin, is working with the electromagnetic sensitivity of people with FMS. She uses specific microcurrent frequencies through graphite/vinyl gloves to treat contractures, spasms, and trigger points. She reports that this therapy helps old injuries with scar tissue as well. This is, of course, just part of the therapy that she utilizes. She also encourages mindwork, bodywork, a balanced and healthy diet, and other methodologies. She can be reached for information at 17214 Division, Ste 2, Portland, OR 97236; phone: (503) 762-0805.

Strange Symptoms

We are usually so busy coping with the disbelief of the medical world that we don't even mention some of the other "minor annoyances" that are distressing us and would have others complaining. Quite often we may not even realize that they may be related. They may seem "crazy." We don't want to detract from the overwhelming pain, fatigue, and other symptoms that seem more "real" and urgent.

These odd symptoms include itchy, cracking, peeling skin; bleeding skin around the cuticles (including peeling of skin on the front of the fingers whenever we have the audacity to look through a card catalogue or a file folder); cracking, bleeding skin on the bottom of the feet; a burning on the tongue; dyslexia of fingers and tongue (how many times have I had to type some of these words!); dropping things and flinging things (and cleaning the resultant messes); forgetting things—it is a list of endless frustrations. Some of the most bizarre symptoms I want to mention here I call "X-File symptoms." But I am not implying that there is something supernatural about them. It's just that we have no idea *yet* why many of them occur. Most haven't been written about, except by me, although some have been explained by Travell and Simons as part of the autonomic system's responses to trigger points. For example, they mention that trigger points can cause areas of the body to feel wet, as if water were trickling on the skin, or to feel as if bugs were crawling underneath the skin.

Some of the bizarre symptoms we share have been explained. For example, there is the condition one person on the FIBROM-L wrote about—"flicker vertigo." "Flickering light such as you would see while driving down a tree-lined highway on a bright, sunshiny day—the speed at which you are moving combined with the light shafts filtering through the trees—causes a type of flicker vertigo that bothers me a lot. If it continues for any length of time it causes me to become dizzy and/or disoriented. The same thing can happen in a shopping mall—especially if there are lots of neon signs." This problem is usually due to autonomic symptoms from sternocleidomastoid (SCM) trigger points—in this case, trigger points in the upper sternal section.

Sternocleidomastoid (SCM) Trigger Points

In addition to creating autonomic system symptoms and referred pain, upper sternal SCM trigger points (TrPs) can affect the eye and the sinuses, including tearing, reddening, or drooping of the eye, and an inability to raise the upper eyelid. These trigger points can also cause visual disturbances, such as blurring of vision. Your surroundings may appear dimmer to you than they actually are. Stripes, polka dots, and checks on fabric can cause dizziness. Sometimes a runny nose and sinus congestion can develop on the involved side. Ringing in the ear and even deafness have been reported

SCM trigger points can be caused by trauma, or by putting too much stress on your muscles. In cases where your body is already stressed, even compression of a tight shirt collar can cause trigger points. SCM trigger points can also be caused by a poorly designed work area, a too high keyboard or counter, a poorly designed chair, or even working when you are tired. Paradoxical breathing can also overload the SCM, which is an accessory muscle to respiration.

Any chronic infection such as sinusitis, any dental irregularity, or any uncorrected vision problem should be dealt with promptly. This will prevent trigger points from occurring or being aggravated. I have found that for some FMS and/or MPS people, a plugged sinus can sometimes be relieved by pressing on the areas behind and below the tips of the ear lobes with the heels of the hands. I have seen what some healers have accomplished with biokinetics, and what other alternate healers do as commonplace, and I am amazed.

A cervical pillow that fits your neck curvature is important. When you turn over in bed, don't lift your head before rolling over. Keep your head on the pillow while rolling. A triple folded hand towel used as a soft collar can guard your neck if you are going over bumpy roads. If you have these TrPs, avoid holding the phone on your shoulder with your neck, or using the crawl stroke when you swim. These particular TrPs cause me more grief than any other.

Clavicular (SCM) Trigger Points

Trigger points in the *clavicular* portion of the sternocleidomastoid muscle system—the collarbone attachment, or back portion—cause other symptoms besides pain. These include dizziness caused by movement, and disturbed balance. Spatial disorientation is common, and can be frightening as you become aware that you are not sure of where you are in relation to the world around you. Vertigo is not unusual, and when you turn your head suddenly, you can even black out. Episodes of dizziness can last for seconds or hours. *Ataxia*, which is unintentional veering with loss of motor coordination, can happen unexpectedly. When you are no longer sure of your steps, and can't trust your ability to walk straight, extreme clumsiness results, as well as close encounters of the painful kind—with door jambs, corners of tables, and any unfortunate thing—or person—in your way.

Because of clavicular TrPs, postural responses become extremely unpredictable. When you look up, you may feel as though you are going to fall over backward. If you look down, you may feel as if you are falling forward. Nausea is common. Climbing into bed can give you the impression that your bed is tilted. When you turn corners in a car you may feel as if you were riding a motorcycle and were "banking" it to the side. When the car stops, you often feel as though you were still moving, especially if a car next to you is moving. You may step on the brake in panic, only to realize that you have been stationary all along. This often leads to a feeling of loss of control. These are all part of what we call proprioceptor disturbances. Unfortunately, they may prompt inadequately educated doctors to send you for a psychological evaluation.

Proprioceptors

Proprioceptors are sensory receptors, or nerve endings, and they are affected by myofascial trigger points. The proprioceptive function of the labyrinth bones in your ears orients your head in relation to the world around you. Neck proprioceptors orient your head in relation to your body. With SCM trigger points, this ability can vanish unexpectedly. You also may lose the ability to judge how heavy an object is in your hand. This can lead to flinging objects you think you are holding securely. (One local group member told me that if meat flinging were an Olympic event, she would have a closet full of gold medals.)

When your proprioceptors aren't functioning properly, eating can become an adventure, as you struggle to keep food on your fork, and get that food to your mouth. You may have to resort to using straws to be able to drink anything without spilling it. You may also experience localized sweating and blanching in the referred pain zones. Going out to eat may be a trial. Life becomes a game in which the rules are changing constantly, and nobody tells you what they are.

Janet Travell and David Simons learned about these proprioceptor dysfunctions as part of the autonomic nervous system trigger point symptoms by listening to their patients. Travell and Simons gave their patients the attention and recognition they deserved, and searched for the reasons behind their patients' bizarre symptoms. As more clinicians learn to believe their patients, more answers will emerge. We don't stand much of a chance to find answers until we look for them. Who knows what new connections remain to be found? I am confident that all of the "way out" symptoms we share will some day be recognized, understood, and treatable. But first we must get recognition for them, and that means that we must find the courage to speak out about them. It isn't easy.

Connections

The integration of the body is a miraculous thing. A stimulus to one area will cause an effect, often beyond perception, in another part of the body. We are just beginning to learn about the interconnectedness of the body's systems. Those of us who have studied Travell and Simons (1983; 1992) have a head start in knowing about referred pain patterns and trigger points. We don't know what other connections lie uncharted. We're learning though.

Those of us with FMS and/or MPS must deal with the complex interactions of our neurotransmitters, inactivity, negative moods, weight gain, carbohydrate craving, sleep deprivation, decreased libido, daytime sleepiness, and Seasonal Affective Disorder (SAD). There is often a seasonal pattern to our symptoms. There may be more important seasonal causal variations than just the amount of available light. We are just beginning to recognize that the body has many biological rhythms. There may be hundreds of potentially relevant neurotransmitters implicated in FMS, and a countless variety of interactions between them and their receptors. The study of these amazing biochemicals is an exciting developing field, and promises hope for future control of some of our symptoms.

Electromagnetic Sensitivity Network

There is a support group for people who have experienced electromagnetic fields in the reverse way—they react to the electromagnetic forces. The director of the group, Lucinda Grant, reports that these may be two sides of the same coin. The network has a newsletter, and you can get information by writing to Lucinda Grant at the Electromagnetic Sensitivity Network at P.O. Box 4146, Prescott, AZ 86302.

Weather

More and more research is being done by courageous doctors who actually hear what their patients say and want to find out why they are suffering. There are now studies indicating that some FMS patients have their symptoms aggravated by stressors such as noise, bright lights, and weather (Waylonis and Heck 1992). Many of us get achy sinuses, or muscle pain, or a pain in the tailbone just before the weather changes. Some of us seem to react to barometric lows. Some of us are affected by cold—perhaps partly due to vasoconstriction of blood vessels. Others feel worse in hot and humid weather. Wind affects some of us. Most of us feel that weather *changes* simply worsen our pain. We don't know why. Studies have shown that the people with FMS who react strongly to weather have more functional impairment (Hagglund, Deuser, Buckelew, et al. 1994) and that there is a strong correlation between their perceptions of pain, stiffness, fatigue, and weather (de Blecourt, Knipping, de Voogt, et al. 1993).

Electromagnetic Sensitivity

There is expanding research in the field of bioelectromagnetics. For example, we now know that the pineal gland in birds is involved in bird migration, and that it is electromagnetically sensitive. In essence, the pineal gland may function as sort of a compass. Pineal dysfunction or dysfunction of the neurotransmitters that affect it may be the reason that so many of us with FMS can't tell right from left.

Also, the pineal gland, which produces the neurotransmitter melatonin, is involved with circadian rhythms. In FMS, these rhythms sometimes seem out of sync. For example, the deepest sleep we often get is in the morning hours, instead of when we first fall asleep at night. We know that NSAIDs can interfere with the synthesis of melatonin. So does bright light. We don't know what else might interfere. The pineal gland is also important in thymus regulation, which, in turn, affects the immune system. This gland, although deep within the brain, reacts to light from the eye via the retina by way of the optic nerve and the hypothalamus.

> ### It Never Rains but It Pours!
>
> If it is just about to rain, but the clouds have not opened up yet, my whole body reacts. There have been times when I have had to just call in sick to work for the morning and sleep. Once the rain comes, I am fine.
>
> I am a barometer! When the pressure hints at rising, the pressure in my head swirls and increases to leave me feeling as though my head will explode. When a high and low pressure system meet, my sinuses feel as if they're going to cave in. And when the pressure lowers, the pressure changes in my head and leaves me feeling that there will be an implosion.
>
> —FMily member

Melatonin and Electromagnetic Radiation (EMR)

Wayne London, M.D., provides some insight on melatonin and electromagnetism. "Melatonin production ... drops under exposure to EMR. ... Some evidence indicates that artificial EMR resonates or interacts with the Earth's magnetic field. This means that the effects of EMR might depend on the latitude of one's city, the seasons of the year, and the position of steel in the construction of a building and the location of appliances. ... Another problem complicating the study of EMR is that the effect might depend on the pattern of the EMR field and not just the strength" (1994, chap. 3, 32). Like music, it may not be just the sound, but the *pattern* of the sound that affects us.

Electromagnetism and Drugs

Recent research has shown that low level electromagnetic fields can either diminish or totally wipe out at least one drug's action (Harland and Liburdy 1997). Melatonin has been shown to inhibit breast cancer cells, but that effect was nullified when the cells were exposed

> ## My Hard Drive Has a Slipped Disk.
>
> Many "wholistic" healers tell us to avoid products with magnetic fields. Others sell them. Some people use screens to block the electromagnetic field of their computers from reaching their bodies. I'd need a huge shield to block my field from fouling the software. I figure that my EM field is stronger than anything the world can throw at me. I emit a pretty tough force. It screws up so many electronic devices and software that I can hardly keep up with it.

to a 12 milligauss electromagnetic field. In the same article, an EPA biophysicist reported that EM fields can "... affect the development of nerve cells when concentrations of nerve growth factor are too low" (Raloff 1997). Are these clues? The study of bioelectromagnetics is in its infancy. What will we learn tomorrow?

Electromagnetism, "Hands-On" Therapies, and the "Chi" Force

Electromagnetic sensitivity comes into play whenever a "hands-on" physical therapist uses a therapeutic modality such as Cranio-Sacral Release (CSR). I have observed that although education is important in this method, the electromagnetic sensitivity of the practitioner is an essential component of the therapy's success.

Cranio-Sacral Release performed by an electromagnetically sensitive individual is akin to magic. It is only marginally effective if the person is electromagnetically null. This is best described in terms of traditional Chinese medicine The vital force, "chi," "ki," or whatever name it is given, must be in balance for optimum health. This is probably also true for other "chi"-related methods such as Reiki and polarity therapy. The sensitivity of the practitioner to this vital force is what I call "electromagnetic sensitivity." Most of us have electromagnetic sensitivity, too, but we need help to find a proper balance of the extra electromagnetic channels we may have developed as a result of having FMS. If we can learn to control this additional sensitivity, who knows what we might be able to do with it?

Electromagnetics and Cognitive Function

Dr. R. Sandyk has found that patients with multiple sclerosis (MS) have immediate improvement in cognitive function and fatigue if they have AC-pulsed electromagnetic fields pulsed across areas of their brain (Sandyk 1997a; 1997b). He has also been able to diminish depression and suicidal thoughts in MS patients using electromagnetic fields (Sandyk 1997c). It has been proposed that these fields work on the magno-receptors in the pineal gland (Jacobson 1994) to moderate neurological conditions in MS, Parkinson's disease, and epilepsy. Might this have any implications for FMS?

Electronic Gremlins

The stories of people with FMS being beset by electronic gremlins are legion. I personally have an incredible history of wreaking havoc on electronic equipment. When I first got a watch, I had to take it to the jeweler to have it "degaussed" (demagnetized) periodically. One woman from England recently sent me a new technique for demagnetizing the body with a hair dryer. How you do it is to run the barrel of an alternating-current hair dryer over your body while the dryer is switched on (setting irrelevant). Hair dryers do emit tremendous magnetic fields.

Some "Shocking" Stories by FMily Members

I cannot wear a watch. My son won't let me in his room, let alone near his computer. I've crashed three computers this summer. I live with two computer experts and they couldn't fix them. One motherboard actually fried itself. We run scan disk and defrag at least twice a week.

●   ●   ●

I also get shocked easily, especially from electrically lit glass display counters in stores. And other small appliances that do absolutely nothing to anyone but me! And the more expensive the watch, the worse the problem. I even got one to run backwards once! No talent, just happened!

●   ●   ●

Many, many years ago I was banned from the computer room of the hospital lab I worked in. Every time I walked in the room all the programs screwed up. I also had to be very careful opening my (metal) locker—sometimes I'd see a flash of electricity jump two to three inches when I reached for the locker.

●   ●   ●

Last night I turned on the computer just by walking past it! I heard it whirring, turned around to see it booting up! I can make analog clocks run backwards! My family thinks I must have some hyper-kinetic powers!

●   ●   ●

I have never been able to wear a "normal" watch. I have to wear a digital watch. Here in the computer lab where I teach part time the technician accuses me of messing up the computers when I come in. An interesting note on the watch thing: my mom says that my grandfather also could not wear a watch. He survived being hit by lightning three times.

●   ●   ●

I have had to change my preferred seat at the kitchen table to create some distance from the cellular phone. We go through a lot of cellular phones. Usually some of the functions stop working shortly after the phones are installed. If I'm in flare, phones, especially cell phones, "beep" as I walk by.

●   ●   ●

I can cause some remarkable effects on this computer and it has developed some totally weird glitches over the year that my husband, with an MS in Computer Sciences, can't figure out at all. And, if I'm really tired, I turn out streetlights as I drive or walk under them. They often come back on and I can turn them out again with my very presence.

PART III

Fighting for Your Rights

Part III covers medical/legal rights and responsibilities. In chapters 10, 11, and 12, you will also learn about communicating with the organizations that may loom large in your life, including HMOs. There is also an informational sheet for your legal representative, should you have need of one, in chapter 11. Chapter 13 will acquaint you with the Social Security Administration.

Part III will prepare you to become a successful self-advocate. Much of how you well you succeed in your medico-legal affairs is directly related to the documentation you get from your medical team, so educate them well. They will need to know what information the legal representatives and organizations in your life require, and in what form they need it. You will learn about that here.

10

Rights and Responsibilities

Your Right to Respect

You have the right to respect. When you need medication for pain, you should not be treated by your pharmacist, doctor, or the doctor's staff as if you were a drug addict. Those of us with fibromyalgia (FMS) and/or Myofascial Pain Syndrome (MPS) have no way of knowing when we're going to hurt bad and need extra medication at a moment's notice. We may want to have something stronger on hand for flares. How do we break through a doctor's reluctance to prescribe adequate pain medication? How to we get a doctor to listen to what we say about how we hurt? It takes time and patience, and when you're hurting, these are both hard to come by. A doctor needs to listen well and take an adequate history and this depends on him/her not having the IAIYH ("It's All in Your Head) attitude.

The field of chronic invisible diseases is no place for cookbook medicine. You have a right to your doctor's respect and trust. Skepticism is a part of medical training that is easy to learn. Compassion, respect, and belief in the patient are not so easy. Your doctor must understand that high-tech diagnostics are useful only if the testing is specific for the condition. Just because the doctor may not be familiar with your medical condition does not mean it isn't real. Unfortunately, those of us with FMS and/or MPS are often required to give doctors some on-the-job training. They must be willing and comfortable with this.

Rights and Responsibilities

You can't have one without the other. Today, the practice of medicine is a battlefield in the ongoing evolution of changing cultural moralities. Whether it's the right to an abortion, adequate pain medication, or physician-assisted suicide, living and dying now have more variables than they had even twenty years ago. The old rules are often blurry and the new rules are not yet codified. On the eve of the medical breakthroughs that the new century will surely bring, the only solid ground on which we stand is formed of ethics and faith.

Your Right to Your Medical Records

The right to obtain your medical records varies from state to state. The original records belong to your physician but, in most cases, you have the right to obtain an exact copy. Don't expect to get the originals. Your doctor needs those for legal documentation. Contact your representative in the state legislature and ask for information on how to get copies of your patient records. If you want to obtain mental health records, as well, be sure to specify that, because many state differentiate between patient records and patient mental health records. If you have been refused access to your records, explain that to the state representative. Be as brief and concise as possible. Your representative doesn't need to know all the details to be an effective advocate for you. Do give him/her names, addresses, and phone numbers. Make it easy for others to help you. Follow up your original inquiries to make sure that any promises made to you are being kept.

The Right to Privacy

You have the right to privacy of records, including ensuring the privacy of your health records in your employee health care plan. In these days of computers and easy access to all sorts of personal records, such privacy is no longer automatic. This is the age of the CPR, the Computerized Patient Record. Security can be compromised and that means confidentiality can be compromised as well.

Ask your doctor what is being done to prevent unlimited access to your records.

Vertical Attention

Do you ever get vertical attention from your doctor, or are you always horizontal before your doctor sees you? That is, are you always half-naked and prone (and vulnerable) on the examining table? Or do you sometimes consult with your doctor while sitting across a desk, or standing upright? Vertical attention can be very important to your self-esteem, and to your doctor's perception of you.

Tape Recording

When you must be examined or interviewed by a hostile force (e.g., the insurance company doctor), tape recording your visit is very important. This may be an adversarial meeting, but you still have your rights. Explain the use of the tape recorder in a nonconfrontational manner, that is, say that you want to be able to provide the authorities with an accurate report of the meeting. If the doctor refuses to do an examination and/or office visit while being taped, ask if you may bring a companion with you. If the doctor refuses taping and/or having your companion present, your attorney can use this against whatever group has called for that examination or interview. When confronted with a "negativity," turn it into a positive force to aid you. People with FMS and MPS must become very creative to deal with life. Use that creativity to deal with adversaries.

Are You Afraid of Your Doctor?

If your doctor frightens you, ask yourself why. Did you shop around for a doctor you feel comfortable with? If not, why not? Do you ask the questions that are really bothering you during a visit? Does your doctor intimidate you? Are you assertive? Does your doctor get impatient with you when you are? Has your doctor ever said, "I don't want to hear that," when you tell him/her you aren't doing well? How did you respond to that brush-off?

You are paying the doctor to hear your complaints, not to make her/him happy. What happens when you bring new information to your doctor? Does s/he read it, within reason (don't take volumes of data) and ask questions, or does it lie moldering in a drawer somewhere?

You have the right to know your rights. It's great when your doctor can be your friend, but not if it's at the expense of your health care. *Expect and demand a healing relationship with your doctor.*

Patient Rights/Doctor Responsibilities

As a patient, you have a right to a doctor who is:

- Nonjudgmental, knowledgeable, and sympathetic

- Attentive and who listens to you and takes you seriously

- Aware that your conditions are treatable, but not curable

- Willing to stick with you through the process of finding out which medications and therapies work best for you

- Accessible by phone (within reason)

- Ready for you when you have an appointment

- Courteous and respectful, and whose *staff* is also courteous and respectful

You also have a right to:

- Responsive and knowledgeable backup coverage when your doctor is off duty

- Feedback on and notification of test results

- Complete and current information concerning diagnosis, treatment, and prognosis, explained in terms you can understand

- Adequate pain relief

- Be believed when you say you are in pain. You are the authority on your pain—the only authority

- Ask for changes in your treatment if your pain persists

- Communicate with other members of your health care team

- A copy of a yearly update from your charts

- Be called by the name you prefer

- Have your questions answered freely

During an office visit, you have a right to:

- An opinion from your doctor without intimidation

- Information, so that you can give your informed consent before any procedure or therapy

- Refuse treatment and be informed of the expected medical consequences

- Respect for your opinions

- Tape record your visits

- Have a friend stay with you during your visit or examination

- Question your doctor without being branded a troublemaker

- Expect continuation of care

- Be educated as to which symptoms you should call about, and which don't require a call

- Reschedule your appointment if your doctor is running late (your time is valuable too)

- Know what medications will be given for a procedure

During a hospital (or similar facility) visit, you have a right to:

- Know the risks, side effects, and benefits of treatment and what alternative may be available

- An investigation of your perpetuating factors

- Examine and receive an explanation of your doctor's bill, regardless of source of payment

- Seek a second opinion or to request a pain-care specialist. (Make sure that such a specialist understands FMS and/or MPS)

- Include your family in your decision making

- Treatment without prejudice from your doctor

- Expect the hospital or similar facility to make a reasonable response to your request for services, within its ability to do so

- Know which hospital rules and regulations apply to your conduct

- Obtain information as to any relationship of your hospital to other health care and educational institutions insofar as your health care is concerned

- Know if a business agreement exists between any individuals or organizations (such as laboratories), who are involved in your treatment

- Be advised if the hospital is proposing or engaging in human experimentation affecting your care or treatment. You have the right to refuse to participate in such research

- Privacy of your records

Visiting Your Doctor

Any visit to your doctor may be anxiety-producing, even if you have a warm and trusting relationship. Just dealing with the logistics of getting to the office, waiting, and getting back home are enough to add excess stress to your body and mind. Do what you can to make the outing as pleasant as possible. For example, if you enjoy reading, bring a good book to read while you are in the doctor's waiting room.

Your doctor should be aware of new developments in the fields of FMS and MPS. A friend told me that if a doctor is "down on" a diagnosis, it's usually because s/he's not "up on it." Your doctor is being paid for expertise. S/he should have it, and not depend entirely on you for information. Your doctor should take time with you, and be interested in you as a whole person, and as part of a family and a community.

This is the era of compliance medicine. You and your doctor are part of a team. It will help the team to function better if you are understanding and responsive to each others' needs. Be reasonable. Your doctor has many patients. Don't waste time. Phrase your questions carefully. Keep a journal or list of your observations and note the sequence of symptom appearances. This will tell you if your symptoms are worsening.

Make the journal legible. List the two or three questions you need answered the most, and have your symptom list handy. Write down your hunches as to what may be the problem. Add any clues. Keep a list of the current medications you are taking. Bring "secretarial" help such as a pen and pad to take notes or a tape recorder to be sure of instructions. It is not necessary that the doctors approve of everything you do. You are the one with the final responsibility to decide what risks are worth taking.

Ask your doctor to avoid blanket photocopying of your medical records. Sometimes, it seems as if everyone in the world has easier access to your health records than you do. Allow copying only of the specific information needed.

Keep detailed records of your needs. For example, if your doctor thinks that you need a special bra for support, make sure the recommendation is in writing, so your medical insurance will cover it. Specify that it is for trigger point prevention, and so forth. Have your goals and "audience" in mind before you put specific plans in motion.

Medical Ethics

Many things that most of us assume to be laws are not. Codes governing the medical abandonment of patients, for example, are not laws, but ethics, and ethics cannot be legislated. A number of medical schools no longer administer the Hippocratic Oath, for example, as parts of it are outmoded (by centuries). Very few of us would swear sincere oaths to Grecian gods today.

Quite a few doctors may be unhappy with some of the AMA's policies and politics, but most of us agree that the AMA Code of Ethics is a just and good code to practice by. It is not, however, legally binding. In other words, a physician cannot be brought up on charges that s/he has violated a part of the code. Power rests at the state level to censure a physician, and to remove or restrict his/her license for serious infractions of good medical practice. Some states have written ethical principles, but many other states simply expect the physician to maintain "professional standards."

Anyone can complain about a physician and bring his/her concern to the attention of the state board of medicine. This usually means that the board is required by law to conduct an investigation of any complaint. You can usually get a form or brochure regarding complaint procedures from the board. The state board of medicine is created by the state legislature, and is usually located at the state capital. The precise name and location of the board is listed in telephone books under state "agencies." Only some members of the board will be physicians. Other members will have no connection to the field of medicine at all. The board is usually appointed by the governor, and it is served by advisory committees. In some states it may have jurisdiction over allied health fields as well as over physicians.

Complaints

To report a complaint to your state medical board, you need to give the name, address, and phone number of the physician, your name if it is different from the patient's name, and the patient's name and your relationship. The board will want to know the dates of treatment, along with significant details about the complaint. Attach *copies* of any supporting documents to your complaint form—*don't ever send originals*. The board will send you a "Release of Information" form. If you are concerned about the physician seeing the complaint, there is usually an 800 number on the Release of Information form. Express your concerns. The board will handle complaints in chronological order. Be specific. Keep a copy of your complaint letter. Note that the state medical board does not handle complaints concerning billing, personality disputes, or general office practices.

Express Your Feelings

If you get the feeling that your doctor dreads your visits, and doesn't want you in his/her care, do you feel fear? Are you afraid that your doctor will get angry at you if you disagree about anything? You can practice ways to converse with your doctor without having an argument.

The American Medical Association Current Ethical Opinion A-97 section E-8.11, "Neglect of Patient," states the following:

"Physicians are free to choose whom they will serve. The physician should, however, respond to the best of his or her ability in cases of emergency where first aid treatment is essential. Once having undertaken a case, the physician should not neglect his patient. [Issued prior to April 1977; updated June 1996 (Part I, Section IV).]

You may need to brush up on your communications skills in order to learn confidence on how to handle delicate and important issues in a nonconfrontational manner. You may not even notice if you are being vague or accusatory. That may be due to having FMS and/or MPS. Remember terms like "confusional or confused," "mood swings," "unaccountable irritability"—are you aware of when those terms apply to your behavior. Also, talk to your local librarian about books on assertiveness. Do you need to learn how to assert yourself more forcefully?

In his book, *Be Sick Well* (1991), Jeff Kane explains the difference between possible perspectives during a conversation: you can have a *view*, a *feeling*, or a *want* or *need* about a given situation. Each perspective will call for slightly different language. For example:

Your *view* of the situation might be, "It's pretty warm in here." Your *feelings* about the situation might be, "I'm uncomfortable." Your *wants* or *needs* might be, "Please turn the heat down." Kane provides exercises to train yourself in communications skills, and he teaches you how to get control of yourself by centering. You cannot get the answers you want and need until you ask the right questions.

Express your feelings as feelings: Don't say, "You're rotten," but it's OK to say, "I think you're rotten because . . ." Think about what you are going to say. Then say it. It's OK to say "no." Your doctor must respect that. In *The Tao of Conversation* (1995) Michael Kahn speaks of the necessity to separate the people from the problem.

It is important, when disagreeing, to focus on your interests, not on your "positions." If you are discussing your opinions, you are not talking about yourself. The visit should be about you. When discussing your feelings, you are talking about yourself. Your doctor needs to know how you feel.

If you have a problem while waiting for or during your office visit, make sure the appropriate person knows about it. Don't scream and yell. You may have to write down your feelings. Discuss it with whomever has accompanied you. As a rule, the best thing is to say that you are upset and ask how the two of you can work it out. You can be respectful without backing down. Discuss what you think may have gone wrong. Remember, it is a triumph of reason to get on well with those who possess none. Take the high road.

Grief, Depression, and Hatred

Your doctor needs to know that, for people with FMS and/or MPS, some amount of grief is normal—as is some amount of reactive depression. There are well-known stages of denial and isolation that most human beings experience when they are confronted with a chronic illness. These are the same stages that we go through when confronting death, and a chronic illness *is* a "little death" of sorts—the death of the old "you."

It is normal for you to have feelings of anger, depression, a desire to bargain, and finally, acceptance. Your doctor should be willing to help you through these stages if they last too long. You may need counseling (the counselor *must* understand FMS/MPS) because feelings of guilt, lack of focus, or listlessness may be due to FMS. An eating disorder may be caused by neurotransmitter a dysfunction. Feelings of worthlessness or even sexual dysfunction may also be attributable to neurotransmitter dysfunction.

If you have been abused by the medical profession, you may have a great deal of righteous anger to handle. Act with reason. Get rid of hate and the desire for revenge. Hate is a destructive emotion. Some of us become consumed by hate and a desire for revenge. Such feelings take over your life, and eat up your energy. When you focus on the person you hate and why you hate him/her, your feelings overpower you. You cannot see yourself clearly as a person without the hatred. Such negativity can color all of your future relationships. You become the hate. You are much more than that. Check out Letting Go of Anger (Potter-Efron and Potter-Efron 1995).

Whenever you lose your physician, you lose the history you share. If you have a good doctor, do what you can to keep him/her. With proper grasp of both patients' and physicians' rights and responsibilities, your interactions with your doctors on your path toward healing should proceed in the most efficient and positive manner.

Doctors' Rights/ Patient Responsibilities

Your doctor has the right to expect you to:

- Keep to the relevant topic during your visit

- Give a complete and truthful answer to his/her questions

- Be respectful and courteous (professionals can also be intimidated)

- Not expect a cure

- Avoid canceling appointments at the last minute

- Be prepared for your call or visit (follow instructions given before a visit, as per fasting, etc., before a test)

- Communicate your feelings and needs—and for you not to expect mind reading

- Tell him/her about any new symptoms

- Understand that it is not necessary that s/he does something each visit

- Not change a treatment plan on your own

- Bring empty medication bottles to new appointments. (This makes it easier for your doctor to remember what was ordered)

- Follow the doctor's directions exactly. If there is a problem, call. If you don't understand or you forget something, call

- Give him/her feedback on medications and therapies

- Show up on time

- Understand that sometimes the answer is "I don't know"

- Report any physical changes or drug reactions

- Use her/his services appropriately and not as a personal support system

- Use one pharmacy for all prescriptions, if at all possible

- Inform him or her promptly if you are on any other medications or therapies

- Indicate what medications and therapies you have tried in the past

- Be honest if you didn't follow previous advice (if you didn't take the medication, didn't take it as directed, etc.)

- Show up prepared for tests and treatments

- Pay bills promptly

- Understand that your doctor has the right to a life. No one can be available twenty-four hours a day, seven days a week

Your doctor also has a right to:

- Give you an advanced warning when more time will be needed, such as for a physical. (Most appointments average 15 minutes)

- Mention issues that you may be too embarrassed to discuss

- Share your concerns

11

Legal Rights and
Advocacy

... ignorance may be bliss, but it's damned poor life insurance.

—Sherri Tepper from *The Family Tree*

Where to Start

The longest journey always begins with taking the first step. Once you're on the road, however, if you want to reach your destination, it's essential to head in the right direction. Travel tips can be invaluable when you are not sure of the direction you need to take. This chapter provides tips for locating helpful resources on the road to financial help and medical recovery.

The United Way, Helpline, and Hotline

I live in a rural area. The closest town (population about 12,000) is in the next state, not too far away. I visited the local United Way/Helpline there, to see what kinds of contacts they could offer in the way of advocacy. The Helpline offered a friendly person with good listening skills, as well as an information-referral service. Their job is to bring people and services together. I found that they provide a very broad range of help. They are affiliated with the

United Way, but their referrals go far beyond the member agencies. The United Way member agencies range from pastoral counseling to credit counseling. They had referral information (addresses, phone numbers, and the names of contact people) about the following services:

- a walk-in clinic (free for those without medical insurance and without a doctor)

- a drop-in center for those who need shelter

- public health services including occupational health

- a Senior Community Service Employment Program (with an annual physical and paid training)

- Home Health Services (including transportation to medical services, home nursing supplies, chore service, and bus service)

- Veterans' services

- VHAP (State of Vermont program to provide health insurance to Vermonters without it)

- a weatherization program

- Community Action (housing, furniture and housewares, adult learning, workforce re-entry)

They also offered referrals to the following:

- local and state vocational rehabilitation bureaus

- Independent Living Centers

- religious groups and service organizations

- local pro bono (free or reduced rate) legal services

- private rehabilitation and vocational rehabilitation

I found that the state offices of human services often go under different titles from state to state, and the Helpline staff were able to give me the names of organizations in the three contiguous states. Check for a United Way, Helpline, or Hotline office in your town.

Financial Help

Once you realize that you have a chronic, invisible illness (or several), it is essential to take an inventory of your assets. Find out what you have in the way of assets. This includes private medical insurance and HMO/CHP (Health Maintenance Organization/Community Health Plan) or other managed care plans. Another possibility might be Personal Injury Protection—the PIP of your auto insurance—if you can prove that an automobile accident contributed to your condition.

Look into the resources you might qualify for, such as welfare, prescription payment assistance, food stamps, Workers' Compensation, Veterans Administration assistance, and Social Security. (Some of these financial-aid organizations are discussed in chapters 12 and

13.) The laws governing welfare are changing so quickly that programs like Aid to Families with Dependent Children cannot be addressed here, because any generalized statements would most likely be false by the time the book goes to press. All of the information in this section is subject to change, but no other laws are changing as quickly as welfare laws.

Do not neglect smaller organizations. Investigate your own community's assistance programs, local fraternal and social associations, and support groups, religious groups, and information and referral lines.

Before things start to get tough, start checking into alternatives. You may need to talk to a financial counselor to discover your options. If one of your bills has been turned over to a collection agency, you are protected by the Fair Debt Collection Practices Act (Code 91 Stat. 874, Public Law 95–109), which became law in 1977, and the amendment to the Consumer Credit Protection Act 15 U.S.C. 1601, which was written into the Congressional Record (vol. 123) in 1977. The collectors are entitled to what you owe, but they're not entitled to harass you. You certainly don't need the added stress. Most creditors will try to work things out before they reach this stage.

Unrecognized and undiagnosed invisible chronic illness can seriously erode your financial condition. How many unnecessary medical tests and procedures were you subjected to before you received a diagnosis. How much medication did you buy and throw out? Our health care system is in crisis. Part of that crisis is directly due to the fact that doctors are not trained in the diagnosis and treatment of FMS and MPS. Write to your congressperson, and send a copy of your letter to your local medical school.

The time to advocate is now, even if you've already received the help you need—*especially* if you've already received the help you need. Those of us who still haven't obtained help urgently need advocates. We are often seriously ill and lack self-esteem. Frequently, we don't know how to advocate for ourselves. If you are already receiving adequate care and services, don't forget the rest of your FMily. Tell your story. Educate others. It is up to all of us to create justice for those who are unable to speak for themselves. For more information, contact:

The Office of the Americans with Disabilities Act
Civil Rights Division
United States Dept. of Justice
P.O. Box 66118
Washington DC 20035-6118
Phone: (202) 514-0301 (voice mail)

Vocational and Occupational Therapy

Some of us will need the services of a vocational or occupational therapist on our health care team. Often, we don't get this help, because we don't realize just what it is that they do.

Vocational Therapists

Vocational therapists are well-named. They help in the work environment by designing ergonomic work stations—that is, they design and arrange things so that people and machines, e.g., computers, interact safely and efficiently. Vocational therapists:

- Find alternative ways for you to accomplish your work tasks without causing any more harm to your health.

- Can deal with any physical, emotional, or mental disability that causes conflict with your work environment.

- Will help you to develop an employment plan.

Be sure that your vocational therapist fully understands that your limits are not just due to pain and fatigue, but to other factors, as well, such as an inability to do repetitive motions, a restricted range of motion, or an inability to be relatively immobile for any length of time.

Vocational therapy treatment varies greatly from state to state. Primarily, vocational therapists can help you to assess your job options in the following ways:

- They will help with career exploration if you need to change.

- They will help you to access community resources.

- In some states, they will take an individual approach, modifying their services to fit the individual's needs.

Some vocational therapy departments include education and training, transportation assistance, worksite accommodations, adaptive equipment, help with transitioning from school to work, and job placement. Start by applying to the Division of Vocational Rehabilitation. You will find it (or a similarly named department) listed in the phone book under state agencies. You will be accepted if they find you have a disability which is a barrier to your employment, but that you would be able to work if you took part in their programs.

Occupational Therapists

Occupational therapists help you with your need to "delete, modify, and delegate" your tasks. They will assist you in adapting life to your specific needs. In spite of their name, you don't have to be working outside of your home to use occupational therapy. They are the "fine motor control" specialists, and their skills are often what we need the most and get the least. Some occupational therapists:

- Can help with perceptual problems as well as with cognitive dysfunction.

- Are specialists in hand therapy.

- Can help with pacing work schedules, and with coping day to day.

- Can help you plan your daily schedule, and teach you how to set limits.

- Can teach you how to lessen your stress burden.

- Can help you learn how to move through your life as easily and as comfortably as is possible.

Occupational therapists can help you learn to use adaptive aids if they are necessary, including helping you to find the adaptive equipment you need to make your life easier. They will also help in the assessment and treatment of work performance skills. Contact your local hospital or the American Occupational Therapy Association, P.O. Box 31220, Bethesda, MD 20824-1220 for the occupational therapist nearest you.

It is important that your occupational therapist and/or vocational therapist understand the limitations of FMS and MPS, including possible proprioceptor disturbances. They must realize that it isn't "all in your mind." The problems that promote sleep disturbance are physiological, not emotional. Stress plays a part, but the stress is often the result of having FMS and/or MPS. Make sure that these therapists get copies of the relevant data sheets from chapter 7.

How to Be an Advocate

Self-advocacy is an art, and like all arts, it must be developed to be most effective. Practice stating your needs clearly and directly, without guilt or apologies. Don't beat around the bush. Don't give in to members of your medical team just to make them happy. Don't automatically assume that medical personnel know what works for you better than you do yourself. For example, today I received an email from someone whose doctor doesn't believe in physical therapy for fibromyalgia or Myofascial Pain Syndrome. In such a case, you might say to him/her:

> I know you don't believe in physical therapy for fibromyalgia. But I am not getting adequate pain relief from the medications, and would like to try some massage therapy or acupressure. Here are three articles from medical journals explaining how good physical therapy is for fibromyalgia. Other people in the FMS support group have told me that Beth at the hospital is very good. Do you have any objections to a trial of physical therapy twice a week for a month? Then we will be able to evaluate how well it works—or doesn't—for me.

Then, start an accurate log of the results of the therapy sessions. Keep the log up-to-date. Create a folder for documents that will provide records to help you obtain future treatment. Stick up for what you believe you need, even if your doctors don't agree. Educate others. Let them know what you know, and back it up. Education and documentation are the two core elements of effective advocacy. They will usually support you and enable you to communicate effectively. Persevere in your efforts. Use the References and Bibliography sections and the other appendices in this book. Don't just copy the material and give it to people. Get them interested in reading it.

Let's help change our health care system for the better, not just by demanding services, but by getting better care through more effective use of *our* money. It is far more efficient to have our medical schools educate our doctors in the first place than to have us pay in pain, energy, and money to educate those few doctors who are open enough to listen to us. The system as it is has failed us. It is up to us to change it. That's what government "by the people" is all about. Whenever and wherever you can, educate.

Know Your Rights

Know what your rights are. Your health care providers are your partners—your equals. Review the section in chapter 10 on rights and responsibilities. Your doctors are people you hire to help you. They are consultants. It is unfortunate that some doctors seem to have taken the course "God 101" in medical school, and that some other doctors act as if they taught the course. Remember, you are the manager of your heath care team. It is your life.

Be Glad for What You Have.

As a child, whenever I saw a figure skater, I used to dream of moving gracefully across the ice, spinning and whirling, dipping and twirling. I am now content to skate a few times around the rink without getting seriously winded. Don't waste your precious energy trying to accomplish the truly impossible. There are always skills that can't be done by everyone. Cherish what you *can* do.

Authority comes with responsibility. Work towards self-reliance and independence. This doesn't mean doing without medications, physical therapy, or any other kind of support. It does mean functioning better with the support you have.

Be Realistic

Before you start to advocate, find out what it is you want or need. Be specific. If you tell your doctor you want to feel better, that isn't specific enough. If you say you need better control of reflux, or you need to get some restorative sleep, your doctor will be better able to help you. Choose realistic goals. Get your facts lined up before you begin advocating. When people warn you that you "can't fight City Hall," remember that it's you and others like you who are responsible for filling that City Hall with people who are responsible and responsive to you. Don't allow yourself to be surrounded by negativity.

Accentuate the Positive and Eliminate the Negative

When you reach an obstacle in your path, don't let it defeat you. If there is a problem, become a problem solver. Figure out what you most need to advocate for, and then focus your strength and energy on that issue. Draw up a specific plan on how to work the change you want to accomplish. Then do it. Stay positive. When it seems as if all the garbage in the world has fallen on your head, you may find it makes excellent fertilizer in which to grow your dreams.

The Do's and Don'ts of Advocacy

- **Don't ever allow anyone to put you on the defensive.** If you cry and lose control, or get angry and lose control, you fail to communicate your needs. Don't get mad. Don't get hurt. Get justice. Keep your cool. Practice how you will handle potential conflicts before they happen. Use the following example as a model:

"Have I heard you correctly? Are you telling me that my symptoms are all in my head, and that I am insane? Is that your professional opinion? May I have that in writing please? If not, please be kind enough to deal with your attitude on your own time. I have taken the effort to come here, and I am paying you for your time and advice. If you feel you cannot help me, I feel you shouldn't be taking my time and money."

- **Don't put up with put-downs.**

- **Learn how to speak effectively.** Do consult the Advocate's Reading List that appears after the Bibliography at the back of this book, or ask your local librarian for some good books on effective speaking. When you advocate for yourself over the phone, find out the name of the person to whom you speak. When people say anything that makes you feel uncomfortable, write down what was said. Talk to them about it. Or write to them. Let them know how their remarks or voice tone made you feel, and that you consider it inappropriate.

- **Do practice advocating for yourself at home.** Work with your significant other or a friend. Shed your tears and vent your frustration learning how to handle yourself *at home*, so that you can interact with dignity and composure when others try to intimidate you.

- **Do be polite at a hearing or appointment.** Don't allow yourself to become rattled. When others become offensive, that will let you know they are "losing it." Don't remain silent either. Stay until the misunderstandings have been cleared up, unless grief or another emotion overcomes you. In those cases, it may be a good idea to follow up with a letter. Write it immediately, but don't send it. Read it the next day. Figure out who should get copies, and remember to keep a copy for your own records. If you get no response to that letter, follow up with another one. Persevere.

- **Do bring you own representation to a hearing, meeting, or appointment.** That is your right. Do make your own tape. If you don't understand something, ask for clarification, and repeat your questions until you do understand. Take notes as well. Some things don't register on a tape recorder, like the disapproving sneers on an interviewer's face. Remember, you are the authority when it comes to your life and your body. Ask for things in writing. Follow up on written requests. Be sure that your legal representative is educated about FMS and MPS.

If you find that you need legal representation in your dealings with aid agencies, copy the following section and show it to your legal representative:

What Your Legal Representative Should Know

You have seen clients with fibromyalgia (FMS) and Myofascial Pain Syndrome (MPS), and you will see more. These clients may have come to you with various symptoms, including overwhelming pain and fatigue. Many have been denied adequate pain relief. Many have been given inappropriate therapies that made them worse, and may have compounded their disability. Most have faced an endless stream of doctors and others who met them with varying degrees of confusion, disbelief, or arrogance. Take the time to listen carefully and patiently to these clients. They may not be used to people actually listening, so you may have to earn their trust.

Each of these syndromes is an authentic, well-documented medical condition, and, to complicate matters, they often occur together. Both are very different, although they are often confused, and they require different forms of therapy. For example, those who have *only* FMS have muscles that can be strengthened, but those who have MPS have muscles with active myofascial trigger points (TrPs), and their muscles cannot be strengthened until the TrPs have been eliminated. If the physician and/or physical therapist cannot tell these conditions apart, your client's health may be compromised. It is worth your time to learn as much as you can about both conditions, and to understand how they interact.

Most medical health workers are untrained in diagnosing and/or treating FMS and chronic MPS. People with FMS and/or MPS often look healthy, and many doctors discriminate against them for having an "invisible" condition. Fibromyalgia and MPS are both major causes of suffering and disability, much of which stems from lack of recognition and inappropriate treatment. Once some lawsuits have been won, insurance doctors and other "experts" will learn the facts about FMS and MPS very quickly. Remember, your client's secondary loss is greater than any possible gain.

By the time you see someone with FMS and/or chronic MPS, it is highly likely that your client has been dismissed, misunderstood, misinformed, undiagnosed, misdiagnosed, and even abused by "the system." They are probably in great pain, and their past experience with the medical and legal establishment may have entailed ridicule and abuse. If you want to help your client and to win your case, there are some things you should know, so that you can review your patient's records and understand where some of the problems originated.

FMS and MPS Are Different Conditions

Fibromyalgia is a "chronic invisible illness." It isn't just a form of muscular rheumatism. It's actually a type of neurotransmitter dysfunction. Neurotransmitters are the biochemicals that the body and brain use to communicate with each other. Fibromyalgia is also accompanied by chronic sleep deprivation. When this is added to the mix of dysregulated neurotransmitters, which control mood, it is easy to see why your client may be unhappy. Be patient. Your client is desperate for knowledge and understanding, and wants only to recover. It will be a great reassurance that you are willing to listen and will help your client to fight for justice.

FMS Is Systemic

It is important for you to understand that fibromyalgia is a biochemical, systemic problem. The patient can't have "fibromyalgia of the back," the neck, or any other specific location. Studies have shown that there is a genetic tendency to develop FMS. Then, it needs a trigger—a severe stressor, such as repetitive work, abuse, or trauma, to develop into full-blown FMS. If your client has a medical chart or an interview form referring to regional types of fibromyalgia, a red flag should go up. That's like saying a woman is pregnant in her right ankle, but nowhere else. It just doesn't happen.

Tender Points

Technically, for a diagnosis of FMS, your client will exhibit eleven of eighteen specific *"tender points."* If these points are pressed, s/he will have pain that does *not* refer pain to any other area of the body. These "eleven out of eighteen" tender points are the criteria for patient inclusion in specific FMS research studies. Having fewer than eleven of the eighteen possible tender points, however, does *not* mean that the patient does not have FMS, because the tender points may vary from day to day.

Myofascial Pain Syndrome

Myofascial Pain Syndrome (MPS) is a neuromuscular chronic pain condition characterized by *trigger points* (TrPs) that *do refer pain to other parts of the body.* It can also cause symptoms such as extreme dizziness, migraines, buckling knee, and calf cramps. Specific regional pain is a symptom of MPS. It can cause small tasks, such as wringing out a washcloth or writing a letter, to become pain endurance sessions.

Chronic Myofascial Pain Syndrome

Fibromyalgia often occurs in conjunction with chronic Myofascial Pain Syndrome. *Chronic* Myofascial Pain Syndrome (MPS) is a musculoskeletal chronic pain syndrome. It is mechanical, not biochemical. It is nonprogressive (although it may seem to be progressive), nondegenerative, and noninflammatory. It is composed of many trigger points, which refer pain and other symptoms in very precise, specific patterns. Chronic Myofascial Pain Syndrome may *seem* to be progressive because each TrP can develop satellite and secondary TrPs, which can form secondaries and satellites of their own.

Trigger Points

Trigger points are incredibly painful areas that often feel like knots, hard lumps, or taut bands of fibers in the muscles. They refer pain to other areas. They can trigger Irritable Bowel Syndrome, irritable bladder, dizziness, weak knees, weak ankles, pelvic pain, dysmenorrhea and painful intercourse in women, impotence in men, and a great many more disruptive symptoms. The tightening and spasming of the myofascia surrounding the muscles can entrap nerves, blood vessels, and ducts. There can be blurring of the eyes, double vision, leg cramps, hypoglycemic-like symptoms, sciatica, hives and rashes, numbness or tingling, mood swings, and confusional states.

Nerve Entrapment

When a nerve passes through a muscle between taut bands of trigger points, or when a nerve lies between the taut band and bone, the unrelenting pressure exerted on the nerve can produce neuropraxia, loss of nerve conduction, but only in the region of compression. This sometimes shows up on EMGs, and is misdiagnosed as nerve damage. The patient often has two types of pain symptoms—(1) aching pain referred from the TrPs in the muscle, and (2) the effects of nerve compression: numbness, tingling, and, sometimes, hyperesthesia. Patients who have nerve entrapment caused by TrPs are often subjected to unnecessary procedures, including surgeries, which serve only to compound the problem.

Some people with MPS cannot be immobile for any length of time, such as during travel, or sitting at a meeting, because their muscles become rigid and extremely painful. Many muscles have multiple TrP locations. The major factor in TrP pain is always mechanical, even if it is triggered by stress. Fibromyalgia and/or MPS symptoms can occur over the entire body, and the usual medical tests will come back negative. Symptoms can fluctuate from hour to hour and from day to day, and often worsen with changes in barometric pressure.

With treatment of the TrPs and the underlying perpetuating factors, TrPs can be minimized or eliminated if they are caught soon enough. Two excellent medical texts are available on myofascial TrPs, *Myofascial Pain and Dysfunction: The Trigger Point Manual, Vol. I* and *Vol. II* by Janet G. Travell, M.D., and David G. Simons, M.D. These texts show the referred pain patterns, tell what causes them and how to relieve them.

Bodywork for TrPs

Appropriate bodywork may provide dramatic relief from pain. But initially it can also promote a feeling of fatigue and nausea, which are indications that trapped toxins and wastes are being released. The patient must be given time to recover, with gentle, brief, non-repetitive stretching when that is tolerated.

FMS/MPS Complex

Fibromyalgia and MPS, if untreated or improperly treated, can form a synergistic, mutually perpetuating FMS/MPS Complex. This is a condition of interconnected symptom spirals that become increasingly worse until the spiral is interrupted. That is, the pain causes muscle contraction which causes more pain which causes more contraction, and so forth. Sometimes, the patient exhibits muscles that feel like cement; this is caused by myofascial splinting.

Tests

As of this writing, there is no simple, specific test to diagnose FMS. Most of the common laboratory tests come back normal. With MPS, as easy as it is for trained fingers to feel the ropy bands and lumps of trigger points, most medical personnel lack the training to diagnose and treat the condition. A normal CAT scan, MRI, or X ray may mean there is no arthritis or herniated disc. It does not mean the absence of a chronic pain syndrome. It takes a doctor trained in diagnosing and treating MPS and FMS to diagnose these conditions properly. Not tests. As stated previously, there is no definitive testing as yet, although research testing has shown definite clinical abnormalities in FMS. Doctors often miss the lumps and ropy bands of MPS, although many patients and physical therapists find them easily. Rigid muscles and even muscular contractures are often dismissed by untrained doctors.

For more about MPS, contact the Gebauer Company in Ohio at 9419 St. Catherine Avenue, Cleveland, OH 44104; phone: (800) 321-9348; and ask for the free monograph, *Myofascial Pain Syndrome Due to Trigger Points* by David Simons, M.D.

The Fourth Estate

When all other attempts at advocacy have failed, remember the power of the press and other media. Write letters to the editor of your local newspaper. Write to magazines. Call in to the daytime radio shows that focus on health issues. If your city supports a municipal TV station, try to get a local reporter interested in doing a story about your support group.

Tell your story, naming names, pointing fingers, and exhibiting documents. Make your story as positive as possible and emphasize what you do to help yourself. Teach others about your symptoms, and what it means to have a chronic, invisible illness or two. Avoid personal attacks; just tell your story and show your documents. Say, "This is what I need. This is what I can't get from the system. This is what I do about it." At the very least, such an approach will get things off your chest and educate others. At the very most, some substantive changes might result.

Those of us with FMS and/or MPS are a great multitude of small voices, working together for change. We *will* change the way things are. Like an avalanche, our efforts will gather momentum slowly. And, like an avalanche, we'll get everything covered, eventually.

> *Lawyers concentrate on winning the case,*
> *judges with interpreting the law;*
> *but who in the system is*
> *directly concerned with justice?*

> —Robert Grudin

If you are among those with FMS, MPS, or FMS/MPS Complex who can no longer work, you will need to investigate the possibility of receiving disability benefits. The "nitty-gritty" of how to go through the process of qualifying for Social Security Income (SSI) is explained in chapter 13.

Disability

In the legal world, definitions are important. Try to understand the differences between these three terms:

- A *disability* is any restriction on or inability to perform an activity of personal care. The inability to dress yourself *or* feed yourself qualifies as a disability.

- An *impairment* is any loss or abnormality of psychological, physiological, or anatomical structure. Chronic pain conditions such as FMS or MPS belong here, although they can also cause other disabilities and handicaps.

- A *handicap* is any restriction on or inability to fulfill your normal role. Examples of handicaps are the inability to work, inability to move freely in your environment, or the inability to maintain customary social relationships.

The Functional Difficulties List

There are overlaps among these three definitions. You will find that many terms dealing with disability are quite broad. Also, each organization defines disability somewhat differently. This tangled web has been woven and interwoven through the years, and it is becoming increasingly difficult to follow a thread. The form below will help you to document your disabilities.

Functional Difficulties List

Name _____ Date _____

Use this form to record functioning problems to report your doctor or therapist.

I am having difficulties with:

- brushing my teeth
- maintaining personal hygiene/bathing/showering
- grooming/getting dressed
- walking/standing/sitting
- sleeping
- writing/computer work
- using my hands
- shopping
- meal preparation
- traveling
- working
- communicating with/dealing with people
- climbing stairs
- lifting
- making love
- driving
- exercising
- doing laundry
- other: _____

There are lots of gray issues. There are many people working on this problem. We pray that there are others who are working on the solution.

The ADA

When the Americans with Disabilities Act (ADA) was made law in 1990, it was designed primarily to provide equal employment opportunities for the disabled. Disability rights are civil rights. The ADA is about the inalienable right of disabled people to work. It is meant ". . . to assure equality of opportunity, full participation, independent living, and economic self-sufficiency . . ." for people who have disabilities (ADA Section 12101(a)(8)). It does not apply to businesses that employ fifteen or fewer employees.

ADA Definitions and Requirements

There are three parts to the ADA definition of disability:

1. A physical or mental impairment that substantially limits one or more of the major life activities

2. A record of such an impairment

3. Being regarded as having such an impairment

That last part is relatively unknown to the public. If you are rejected from a job because of the myths, fears, or stereotypes associated with FMS and/or MPS, you may have suffered illegal discrimination. Some employers may feel that anyone with FMS is too fatigued to work, or they may hold some other misconception that will result in your rejection for employment. If you suspect that is the case, talk to the prospective employer. Tell him/her that each of us is different in our capabilities and symptoms, and be clear about your abilities and limitations.

According to the ADA, physical or mental impairment is defined as any condition that affects one or more of the following body systems: neurological, musculoskeletal, special sense organs, respiratory (including speech organs), cardiovascular, reproductive, digestive, genito-urinary, blood and lymphatic, skin and endocrine; or any mental or psychological disorder, such as emotional or mental illness, and specific learning disabilities (29 CFR 1630.2(h) (1992)).

Existence of an impairment is determined without consideration of the use of medications or devices that may lessen the impact of the impairment. For example, if your ankles buckle unless you use a walker, you are still disabled, even though you may be able to walk with the walker.

An impairment becomes a disability when it substantially limits a major life activity, which includes caring for oneself, performing manual tasks such as shopping or picking up your mail, walking, seeing, hearing, speaking, breathing, learning, and working. Other major life activities include sitting, standing, lifting, and reaching (29 CFR 1630.2(i)). You are disabled if you are unable to perform a major life activity that the average person in the general population can perform, or you are significantly restricted as to the condition, manner, or duration under which you can perform a particular major life activity as compared to what the average person in the general population can perform of that same activity (29 CFR 1630.(j) (1991)).

If you are prevented from performing a broad range of jobs, you are substantially limited because your condition eliminates entire fields of jobs. Two or more impairments that significantly limit a major life activity because of cumulative effects are also considered disability. For example, a person may have osteoarthritis of the wrist and hands, as well as TrPs in the hands, fingers, and arms. Alone, these are not disabilities, but the arthritis is a perpetuating factor of the TrPs, and the TrPs may prevent reliable grip strength and undermine dexterity and fine motor skills, which will be considered disability.

Title I of the ADA entitles you to "reasonable accommodation" that does not impose "undue hardship" on your employer. For example, if you were employed as a proofreader and suddenly became blind, you couldn't expect your employer to hire someone to read aloud to you so that you could continue your job. However, you might be able to work elsewhere in the firm, without causing "undue hardship" to your employer. Sometimes, your needs can be met with job restructuring, modification of work schedules, or modification of worksites for accessibility.

To *Get* Your Rights, You Must First *Know* Your Rights

Your employer's duty to make changes to accommodate you does not begin until s/he knows about your disability. This notification must be in writing. You will have to schedule a time to discuss your specific limits and needs with your employer—and be sure to bring a written summary to the meeting that describes potential accommodations. Try to make the accommodations easy for you both.

"Undue hardship" requires significant difficulty or expense considering the nature of the workplace, the nature of the work, the number of employees, the financial resources of the employer, and the effects of the accommodations on the resources and the workplace. Employers may be eligible for tax credits toward the accommodations. But reassignments may violate union bargaining agreements. If you don't understand what might be involved, ask. Strive for compromise.

Negative impact on the morale of the other employees does *not* constitute undue hardship. Expecting other workers to carry some of the burden of your job responsibilities *is*. Employers are allowed to hire someone else if s/he is more qualified than you are. They may *not* refuse to hire you if you are the most qualified person for the job. You must, however, be able to perform the essential job functions. Study written job descriptions very carefully.

A job application cannot legally ask whether you have a disability. The form cannot ask for or contain a list of impairments. An employer can ask you if you will be able to do the job, and how well. The employer can require you to take a medical examination if all employees for the same job are required to take it.

If you have a job, you are entitled to equal treatment. This includes equal wages for equal work, equal fringe benefits, and so forth. Many state laws are even more extensive than the ADA, so you should inquire about your state civil rights act. State laws vary from state to state the way that trigger points vary from person to person.

If You Suspect Discrimination

Get it in writing. Document everything. Get eyewitnesses to what you can't get in writing, and get *their* statements in writing. Take photos of inaccessible areas. Keep a file at home. Keep all of your job evaluations and other pertinent material. Be sure to keep periodic updates of your personnel file. Update your medical file and keep all documents so that you can prove you are a qualified person with a disability. If you lose your job, document your attempts to find another job. If there is a problem, don't delay in dealing with it—and remember to file all complaints in writing and keep copies.

You can request a complaint form from the EEOC. Contact:

Equal Employment Opportunities Commission
1801 L Street NW
Washington, DC 20507
Phone: (202) 663-4900 (voice mail)

When you send in a compliant, send an extra copy to be date-stamped, along with a stamped, self-addressed envelope. Use sufficient postage on the self-addressed envelope for the stamped copy to be returned to you. It is often wise to seek legal advice at the same time. It is good to have a strong voice to add to yours and, in most cases, employers and prospective employers find the voices of lawyers to be exceptionally strong.

Note that there is a statute of limitations on discrimination charges. They must be filed within 180 days of the specified discrimination.

You can be discriminated against by insurance companies, too. Check your state laws if you have difficulty obtaining insurance. Get everything in writing and read everything, or have someone whose judgment you trust read it for you. If your insurance company denies you coverage or benefits that you believe are yours, check to see whether you have any legal recourse. Ask for the reasons for their denial in writing.

The Family and Medical Leave Act

The Family and Medical Leave Act (FLMA) covers employers who employ more than fifty people, and some states are considering legislation that would lower this to twenty-five employees. Medical leave must be made available to employees for serious health conditions, under Federal Regulations Part 825, The Family and Medical Leave Act of 1993.

Under FLMA law, a "serious health condition" is a condition that leaves you unable to perform your job, and requires inpatient care at a medical care facility, or continuing treatment by a licensed health care provider. Serious health conditions resulting in workers' compensation coverage are included within this definition.

The FMLA allows you to take up to twelve weeks of unpaid leave to care for yourself, your sick child, spouse, or parent without losing your job. Companies who qualify must have a written family-leave policy, and information explaining it must be made available to you. Your employee policy brochure should describe your rights to employee benefits during your leave of absence, as well as your responsibilities. For example, you may be required to provide certification by a licensed health care provider that you require such leave. You may even be required to give your employer a specific description of your treatment regimen during the leave period.

When your period of leave is over, the FLMA requires that you be restored to your "original or equivalent position with equivalent pay, benefits, and other employment terms." There are exceptions allowed by the law. Study the policy. Ask what will happen if your job no longer exists when you are ready to return to work.

Think over the possible consequences of taking a leave. Is there a chance that you may not return to work? What would happen if you are paid benefits during the leave time, and then are unable to return? Read your company policy statement thoroughly, and understand it. Inquire about your options. You may be able to take intermittent leave, a few hours at a time, to take care of an ill family member.

The FLMA does not affect any federal or state law prohibiting discrimination, such as the ADA, or supersede any state law, policies, or labor agreements providing greater family or medical leave rights, and/or benefits.

The Veterans Administration

Many veterans coping with FMS and MPS have told me that the Veterans Administration (VA) has saved their lives. I have always heard that they treat veterans with respect. Veterans often struggle with Post-Traumatic Stress Syndrome and this syndrome may be an initiating trigger for FMS or MPS. It is important that your VA contact understand that these three syndromes all require different treatments, and that they will perpetuate each other. Veterans Administration benefits include disability compensation, education benefits, vocational rehabilitation, home loans, burial benefits, dependents' and survivors' benefits, health care, home care, and life insurance. Some of these benefits are also available to dependents. The military VA codes are 6399 and 6350, respectively, for undifferentiated connective tissue disease and fibromyalgia.

The Veterans Center Outreach and Assistance will get you started. Benefits counselors can be reached at (800) 827-1000. You can also contact them through the American Veterans National Service Program at 807 Maine Avenue SW, Washington, DC 20024.

I Used to Be a Doctor

by Harry Hlavac DPM

I used to be a Doctor, now I am a Health Care Provider.
I used to practice medicine, now I function under a managed care system.
I used to have patients, now I have a consumer list.
I used to diagnose, now I am approved for one consultation.
I used to treat, now I wait for authorization to provide care.
I used to cure patients, now I am dared not to cure them by insurance carriers.
    I use up the authorization, I lose the patient.

I used to see patients on referral from doctors, patients, and friends,
    now I must be listed in their Providers Manual.
I used to see patients who traveled to see me,
    now I am considered out of their approved geographic area.
I used to be paid a Usual, Customary & Reasonable (USR) fee,
    now I don't have a usual fee; now there is nothing customary,
    only managed competition; now who is reasonable?

I used to get paid,
    now I accept the allowed charges as payment in full for covered services.
I used to be paid for professional services,
    now I am not paid either for time, materials, or nonallowed services.
I used to be an independent specialist,
    now I am a dependent ancillary care provider.
I used to provide charity care,
    now since I am not an authorized provider, I am not permitted to provide charity,
    or to barter, or to offer advice.
I used to consider the insurance company as a third party carrier,
    now insurance is a fiscal intermediary between the provider and the consumer.

I used to care for patients by appointment,
     now the patient requires authorization to make an appointment.

I used to provide hands-on care,
     now I provide hands-off, gloves-on procedures,
I used to use words to describe my care,
     now I must fill in all the boxes with appropriate code numbers.
I used to provide necessary services, now I am unnecessary.
I used to have a front office coordinator,
     now triage is performed at the front line.
I used to have a clean office, now I am certified by OSHA.

I used to have a practice, now I am employed to provide services.
I used to have a successful "people" practice, now I have a paper failure.
I used to spend time listening to my patients.
     now I spend time justifying myself to authorities.
I used to have feelings. Now I have an attitude.

Now I don't know what I am.

12

The Medico-Legal Jungle

Health Maintenance Organizations and Community Health Plans

Today the practice of medicine is in transition. The days of the doctor who made house calls at all hours are long gone. This is the era of managed health care—Health Maintenance Organizations (HMOs) and Community Health Plans (CHPs): networks of health care providers with long lists of pre-approved doctors, nurses, and medical facilities booked on a prepaid basis. Medicine has become big business where as much attention is paid to the bottom line as to new wonder drugs. Currently, there are several terms in use for managed care. In this chapter, the term "HMO" is used to indicate any managed care organization, because it is the most familiar.

In a speech made on November 10, 1997, to the Vermont House of Representative's Health and Welfare Committee, former Surgeon General C. Everett Koop warned that good medical practice is being overshadowed by the financial pressures imposed by managed care insurance networks. "Now I think too many managed care companies seem . . . too interested in managing costs and only secondarily in managing health." Instead of being networks, in which a single physician directs all of a patient's care, they have become economic entities controlled too often by people who are more concerned with the bottom line than with patients' well-being. Dr. Koop said that this, "threatens to eradicate what trust remains between doctor and patient" (*The Brattleboro Reformer*, Nov. 11, 1997, page 3).

Capitation

When you are enrolled in an HMO, you no longer hire your physician, the insurance carrier does, and HMOs do things differently than insurance companies. For example, if you belong to an HMO, check to see whether your physician is "capitated." This means that your doctor is working for a salary, not for a fee-for-service. Often, the income of a capitated doctor increases if fewer rather than more services are provided to the patient. Think about that. The reverse used to be the case. It is now in the financial interest of these physicians to provide less care. (If your doctor is capitated, a loud alarm should go off indicating "Danger! Warning!")

In some HMOs, the doctor loses money for every test s/he orders. But no one can check for hidden perpetuating factors or provide documentation for an invisible chronic illness with a Ouija board. Tests are needed. As far as the patient is concerned, such a doctor might as well be decapitated. (And the patient will be the one wanting to make heads roll.)

If you are in this situation, see whether you can make an arrangement with your doctor to work around this impasse. Find out what the penalties are if you choose to consult a doctor who is not in your HMO, or if you request tests which your doctor has not approved. You may be required to pay the full costs yourself. This can result in tricky legal complications if the tests should prove positive, or if the consulting doctor disagrees with your HMO physician.

It may be invaluable to discuss your options in detail with the HMO. If possible, get their reply in writing. When you talk with their representative on the phone, make note of the name of the representative with whom you talk, what is discussed, and what is decided, as well as the date and time. Send the HMO a follow-up letter, naming the person with whom you talked and briefly outlining the discussion. Be sure to keep a copy of the letter. Remember, documentation is very important.

Every HMO is governed by a board of directors and the doctors on that board determine the quality of care. If those doctors think that fibromyalgia (FMS) and Myofascial Pain Syndrome (MPS) are nonexistent, "wastebasket" diagnoses, patients in that HMO have a *big* problem—the HMO may not approve tests and/or treatments *the board doctors* think are unnecessary. If you are enrolled in an HMO, find out the board's official stance on FMS and MPS. If those doctors think they already know all there is to know, don't give up. You have a lot of useful scientific documentation in the References and Bibliography sections of this book to refute such injurious attitudes. Go higher. Ask for a meeting with the Director of the Board, or the CEO of the hospital corporation.

If you are granted a meeting, bring your tape recorder and keep it running. When the HMO authorities see that you are documenting their position, they might be less likely to engage in obstructive or delaying tactics. If they know that you might sue, that knowledge might force them to soften their position and to be more receptive to tests and treatment options.

I have a friend who is an FMS- and MPS-aware physiatrist. He is appalled at what is happening to the health care system, and is currently writing a book about the dangers we face. He has kindly allowed me to quote this message that he posted to an Internet support group.

These problems are medical, not political, and your primary concerns should be with caregivers, not with attorneys and elected officials. Unfortunately, medicine has become political. Even worse, it has become a business instead of a profession. . . . Insurance companies are your enemy. Don't ever forget that. They make profits only by selling premiums, never by paying off claims. Remember, a payment of a claim is classified by them as a "loss"; that should always be a clue as to how they regard you. HMOs now classify money spent on patient care as "medical loss." If the HMO system was a race horse, it would be named Ripoff, out of Duplicity, by Greed. . . . The American health care system is the ultimate oxymoron; a successful failure. It is a system with a reputation for efficacy that is unsurpassed, a capability that is overwhelming, an attention to detail that is stunning, a disdain for cost that is positively regal, a determination to Do Good that arguably merits canonization, and a presumption of infallibility that is ubiquitous. . . . It is unreservedly proclaimed by those whose rice bowl it fills to be the envy of the civilized world. One small flaw; it is now a wholly owned subsidiary of the insurance industry, which has changed its role from healer to cash cow.

—Kenneth Hoelscher, M.D.

Deselected Doctors

There are many doctors who are very unhappy about having to deal with HMOs. They feel that they now have all of the responsibility of patient care (including payment of malpractice insurance), without any of the authority that proper care entails. Doctors who don't comply with HMO regulations can be "deselected." If you are covered by an HMO that has deselected your doctor, that means you can't be treated by that doctor anymore, no matter how helpful that doctor may have been for you, unless you can afford to pay her/his bills completely out of your own pocket.

Gatekeepers

In managed care, each patient has a "gatekeeper." That person doesn't work at the doctor's office as a secretary or assistant. Gatekeepers work for HMO administrations, at HMO offices. They decide what care a patient may receive, and what specialists that patient may see. As an employee of the HMO, the gatekeeper decides what the plan will pay for, along the lines dictated by the HMO, according to policies set by the HMO's board of directors. In some HMOs, your primary physician is hired to be your gatekeeper.

Doctors can no longer make independent judgment calls. To practice medicine they have to first deal with an administrative bureaucracy. There have been cases where a doctor wanted to argue with a gatekeeper about the necessity of a test or treatment, and the HMO administrators were not available for consultation because it was "off-hours." Unfortunately, the need for urgent care often occurs outside of bureaucratic hours.

The sicker the patient, the more unprofitable that patient is to the HMO. Services are now being denied because they are not considered "basic health care," necessary for the health of the patient. The newspapers have been full of stories about people who were denied medical care they needed to survive. In our national scramble to create an affordable health care system, the needs of patients are often unmet, and millions of people are still uninsured. Clearly, there are no easy answers.

HMOs and Gag Clauses

Many HMOs have instituted a "gag" or confidentiality clause in their contracts with the doctors on their approved lists. These clauses expressly prohibit physicians from saying anything that could harm the patient's confidence in the HMO's policies and coverage. Doctors also are instructed not to refer patients to specialists outside of the organization nor to "identify," or even *mention*, any available, but noncovered, services to the patient. This means that if your doctor thinks it would be good for you to see a chiropractor, and your HMO does not cover chiropractic therapy, the doctor may not mention it to you, even if you would be willing to pay for it yourself. Due to the bad press this generated, not to mention the fact that many physicians gagged on this gag clause, recently, a few HMOs have reversed their stance on this clause.

Lately, however, some HMO physicians are receiving *oral* gag orders. This means that if a doctor tries to arrange a referral to someone outside of the "Preferred Provider Organization," or mentions chiropractic or physical therapy options that are not covered, or discusses any complementary medical options available in the community, that doctor will receive a phone call from someone in the HMO administration and will be firmly "reminded" not to "identify" noncovered services. Some doctors have fought back by forming PSOs, which are Provider Sponsored Organizations—HMOs that are owned and operated by physicians and hospitals, rather than by an insurance entity.

The AMA's Code of Ethics

I have never been a big fan of the politics of the American Medical Association, but they authored a Code of Ethics that is a vital part of the medical world. To their credit, they have been in vocal opposition to gag clauses. They state: "The physicians' obligation to disclose treatment alternatives to patients is not to be altered by any limitations in the coverage provided by the patient's managed care plan. Further, patients cannot be subject to making decisions with inadequate information as this would be an absolute violation of informed consent requirements" (AMA Statement on Gag Clauses, Charles W. Plows, M.D., Chair, AMA Council on Ethical and Judicial Affairs). This statement was posted on the website of the American Academy of Family Physicians. The page was last modified on July 19, 1996. The Internet address is:

http://www.aafp.org/family/managed/gagrule.html

Legislative Opposition to Gag Clauses

In addition to the AMA's opposition, many state legislatures have stated that the gag clause is unethical and undermines physicians' abilities to properly care for their patients. Massachusetts has enacted a "Patient Confidentiality Bill" that bars HMOs from writing gag orders into the provider's contracts. Other states are following suit. According to the American Academy of Family Physicians, some states now require HMOs to disclose any financial incentives or penalties that are intended to encourage minimization of provided services. If you want to know where your state stands on the gag rule you can check it out by logging on to this web address: http://www.aafp.org/family/managed/gagrule.html.

Changing the Rules

The rules are long overdue for changing. People are asking, "If a doctor can be held responsible for a decision, and sued for malpractice, why not an HMO?" A bill called the Patient Access to Responsible Care Act of 1997 is now before Congress. It would enable patients who were refused treatments by their HMOs to appeal those decisions. The charge of "denial of care" would be reviewed first within the health care company, and then, if necessary, by an outside panel. Patients would also be granted the right to a reasonably large choice of doctors, and the right to know more about their health plans. The HMOs would have to provide access to specialists when such care is medically indicated in the professional judgment of the treating health professional. Furthermore, HMOs would no longer be allowed to discriminate against enrollees on the basis of socioeconomic status, age, disability, health status, or anticipated need for health services.

Of course, there are some members of Congress who are dedicated to gutting the provisions of this bill. But, eventually, such a bill *must* pass, especially if we keep badgering our congresspeople about the need. Under this bill, patients would still have to choose their doctors from a pre-approved list and still have to deal with the "gatekeeper" bureaucracy. But they would be given the right to payment for emergency room visits—even if the visit turns out not to be an emergency—as long as a "prudent layperson" in the same situation would have believed his or her health was in danger. In addition, this bill would outlaw gag clauses.

> **AARP Brochures**
>
> When I joined the American Assoication of Retired Persons (AARP) they offered some free publications. Among them were *Checkpoints for Managed Care: An AARP Guide for Medicare Beneficiaries*, and *Know Your Managed Care Rights*. AARP does a good job of educating its constituencies. For information, contact their Managed Care Editor, AARP Bulletin, 601 E Street N.W., Washington, DC 20049.

Congress is also investigating many other HMO (and insurance) practices. One practice that has a heavy impact on us is the concept and use of the "pre-existing condition." Insurance companies have used this blanket phrase to choose only the healthiest applicants for their clients, excluding people who are more likely to need expensive medical care. Let's face it, *life* is a pre-existing condition for disease and death. Some other medical issues currently under consideration by Congress are these:

1. Instituting an ombudsman's office to help patients deal with the health care system.

2. Providing insurance equality for mental health coverage.

3. Creating lifetime coverage caps.

4. Providing access to medical records.

5. Creating lists that would provide coverage and costs comparisons among health care providers.

6. Instituting variable rate coverage. (Variable rate coverage allows an insurance company to charge different rates for the same coverage, depending on how healthy the insurance company believes the client to be.)

Many of the concepts presently in use by HMOs seem as if they've been with us forever. Others seem to have crept into our lives unheralded, and are only discovered when we run head on into them and crash and burn. Some of us have no other options but to join an HMO if we want any medical coverage at all. Those of us who do have a choice often don't investigate the options we have. One thing is for sure, HMOs are forcing us to look long and hard at the unhealthy state of health care coverage.

Workers' Compensation

If you experience a precipitating event on your job, such as a fall or another type of accident, you may qualify for workers' compensation. This benefit is federally mandated insurance that your employer is required to carry for employees' work-related injuries, including repetitive-strain work injuries. The benefit may include payment for medical bills and, in some cases, payment toward job retraining. The workers' compensation laws state that nearly all employers in the U.S. must have this coverage in some form. Civilian employees of the federal government, railroad and shipyard workers, seamen, agriculture workers, domestic and "casual" workers, and home workers are the only exemptions.

If your diagnosis is "post-traumatic fibromyalgia" (FMS) or Myofascial Pain Syndrome, the FMS and/or MPS is *not* the qualifying injury. The injury may have led to the FMS or MPS, but the qualifier is the initial injury. When it comes to repetitive-strain work injuries, the laws are inconclusive and often contradictory. Also the rules that govern Workers' Compensation are constantly changing. Every year in practically every state new statutes are written to regulate how worker's compensation benefits are handled. Each state is different. This might work in our favor, eventually, because the people who interpret these laws don't know much about either FMS or MPS, but they can be educated—no matter how much work it takes. And it will take work.

If and when you apply for workers' compensation, it is vital that your doctor and physical therapist understand and be able to articulate the differences between FMS and MPS. It is easy to document the relationship between repetitive-strain work, the resultant trauma, and the subsequent myofascial trigger points. The medical articles are legion. With fibromyalgia, it is a different ball game entirely. Here, again, you may have to pay for the lack of training on the part of your doctors.

Dealing with Bureaucrats

In many cases, workers' compensation will pay your medical bills and a percentage of your lost wages. These benefits are usually more comprehensive than other job-related insurance. They cover the claimant for a longer period of time, although the administrative staff will push for "closure." It is difficult, however, to obtain permanent disability from workers' compensation for soft tissue damage.

It is essential that if you have an accident that causes a specific injury, you must fill out an accident report immediately. If you need emergency care, call your supervisor as soon as you have received the care. Then fill out the form and register it with your employer as soon as possible. Make sure that the form is signed by your supervisor. You may have to see the insurance company's doctor right away. In this case, time is money. If you are instructed to stay home from work, you will need a doctor's written statement.

You may find out that the insurance company you deal with is not really the "carrier." Your employer may be self-insured and use the insurance company only to "administer" the policy. You may not have a written record of the contract between your employer and the administrative service. Since your medical insurance is an employee benefit, you may have no legal recourse to get access to the insurance company.

At worst, this may mean legal complications, as you may be put into the situation of having to sue your employer (rather than the insurance company) to obtain what you believe are your rightful benefits. At best, you may have to ask your employer to help you convince the insurance company (or administrative service) to spend more of your employer's money to pay you the benefits to which you are entitled. This is true in both workers' compensation cases and other insurance reimbursements. To complicate matters even further, workers' compensation laws prohibit lawsuits by injured employees against their employers. The resulting tangle may take more energy than you have to undo.

A True Story

When I started planning this book, I sent out a call to my Internet FMily for stories they wanted told. I was sent a tape of a workers' compensation interview that is a prime example of wasted and misguided effort on the part of the insurers. They may have felt as if they offered a lot, and they did expend a lot of effort, but they sure didn't help the patient.

The insurer arranged for the implantation of an electrical stimulation device to help block the patient's pain. They arranged for the patient to stay at a hotel in the doctor's vicinity, so that the device could be adjusted after implantation. What they didn't arrange for was transportation for the doctor to the hotel, although it was more than a mile away. The patient couldn't afford to pay, and the insurer wouldn't. She was not able to walk that far and she didn't get the stimulator.

This same patient wanted the insurer to pay to rewire the hot tub in her backyard. They were willing to pay the cost of visits to a spa hot tub and for ongoing transportation to and from the spa, although the pain of the travel nullified most of the therapy. The relatively cheap rewiring of the patient's hot tub in her backyard (an easy walk) was not listed as a possible expenditure, and so the workers' compensation agency refused to pay. Bureaucracies learn slowly, if at all.

It was very hard for me to listen to this interview, which ranged from mild to derisive interrogation and then to downright belittlement. Dealing with the background materials I used for this book was an ordeal, because I understood what these patients had endured at the hands of thoughtless and often cruel bureaucrats. If this book allows some of you to win some of your battles with the establishment, it will have been worth all the effort of writing it.

Rehabilitation Benefits

Workers' compensation may provide benefits for occupational rehabilitation at your employer's expense, unless your employer feels that you are not entitled to compensation. Again, you may have to fight for it. Just because your employer pays for rehabilitation doesn't mean that s/he admits to liability in relation to your compensation claim. Your employer may claim that s/he paid for your rehabilitation out of compassion. The fact that you had to take the employer to court, however, may speak to the validity of that claim.

Write to your congressional representatives. Let them know how tough the process is. You elected them, and *may or may not do so again.* Be polite and clear. Ask for strict penalties for insurance companies if they don't respond to letters or inquiries in a timely manner. If insurance companies had to pay a premium interest rate on claims when they settled a claim with an individual, it would be in their interest to speed up the grievance and appeals process. Ask for a streamlined procedure for the grievance and appeals processes to be created. They need to be simplified and made more intuitive. Right now, filing a grievance or an appeal is a lengthy and complicated obstacle course designed for the ease of lawyers.

Disability Insurance

Sometimes it seems that you buy "insurance" solely for the benefit of the insurance company. You pay the premiums, and they are happy. Yet when you need to use your insurance, the company doesn't want to know you. When it comes to invisible chronic conditions, dealing with disability insurance can be a nightmare.

Know Your Policy

Read your policy. I know, I know! Those of us with FMS and/or MPS are allergic to forms, and small print is confusing and daunting. *Persevere.* When you read your policy, try to understand how it could be interpreted *against* you, as well as for you. Write down your findings. You may find it helpful to go through it with at least one other person, reading it aloud, one paragraph at a time, and interpreting its meaning. If you enjoy science fiction, look upon it as trying to crack an alien text.

Summarize your policy, citing specifics. Become familiar with the procedures that must be followed for physician and other referrals, as well as with the grievance and appeals processes. Document. Then organize your documents. Write simply, clearly, and as briefly as possible. Taking notes is of no use if you can't read them later.

The best way you can prepare for appealing a health insurance refusal is to educate yourself about your condition, as you are doing when you read this book. Talk to your doctor, insurer and/or HMO. Be polite and courteous, and assertive. Don't give up.

Be Cautious

When you make a claim, or appeal a denial of a claim, it will seem that everyone wants a copy of your medical records. You have the right to privacy of records in your insurance coverage (see chapter 10). Don't allow blanket photocopying of all your records. The insurance company doesn't need to know your whole life story. Allow them access only to what they need. Your records could wind up in the wrong hands, and nonessential and unrelated parts could be used against you.

Be careful. Someone may be watching you and it's not the cat. Some insurers will stake out a client who has filed a claim and then secretly record videos of that client's actions during his/her daily life. They'll use whatever they can get in any way they can to discredit you. Some of these agents seem to have been trained by the FBI or a Hollywood studio. They can be ruthless. If you think you are being shadowed, talk to your lawyer and your doctor. See if you can make a video of them recording a video of you. It will drive them wild. Even if you can't, it's fun to think about it.

It can be difficult to explain why you may be able to do a task well, once, for about ten minutes, although you know you will pay for it with pain afterwards. It is hard for them to understand that if you had to do the task a second or a third time, the pain would become unbearable. They will have the proof that, at one time, you did do that task. To them, that means that you can *always* do the task. You may have to pay for a lawyer to fight this one, when you suddenly lose your benefits and your income. Their attitude can drive you to paranoia, and then they've got you for something else. Before you know it, they'll be coming to take you away. *Harassment is illegal.* We must work to curb abuses.

Treat Your Allies Well

Find an ally who is a medical professional. Don't waste his or her time, and make contact only when you *need* to. Medical people do burn out, and we can't afford to lose even one knowledgeable advocate. Find someone who is willing to go head to head with the bureaucrats. Each of us has our own skills and roles to play. *Don't* ask people to do inappropriate things.

I have had sincere and needy patients dump five hundred pages of medical records in my mail for review. Patients have called and asked me to get a book, read it, and then tell them whether it's worth reading. People send me books, videos, and personal diaries to review. Of course, after doing so, I am to send their materials back at my own expense. I have had people call me to "fix their lives"—talk to their estranged wives, employers, and so forth. People have called me from other countries to ask me to solve their local problems with housing, employment, family relationships, and so forth!

When cultivating compassion, saying "No" and remaining positive takes enormous spiritual balance. Saying "No" without causing the needy person to feel abandoned takes a state of grace. I try, but I know I often fall short of the mark.

When life becomes overwhelming, and when you are dealing with medico-legal issues, it does so with a rapidity that can make your head spin. Then, there is a temptation to grab for help like someone who is drowning. That's because you feel as if you *are* drowning. Nevertheless, when you are weighed down by so many burdens, there is a good likelihood that if you reach for the wrong person, you will just pull that person down with you. Even an Olympic swimmer can be pulled down by the weight of many.

Do a little research before you contact someone. It will pay. The question you want to ask may simply be, "I want to do so and so and don't know where to start. Do you have any suggestions?" This simple question is likely to be met with a positive response, and then you can get some guidance and be on your way to achieving the goal of your quest.

I Can't Have a Crisis Today, My Schedule Is Already Full.

One day, in desperation, and on the advice of my counselor, I wrote a form letter explaining that I could no longer answer letters personally. I was overwhelmed with correspondence and work on a book. Among my responses was a letter that told me this option wasn't going to work. The writer told me that, if she didn't know better, she would have thought that letter had been sent by someone else. After all, I had answered four of her very long and detailed letters personally and in depth in the past two months. She also knew I had no office help, and had severe FMS/MPS Complex. A spiritual "skyhook" and a well-developed sense of humor can be a lifesaver at such times. Most overburdened medical personnel may not have those handy at the moment you ask for help. Don't take it personally.

Lawyers: Friends or Foes?

Lawyers can be tremendous allies—*your* lawyers, that is. Fighting the bureaucratic battle takes tremendous reserves of energy and perseverance. Just to learn that the insurance company has denied your first appeal may take weeks of waiting and dozens of phone calls, many of them long-distance. Waiting on "hold" is like treading water; you can do it for only so long before your endurance fails, and you go down. Insurance company personnel and their lawyers are healthy. They are well paid. It's their job to help the insurance company—not to help you.

Don't make the mistake of looking upon insurance lawyers (and insurance doctors) as disinterested parties. They're not. Many are professional bullies. They are trained in the art of intimidation, and they use it very effectively. That's what they're paid for. Get your own enforcer to play smash mouth with the bad guys. Make no mistakes here. The medico-legal game is rollerball. Don't let yourselves get caught under the wheels.

COBRA

COBRA stands for the Consolidated Omnibus Budget Reconciliation Act. It is an amendment to ERISA, the federal Employee Retirement Income Securities Act. COBRA applies to companies with twenty or more employees. If you lose your job because of downsizing or through no fault of your own (gross misconduct disqualifies you for COBRA), or if you retire, or lose insurance coverage because of reduced work hours, you may be able to continue group health insurance coverage for about a year. If you are entitled to COBRA benefits, your health plan must give you notice, stating your right to choose to continue benefits. *You have sixty days to accept, or you lose all rights to the benefits.*

Once you choose COBRA, you will probably be required to pay for the coverage. COBRA covers inpatient and outpatient hospital care, physician care, surgery and major medical benefits, prescription drugs, and other medical benefits such as dental and vision coverage. It does not cover life insurance. If you become eligible for Medicare, your spouse may qualify for COBRA. If you are covered by a spouse's health insurance, COBRA will also cover you through a specific time period specified in a divorce or legal separation from the covered employee, or after the employee's death. It will also cover a dependent after the loss of "dependent child" status. There are special rules for individuals who qualify for Social Security Disability benefits that can extend COBRA coverage. For further information contact the U.S. Public Health Service, Offices of the Assistant Secretary for Health, Grants Policy Branch (COBRA), 5600 Fishers Lane, Room 17A-45, Rockville, MD 20857.

13

Social Security and Medicare

This chapter contains some material from my first book (Starlanyl and Copeland 1996) on how to begin to apply for Social Security and provides a great deal of new information on how to navigate through the claims and appeals processes. It also gives you some suggestions on how to advocate for yourself during the process. Always remember that the SSD (Social Security Disability) and SSI (Social Security Insurance) claims process is *adversarial*.

During the process, which seems to take forever, you will try to prove that you need benefits, and they will try just as hard to prove that you don't. They may send you to doctors who work for SSD or for insurance companies. These doctors may have no training either with fibromyalgia (FMS) or Myofascial Pain Syndrome (MPS). The disability determination board is comprised of people appointed by the governor, and the board is under contract to the federal government. Some of the people on the board are not even doctors.

Recently, I have seen the rise of a set of doctors who are opposed to the recognition of FMS, MPS, and other "invisible" chronic conditions. In the face of all the mounting evidence, they persist in believing that these conditions literally do not exist. There is also a second set of doctors who believe that FMS and MPS do exist—and that they are disabling—but these doctors also believe that the system cannot *afford* to take care of those who have been afflicted.

This second set of doctors has gone over to the "dark side," frequently attacking the doctors who are dedicated to helping us. Often, when you read the papers they write, you find that they've done financial studies demonstrating how much it costs the system to take care of FMS and MPS patients. I even heard one doctor say, "God knows, these people need

Social Security Disability, but we can't afford to let them have it. Do you realize what that would do to the system?"

He, and others like him, have forgotten that those statistics stand for real people. The numbers refer to real patients whose tears are conveniently hidden from view. Those doctors have forgotten, if they ever knew, what FMS and MPS cost those who are afflicted with them. Most of this cost can be attributed to our malfunctioning medical system, which does not train its doctors in early diagnosis and treatment of these conditions. I challenge those doctors to remember their vow to "do no harm." Rather than kicking us when we're down, why not put your energies into fixing the system?

The people who work for the Social Security Administration (SSA) also do their best to protect the system. That's their job. Unfortunately, the system is not set up for the person with FMS and/or MPS disabilities. However, there are ways to help the system work for people who have these conditions, and you will find them in this chapter.

Some disabled people have managed to get advocacy aid from their congresspeople. It never hurts to educate your legal advocates, which is exactly what you elect your senator and representatives to be. If you decide you need an attorney, be sure you select one who specializes in SSD cases. Only someone familiar with the SSD jungle should be your lawyer.

Applying for Social Security Benefits

You start the process of applying for disability insurance by making your claim at the local SSA District Office, in person or by telephone. This agency will need to know the nature of your medical condition; your physician's (or physicians') name(s), address, and telephone; and your job background and education. When you call, the agency will set up an appointment for an interview. They will also send you a packet with information and forms.

You must make the SSA understand what kind of problems you have. Describe your problems with fingering, dexterity, depth perception, changing vision, sensitivity to fumes and dust, and so forth—things that they have some familiarity with. See the Fibromyalgia and Myofascial Pain Syndrome Functional Questionnaire in Appendix D.

The Forms

The SSA likes forms. They want you to fill out lots of them. It doesn't matter if writing is excruciatingly painful for you. It doesn't matter if the forms are biased against chronic pain patients and completely irrelevant for FMS, MPS, or FMS/MPS Complex patients. That is why the Fibromyalgia and Myofascial Pain Syndrome Functional Questionnaire form in Appendix D, which is based on the Fibromyalgia Impact Assessment form, is so important to you. Its questions are meaningful to the person with FMS, MPS, or FMS/MPS Complex. You are allowed to add many pages of comments, but the people at SSA go by the forms.

The Interview

There is one rule you should always follow, whether you are having an initial interview, a follow-up interview, or appealing your claim: Take a tape recorder with you. Your interviewers will probably tell you that you can have a copy of their tape, but that may take quite a while to get to you.

The Review Process

The request you make triggers an in-depth investigation of your problem and disabilities. The SSA also investigates your medical history: the initial description of your condition, including your capacity for lifting, walking, standing, and sitting; your job history—the date you last worked and a description of past work; and proof of citizenship and insurance status.

You must be examined by a physician working for the Disability Determination Service. "Frequently, waits are long, examinations are brief, and medical records are not available for review by the SSA physician, who is paid approximately $88 for the examination and report" (Potter 1994). A number of insurance doctors have licenses to practice in ten or more states, just so they can work for insurance companies. No bias at all there. Right?

In addition, be aware that the physician-reviewer who is part of the reviewing team is usually not a practicing physician and probably knows little or nothing about FMS or MPS.

To receive a response after this review may take six to eight months. (How the people filing for SSI are supposed to eat during these months is a mystery.)

Qualifying for Social Security Disability Benefits

One of the major factors in our uphill battle for benefits of any kind is that, as of this writing, there are no specific codes used by the SSA, HMOs, or insurance companies to define either FMS or MPS. Medicode ICD-9CM is the definitive listing for diagnostic codes.

Medicode ICD-9CM Codes

729.0 is the code for Rheumatism unspecified and Fibrositis (they do not use the name fibromyalgia).

There is no code for Myofascial Pain Syndrome.

729.1 is the code number for muscle pain, myalgia, and Myositis—unspecified.

An experienced nurse once told me, "For myofascial pain (and also for FMS) you can code the pain by site. I do this for some insurance companies. If I use FM (729.0), they [the insurance company] will 'down code' the procedure, or pay for only a brief visit. If you use the code for lumbosacral pain, however, they will not down code and will pay the full amount. Some of these codes cannot be used with Medicare, they will not take a nonspecific code. But private insurance companies will still pay on them."

Other Diagnostic Codes

728.8 Other disorders of muscle, ligament, and fascia
728.85 Spasm of muscle
729.4 Fascitis unspecified
729.5 Pain in limb
729.9 Other and unspecified disorders of soft tissue; Polyalgia
625.9 Broad ligament pain
724.2 Lower back pain
724.6 Sacroiliac pain

According to "the system," we don't fit into any defined slot too well. That's another reason why we must make some changes. Bureaucracies don't take change well, especially with something as varying and invisible as these chronic conditions. It won't be easy—but it must be done.

Do You Qualify?

To determine whether you qualify for any government-run programs, you first must establish whether you meet the particular agency's definition of "disabled." In most cases, this means you must be incapable of performing *any* work, although this rule has more flexibility if you are age fifty or older. When you file for SSD, you must be prepared to prove that you haven't been able to perform "substantial" work for at least a year. Be specific about what you cannot do, what you cannot do well, and what you need help to do. Remember, most work requires regular attendance and the ability to concentrate and follow instructions. If you cannot meet those criteria, let them know that.

If you are working and making more than $500 a month, it is very unlikely that you will be considered disabled. It doesn't matter how much pain you are in, or how much you cry at the end of each day, or how much your home life has been destroyed. All they will consider is your tax statement. It is proof that you can work. You must be able to prove your condition is severe, and that you can't do the work you previously did—or any other type of work.

Personal Estimated Benefits Earning Statement

Contact your Social Security office and ask how to obtain your Personal Estimated Benefits Earning Statement ("PEBES"). Social Security is insurance you've paid for throughout your working life. You are given credits based on how much you have earned, up to four credits per year. Your PEBES will tell you how many credits you've earned. The amount of credits you need to be "insured" under Social Security is based on your age. From this statement, you will be able to figure out approximately how much your SSD monthly check will be.

When to Apply

As soon as possible after you become disabled, apply for benefits. Don't wait until you are destitute. It takes at least sixty to ninety days to process your initial claim. If you are eligible you will not be paid anything for the first five months after you apply for SSD. That is, if you file your initial claim in January, and you are approved, you will not see your first payment until the sixth month after you file—in this case, June. It may be wise to file for both SSD and Social Security Income (SSI) at the same time because if you are found to be eligible for SSI, they will pay retroactive benefits for the first five months after your claim is filed, although the benefits package will in all likelihood be much smaller than it is for SSD.

A Social Security Administration (SSA) worker will help you fill out your application. As you know, forms are generally not easy for us. When you apply, you will also need a W-2 tax form. You can file for SSD by phone or by mail.

At that time, or beforehand, ask for a copy of the *Pocket Guide to Federal Help for Individuals with Disabilities,* published by the Office of Special Education and Rehabilitation Services. This pocket guide will give you information on special disability groups, vocational rehabilitation, educational rights, library services, financial assistance, and much more. Call (800) 949-4232, or write to the Department of Education, Room 3132 Switzer Building, Washington, DC 20202-2524.

Caution: When you file for SSD, if you are already covered under private medical insurance, be sure they don't charge you for Medicare. It isn't unusual to find that your first SSD checks will have had Medicare costs taken out, even if you did not request it, and it takes time (and your money) to get this straight. If you do need Medicare, make sure to apply for it within the required time period (see the section on Medicare later in this chapter).

Appeals

You can appeal if you are denied benefits at this stage, and you usually will be. *Initial applications for disability are routinely denied.* Don't let the denial throw you. No matter how well you have prepared yourself for the denial, it will come as a blow. It is meant to discourage you. Don't let it. If your needs are just, you deserve benefits.

Your appeal will be reviewed by a different set of people than the ones who first reviewed your case. Again, they will probably not know a thing about FMS or MPS. If you are denied a second time, you can ask for a hearing with a judge. At this stage, it is recommended to look into employing legal representation. It may be useful for you and your representative to thoroughly check the Social Security "bluebook" of recognized disabilities to see how many categories into which you fit. You may be denied on the basis of one condition, and be approved on the basis of another. The combined weight of several conditions may make it easier for the SSA to grant you disability benefits.

Not only are there lawyers to help you through the SSD maze, but today there are more and more consultants working to do the same. Make sure your representative has a thorough knowledge of the SSA system and understands FMS and MPS, and any other condition you may have. There are also business firms that will help you get your disability benefits, such as National Disability Consulting. Their address is 5720 SW 72 Street, Suite 219, Miami FL 33193-3136; phone (305) 957-7527, fax (305) 383-7395. Or you can contact them at their website NationalDisabilityConsulting@worldnet.att.net

(Their representatives are very knowledgeable concerning FMS, CFIDS, and Gulf War Syndrome, but when I contacted them they didn't know about MPS.) For their fee, these firms take a percentage of your initial disability payment. It takes so long to qualify for disability benefits that this initial payment is often substantial—and so is the fee charged.

Communicate During the Appeals Process

Let the Social Security representatives know how you feel about how you are being treated. Do so politely. Let them know that you can't afford help to keep your house clean, and you can't do it yourself. Let them know that you can't afford physical therapy that would enable you to work, or to do more work with less pain. Help them to understand what your limitations are.

The Hearing

At your hearing, a vocational expert may be present to testify. You will be given the opportunity to review your file, but you must arrive thirty minutes before the hearing to do that review. At the hearing, you will have a chance to testify and tell the judge about your case. The judge will question you and other witnesses under oath. It will be recorded. Based on his/her findings, the judge will issue a written decision, and you will get a copy. Be prepared for additional stress. You may need additional medication because the stress of these encounters may send you into flare.

The Appeals Council

If you are denied benefits after a judicial hearing, you can appeal the judgment. Then your case will be brought before the Appeals Council. You can also appeal their denial ruling. By then, you will be exhausted mentally, physically, emotionally, and financially. That's the idea. The system tries to wear you out. If you get discouraged and quit, they don't have to pay you. I continued my efforts because my SSA agent encouraged me to continue. I, too, encourage you to continue. You may feel like David doing battle with Goliath. Remember, David won. Information is your slingshot, and you are not alone.

The United States District Court

Your next step is to go before the United States District Court. If they rule against you, you have sixty days to file an appeal. *You must obey this time limit.* If you don't, any future appeal will be barred, you will have to begin all over again, and it would be unlikely that your case would *ever* get anywhere.

Supplemental Security Income

Supplemental Security Income (SSI) is a form of federal welfare. It is very different from SSD. It is a needs-based disability program for people with very low incomes. The program is restricted to disabled people or to people over sixty-five-years old with very limited incomes or no income at all, and who own little in the way of assets. For example, to be eligible for SSI, a single person may not have assets over $2000, although certain assests such as your home, your car, your personal jewelry, and other personal items may be exempt.

Applying for SSI

You apply for SSI at your local SSA office. You will need your Social Security card, or an official document of some kind with your Social Security Number on it. You will also need your birth certificate, financial information about your home, tax or payroll records, bankbooks, and proof of assets (or lack thereof). Note that you don't require work credits to qualify for SSI as you do to qualify for SSD.

You are not allowed to receive both SSI and Aid to Families with Dependent Children. However, you may qualify for Medicare and food stamps in addition to SSI, although eligibility requirements for these programs are in flux. Medical requirements for both SSD and SSI are the same, and personal disability is determined by the same process. For information packets about these programs, call your local Social Security office or (800) 772-1213.

possible, but it is still painful. At my hearing I let the judge know that I had plans to return to work. I planned to use the SSD settlement money to set up an ergonomic workstation to enable me to function as an author. I told him I thought I would be able to refuse benefits within a year. (It took nine months. I wrote to the judge and let him know that.)

The Importance of Documentation

The most important element in all benefit claims is the amount and quality of the documentation. Be prepared for dealing with innumerable bureaucratic forms. I don't know who decides how long it is "supposed" to take to fill out the forms, but the time frame is entirely unrealistic for those of us with FMS and/or MPS. Let them know how long it takes you to comply, and that their stated times are the estimates for healthy people. It often takes one of us an entire week to fill out what they say "should" be filled out in thirty minutes.

They will want exact dates for all the visits you have made to your doctors, sometimes going back for many years—fibrofog notwithstanding. The added stress of dealing with the "system" will not enhance the quality of your life. Let them know how this affects you. This is an important aspect of your disability, and they should be made aware that they are adding to the burden of symptoms you must endure. Your doctor may need to give you extra medication to withstand the stress of meeting with the SSA's representatives. Let them know this as well. It is important that they understand the depth of your disability.

Dealing with Forms

If possible, type most of the forms. You can even paste the typed forms onto the forms they give you. Many of us find writing painful, and the results are often illegible. Most SSA investigators will encourage you to continue to send them additional information as soon as you receive it from your doctors. If you ask your doctors to send additional information directly to the SSA, make your request in writing, ask for it to be done in a timely manner, and keep a copy of your written request. Also, be sure to ask that a copy of your doctor's reports be sent to you. Follow up on this. Papers get lost, and doctors, and their office staffs, forget.

The SSA now has many of its publications, documents, press releases, and statistics on the Internet. There are more than one-hundred publications in English and in Spanish. There is a list of frequently asked questions (FAQs) with answers. Some of the documents have imposing titles, such as "Your Right to an Administrative Law Judge Hearing and Appeals Council Review of Your Social Security Case," and "How Social Security Can Help with Vocational Rehabilitation." There are even information booklets on what you need to know when you get disability benefits. The local SSA people will help you understand them.

Let Them Know What You Cannot Do

As you go about gathering the necessary documentation, remember that the SSA needs to know what you *cannot* do. Your focus must be on establishing and proving you have a medically determinable condition that prevents sustainable gainful employment. Your job will be made much easier if your doctor's notes contain statements like these:

- Patient's previous work required occasional lifting, climbing stairs, ability to work every day with a sustained eight hours of work and considerable multitasking.

- This patient cannot perform sustained work daily, but needs several days and additional physical therapy to recover from a few hours work.

- Even a few hours of work leaves the patient exhausted and in pain. The pain and medications often lead to confusional states wherein the patient cannot concentrate.

If the doctor's statements consist of brief, unexplained notes such as "Saw patient. Still overweight. Ongoing pain, fatigue. Continued medication," your doctor is not doing his/her job adequately for you, and it is likely that the SSA will dismiss your claim. Your doctor's understanding of FMS and MPS is being tested here, and you are the one who will pay for lack of knowledge. *Your claim depends on the accuracy and thoroughness of your doctor's notes.*

Your Doctor's Report

Your medical charts should include an explicit narrative report. As a rule, your likelihood of getting disability benefits will depend on your doctor's ability to take a comprehensive medical history and complete office notes. Ask her/him to include lists of all your medications and their side effects, physical therapy evaluations, and what happened with sustained efforts at work. The notes should include specific activities that worsen pain, and information on your doctor's experience in the field of FMS and MPS. They should include a clear statement that you are *not* malingering. (See Appendix D: "The Functional Inventory Assessment" for an example of what should be included.) Your doctor's report may need to be only three-pages long, but if it is specific and detailed, so much the better.

The SSA reviewers will get lost in pages and pages of "I saw so and so, no change." It will help if you include the relative age of listed disorders, such as "Symptom so and so appeared on such and such date." It will also help if the actions that contributed to or triggered the symptoms are described (e.g., due to lifting, carrying, pushing, pulling, such and such took place). Give specifics on the kinds of movements and tasks that your job required. Include information on the weights of files and small tools that needed to be carried, handled, and fingered. Add facts about balancing, climbing, and stretching. Your doctor's notes should include information on how you cope with stooping and bending, working outside, or extremes of cold or heat. They should also include information on how your body reacts to temperature changes, wet and humid conditions, noise and vibration. What happens if you are exposed to fumes, odors, or dust. The doctor should list any problems you have with eating, dressing, ambulating, "toileting," bathing, continence, grooming, communicating, reading, cooking, cleaning, shopping, doing laundry, climbing stairs, using a telephone, managing medication, managing money, and your ability to travel.

Your Report

If you've kept a pain diary, it may help to include some pages from it as examples of your day-to-day difficulties. If you have not kept a pain diary, perhaps you should start one now. In your diary, list all of your symptoms, and be specific. Describe how they force you to make changes in your life. Observations such as the following will help:

Due to FMS and/or MPS:

- I stay at home most of the time. I change position frequently to try to become comfortable, and I never quite succeed.

- I walk more slowly and only for short distances, and I use a handrail or a cane (or have to use elevators).

- I lie down and rest more often, and I have to hold on to something to help me stand up.

- I try not to kneel down or bend much. It hurts too much.

- My hands are painful almost all of the time, and it takes me four sittings to write a one-page letter. Sometimes I can't do even that.

- I have trouble putting on socks, need help to get dressed, and I can't wear clothes with buttons, because I can't manage them.

- I'm more irritable due to the pain and fatigue. I hurt much worse when a storm is coming in.

Describe your efforts. Most of us are hard workers, and we push ourselves harder than we should. We're stubborn and independent. Many of us try to avoid having to collect disability benefits, and we often don't seek a doctor's help for getting them until the symptoms are unbearable. We are then frequently undiagnosed/misdiagnosed for some length of time, and the symptoms multiply because we don't receive adequate and appropriate care. We have often been run to the ground by our caretakers, and put through inappropriate physical therapy. Our bodies have been ruined by assorted inappropriate medications and we are emotionally, physically, and financially exhausted. Then we must face the ordeals and delays of applying and qualifying for disability benefits. Explain all of this. It is important.

Know Your Rights

Know your rights. If you object to any issues the SSA officials stated as reasons for your denials, you must tell them in writing why you object, and as soon as possible. You may submit additional evidence. You may request a subpoena to require someone to submit documents or to testify at your hearing. If this is necessary, submit a written request to the judge, identifying the necessary documents and witnesses and stating why you need them and can't get them without a subpoena. Help them to help you.

If you do qualify for benefits, the struggle isn't over. There will be reviews and more forms. Be aware that "failure to cooperate" can disqualify you from continuing to receive your benefits. Make sure you understand what that entails. Call your local SSA office if you need help.

The Future of Social Security

You may have heard lots of talk about SSA going bankrupt. There are serious long-term financial problems. Most of the money collected in FICA taxes hasn't gone into entitlement programs. This is the money we are "entitled to" when we become disabled or retired. It is ours. Yet the government has been "borrowing" from the Social Security trust fund for more than twenty-five years to conceal the true cost of the federal deficit. Check out the book, *America: Who Really Pays the Taxes?* (Barlett and Steele 1994).

The problem has to do with a change Lyndon Johnson made in 1968, which he called a "unified budget" plan. President Johnson combined Social Security, Medicare, and other trust fund accounts into what he called the "general fund revenue." This started a "surplus" that the federal government has been dipping into ever since.

The Social Security monies went down fast. The surplus was 4.8 billion dollars in 1969, and dropped to 400 million dollars in 1973. At that point, they started raising Social Security taxes (FICA). As I write, workers pay 6.2 percent of their earnings up to $65,400 in FICA taxes, and the employer chips in the same percentage. Those of us who are self-employed pay 12.4 percent of our incomes in FICA taxes.

Social Security Administration disability benefits range from $350 to $1000 a month. The Social Security laws are being changed as this chapter is being written, but for now, Supplemental Security Income is payable from the date the application is filed.

The Changing Face of Social Security

The SSA rules are in flux. They are constantly changing. Everyone is tightening the belt, and the belt often becomes a noose for folks suffering from "invisible" chronic pain conditions. As I write, there are a number of "rulemaking edicts" being issued that could impact adversely upon our lives.

The 62 Federal Register 50279 (September 25, 1997) contains a proposed rule that would weaken our Social Security benefit rights. If passed, it would require the administrative law judges and the Appeals Councils that hear SSA disability cases to give more weight to the "opinions and findings by nonexamining state agency medical personnel and the medical experts they utilize." In other words, the opinion of a doctor who hasn't examined you and may not know a thing about FMS and MPS could be considered more valuable than the opinion of an expert you hire to examine you. It would be one more way to save the government money, at the expense of those who legitimately need help. So much for justice. If this law is passed, I don't believe it will hold up to a constitutional challenge.

Returning to Work

If you are receiving Supplemental Security Income or Social Security Disability and want to return to work, you can use the government money to help yourself build a bridge on the way to gainful employment. You may be afraid to try, for fear you won't be able to continue, or that you might lose your benefits. There are SSA work incentive rules that may help, and an SSA agent will be glad to help explain them to you. Be very careful. If you tell the SSA to stop your checks, you may have to fight to keep any federal money sent to you after that time, even if you do not make enough money to disqualify you for SSD. This will require a waiver, more forms, and much grief, as the system is not used to people voluntarily quitting SSD when they still have a chronic medical condition.

Trial Period

If you return to work, there is a trial work period of nine months in a sixty-month period, during which time you may receive Social Security checks. They need not be consecutive. After nine months, the SSA does a work review to see if you should be allowed to continue receiving benefits. For at least thirty-six months after the review, you may be entitled to income if your earnings fall below $500 a month.

Medicare Benefits

If your Social Security checks are discontinued because you are earning a substantial amount of money, Medicare benefits will continue for at least thirty-nine months after the trial work period. Even after that, you can purchase Medicare coverage. If you have a very low income, your state may help you to pay for this. If you lose your job within the extended period of eligibility, it will not affect your Medicare benefits. You will not be required to undergo a waiting period nor have to reapply.

Work Retraining

If you were to become unable to work because of your disability, you would have to reapply for Social Security benefits. The State Rehabilitation Agency and the SSA will pay for work retraining. You will continue to receive benefits while training. Most of the scholarships or grants used to pay for tuition, books, and so forth may not count as income. You may also be able to deduct expenses for items that enable you to work, such as prescription medications, special keyboards, or other work equipment. Ask your local Social Security office to send you the leaflet *Medicare Savings for Qualified Beneficiaries* (HCFA Publication 02184), or call the Medicare hotline at (800) 638-6833.

Medicare

Medicare is a type of health insurance that you have paid for with your Social Security taxes. It's a form of joint national health insurance for people who are entitled to Social Security benefits, administered by the federal and state governments. Qualified individuals can enroll at their local Social Security office.

What Medicare Will Cover

Medicare Part A covers inpatient hospital services, skilled nursing facilities (*not* custodial care, such as nursing homes), home health services, and hospice care. Medicare Part B covers part of the costs of physician services, outpatient hospital services, medical equipment and supplies, and other health services and supplies. Part B must be purchased, just like a private health insurance policy, but the premiums are relatively small. If your income is low enough, your state may pay for the premium, or for part of it.

If you are confined to your home and require skilled care, Medicare will pay for care provided by a home health agency. Your physician should provide the home health agency with a plan of treatment. The services may be provided either on part-time or intermittent bases, but they do not cover full-time care.

The Medicare program is run by the Health Care Financing Administration (HCFA). You can address any advocacy concerns to them at the Humphrey Building, 200 Independence Avenue SW, Washington DC, 20201. You can also obtain single copies of any of their publications by calling the Medicare hotline at (800) 638-6833.

Medicare does *not* pay for most prescription drugs, examinations for prescribing or fitting eyeglasses or hearing aids, hearing aids, or routine eye exams. Medicare helps pay only for chiropractic manipulation of the spine to correct a subluxation that has been demonstrated by X ray.

Medicare Availability and Coverage Limitations

Neither all hospitals nor all doctors take part in the Medicare plan. Check to see that your hospital or doctor does before you use their services. Ask your doctor whether s/he participates in Medicare. Also, the names and addresses of Medicare participating doctors are listed (by geographic area) in the Medicare-Participating Physician Directory. Medicare is limited, so also check to be sure of what services are covered.

Medicare and Medications

Unfortunately, Medicare will not pay for all medications, especially new ones. In conditions such as FMS and MPS, patients experiment with new medications all the time. This is very hard for the "system" to understand. Medications that help one person will have no effect on another. This is another reason why the Bibliography and Reference sections are so extensive. Use them as educative tools whenever possible. Whenever you educate someone, you are helping others to avoid the endless grief that those of us breaking new ground have endured. It's a long road we are building, but, at least, it's a road already under construction.

Medicaid

Medicaid is different from Medicare. It's an assistance program. Medical bills are paid from federal, state, and local tax funds. It serves low-income people of every age. As a rule, patients pay no part of the costs for covered medical expenses; however, in recent years, a small co-payment is sometimes required. Medicaid is a joint federal-state program. It varies from state to state. States determine the amount and duration of services offered under their Medicaid programs, working under broad federal guidelines.

Medicare and Managed Care

Medicare Health Maintenance Organizations (HMOs) do cover a broad range of preventive health care services, including routine physicals. In these HMOs, there is provision for people on Medicare. You must still pay the Medicare premium, and the HMO premium, but you do not pay medical deductibles and coinsurance, which are paid by the HMO. Generally, you must receive all of your health care from the HMO organization, but you may be able to receive such benefits as dental and eye care free. Check your HMO policy thoroughly. To find out more about these plans, request a copy of *Your Medicare Handbook* from the U.S. Department of Health and Human Services, Health Care Financing Administration, 7500 Security Blvd., Baltimore, MD 21244-1850.

National Medicare managed care plans must give you a receipt of notice—in writing—if they deny, reduce, or terminate any service. They also must contact you within sixty days after you have requested services (do it in writing and keep a copy), or within sixty days after you disagree with the reduction or termination of any service. If you request that a decision be "expedited," that indicates you need a response within seventy-two hours, because you believe that a delay of up to sixty days could harm your health. If you have a difference of opinion, they will probably want you to ask for an internal review. That, more or less, means that they will review themselves, and guess who they will side with? Don't go for it. Ask for a "PRO—peer review organization review." (The PRO is a state Medicare board, which will provide an unbiased peer review. Every state has a Medicare peer review organization that is physician-directed, not run by the state.) You can also file a grievance with your managed care plan.

The Health Care Financing Administration (HCFA) (800-638-6833 or http://www.hcfa.gov) administers the Medicare managed care system. Contact the Medicare Rights Center at 1460 Broadway, New York, NY 10036, for publications and Medicare advice. The PROS Medicare Hotline at (800) 638-6833 investigates complaints about the quality of care people receive. You can also contact your State Department of Insurance under your state government in the yellow pages of the phone book.

Medicare and Managed Care: The Good and the Bad

Some advantages of Medicare's managed care plans include the following:

- Additional benefits not covered by Medicare, such as drugs and eyeglasses

- Smaller premiums than those of the free-standing Medigap plans

- Less paperwork

- Coordination of medical services;

- An emphasis on preventive care

Some disadvantages of managed care plans include the following:

- The inability to go directly to specialists for services. (This is because you need a referral from your primary care physician. It can take up to thirty days to disenroll and until your disenrollment is implemented, you must continue to use the medical services provided by your managed care plan.)

- A smaller network of providers. (When you join a managed care plan, your current primary care physician and other health care team providers may not be in the plan's network; and there may be limited coverage outside of a particular service area.)

Medigap

"Medigap" is the term used for insurance policies that people can buy from private health insurance companies. It's a form of private Medicare supplemental insurance that was created because Medicare pays less than 100 percent for some services. In some states, insurers are required to offer Medigap insurance to people who are disabled and on Medicare, even when they are under sixty-five, but this varies, so check to be sure. They don't always tell you.

A Medigap policy pays for Medicare-approved charges that are not paid by Medicare because of deductibles or coinsurance amounts for which the beneficiary is responsible. The cost of Medigap policies varies from company to company and from plan to plan. You need to contact the private insurance companies to find out the costs of their policies, although sometimes the states will provide a listing, with a comparison of rates. For more information, see HCFA's publication, *Guide to Health Insurance.*

State Information, Counseling, and Assistance (ICA) Program offices can provide beneficiaries with general information about Medicare, Medicaid, managed care plans, and the various types of health insurance available to supplement Medicare, including Medigap and long-term care insurance. Counselors can also help you with questions about your medical bills, insurance claims, and benefit explanation forms. The services are free. Ask the HCFA how to contact the offices in your state.

A Note to the Reader

As I did the research for this chapter, it was very common for case workers and SSD interviewers (including judges) to express concern about the overuse of medications. There was also frequent mention of a desire to get patients back to meaningful work, so that they could "forget about" their chronic pain. This indicated to me that these people have no idea of the pain load we carry. If you can get them to understand this—and you should be able to if you use the Bibliography, References, and other parts of this book as teaching tools—you will have come a long way in your quest for benefits. One of these days, FMS and chronic MPS will be on the list of disabling impairments. Full-blown FMS and MPS will also be much rarer, as physicians learn how to diagnose them early and deal with them appropriately.

PART IV

Dealing with Your World

Life can be enjoyable in spite of having FMS and/or MPS, or it can be a burden—a truly heavy load. How you deal with the issues discussed in Part IV can make the difference. Chapter 14 provides suggestions for discussing basic matters of rights and responsibilities with the important people in your life and offers helpful tips on overcoming loneliness and isolation. Chapter 15 has useful information on dealing with change and conflict and provides some helpful exercises to learn how to better resolve interpersonal conflicts. Chapter 16 covers the special issues of childhood, pregnancy, menopause, and old age as they relate to FMS and/or MPS.

14

Family and Friends:
Rights and
Responsibilities—
Isolation and Loneliness

Personal Rights

You know you have civil rights, but have you ever stopped to examine and define your rights (and responsibilities) as family members, friends, consumers, and employees? In all your roles in life, you have rights and responsibilities and, all too often, you can slip into unhealthy relationships. When chronic pain is also an issue, these issues can be compounded.

In his book *Belonging: A Guide to Overcoming Loneliness* (1994), William R. Brassell provides a framework in which to examine our rights as members of families. He also provides an exercise, which he has kindly allowed me to reprint here, that will enable us to assess the status of our family rights and responsibilities. If you haven't been keeping a journal or notebook, this is a good way to start. Using these lists will help you to reassess the parts of your life that you may have been taking for granted—parts that may be overdue for a change. It may be time for you to advocate, without guilt, for your own personal rights.

Your Rights as an Adult Son or Daughter

- To decide how often you should visit your parents

- To dislike and avoid relatives who are unkind or unfair to you

- To be free from guilt should you decide to spend holidays away from your parents

- To make your own decisions, even when they conflict with the desires of your parents

- To rear your own children by your rules, rather than your parents' rules

Your Rights as a Friend

- To expect friends to share the costs of mutual activities

- To expect items that have been lent to be returned promptly and in good condition

- To expect friends to be on time—most of the time

- To expect friends to share in planning time together

- To expect friends to listen as well as talk

Your Rights as a Consumer

- To refuse to listen to sales pitches if you so choose

- To expect items you've bought to be replaced or repaired when they don't fit or operate properly

- To be treated courteously and respectfully

- To be served promptly

Your Rights as an Employee

- To be paid fairly for the work you do

- To be treated with dignity and respect

- To have pleasant, safe surroundings

- To have adequate materials, supplies, and space

- To have the support of your supervisor

- To be granted time off graciously

- To receive clear instructions about your duties

- To receive feedback about the quality of your work

- To be free from harassment of any kind

Your Rights as a Spouse

- To have a share in making decisions that concern you

- To be listened to as well as to listen

- To be treated respectfully and affectionately

- To ask to have sex or to turn it down if you're not in the mood

- To not be blamed or criticized unfairly

Exercise: Identifying Your Roles and Rights

The purpose of this exercise is to help you recognize the areas in your life where you can begin to use assertiveness to get what you need and deserve.

1. In your notebook, make a list of all the roles you play in your life. Remember to include minor as well as major roles.

2. Now, taking each of your roles in turn, think about what your rights are in that role. Don't analyze too much; this is a brainstorming exercise. Just list all the rights you can think of, without stopping. When you run out of rights in one role, pick another of your roles and list the rights for that one, and so on until you exhaust all your roles and rights. Note that you probably will list the same or similar rights for several roles.

3. Review the rights you listed. Place a check mark beside each right that *isn't* currently being honored.

4. Review the *checked* items, and circle the five that are most important to you. Then give each of those items a number from 1 to 5 to indicate its level of importance to you, with 1 as the most important.

5. At the top of a new page in your notebook, write "I have a right to _____" and then list the most important of your rights that currently are not being honored.

6. Beneath that line, draw a vertical line down the center of the page. Title one side "Who" and the other "Where." Then, under the Who column, list the people who disregard that right. In the Where column, list the situations in which the right is commonly disregarded.

Self-advocacy and assertiveness are essential aspects of learning how to take care of yourself without feeling guilty. Once you have identified the people and the situations where your rights are not honored, you will have taken the first step toward self-advocacy. The second step requires you to speak up for yourself the next time you are in that situation. You don't have to get angry, but you do have to let that person know you feel the way you do—that your rights are being ignored or otherwise devalued. Ask that person for a few minutes of uninterrupted time and quietly, but firmly, say what you are thinking. Then, listen to the response without interrupting the other person. If the response is not satisfactory, try again. If you both start to quarrel, take a "time-out" and reschedule another talk. You will be surprised at how much better communicating with others becomes when you start standing up for yourself.

Talking with Your Family

If you haven't had a family meeting on fibromyalgia (FMS) and/or Myofascial Pain Syndrome (MPS), perhaps this is a good time to initiate one. A frank discussion about your condition(s) and the impact it has on you and your family may help clear the air, and give your family a chance to ask questions. They may have fears you don't know they have. They may be worrying about matters like these: "What will this illness do to you? What changes will take place? Will our relationship change? How will this affect me? What can I do to help you feel better? Is it hereditary?"

There may be disbelief and anger, especially if there has been a long period of illness before your proper diagnosis was made. You may want to explain that although you can't do everything you want to do, you can give them either/or choices, or attach conditions on the things you can do. For example, you might say:

- We can either go to the movies tonight or go to the play tomorrow, but I won't be able to manage both.

- We can go for a walk this afternoon or I can help you with that term paper, but I'll only be able to do one of those things today.

- I can bake cookies for your class—if you help me make them—including cleaning up.

Grief and Other Emotions

When a chronic illness strikes you, your kids and significant other also grieve—they experience the grief cycle that was first identified by Elisabeth Kübler-Ross. This means that the change in your lifestyle caused by chronic illness will likely be met by your family first with denial, and then with anger, bargaining, depression, and, finally, acceptance of that which is—that which cannot be changed and must be accepted.

Elisabeth Kübler-Ross is a pioneer in the field of hospice care. Neither fibromyalgia nor Myofascial Pain Syndrome is a fatal condition, yet those of us who have them undergo what in hospice care is called a "little death." We lose the self that was—the active self who could do so many things without having to deal with the consequences that FMS and MPS impose on us. Stephen Levine, in his book, *Who Dies?* (1982), describes this grief cycle as the stages of converting tragedy to grace. The stages do not necessarily follow the order described.

As a rule, though, denial is commonly the first response. You, or one or more members of your family, will refuse to accept that you have these very real conditions that impose such very real limits on you. But this denial can make your condition even more limiting, as you cannot deal with what you don't accept, and the quality of your life will not improve until you deal with the conditions. Although the emotions that characterize this cycle of grief are normal, if any one of the stages seems to be taking over your life, or the lives of any family members, please seek professional help.

Some members of your family may be jealous because you are getting more attention from everyone. Different relatives may feel different emotions, such as embarrassment, shame, grief, and depression. Talk it out. These responses are normal, and you can work through these feelings together. Make your family a part of your healing—not a part of your illness. Be sure your children understand that your illness is not their fault. Watch your children carefully and stay tuned in to their needs. If they know you are responsive to them, that will ease their anxieties considerably.

In general, children will deal with chronic illness the same way their parents do. You are a role model, as is your significant other. Observe the children carefully for signs of rebellion, or depression. Pay attention to any changes in school grades. When their parents are ill, some children do well in school, and even improve their grades, but they may still be very depressed. They might be trying to lose themselves in schoolwork. Keep an eye on them. Keep the lines of communication open. Pay attention to their habits and routines. Are they are eating or sleeping too little or too much? Expect the unexpected. If they are young, there may be obvious regressions, such as bedwetting. Involve your parents, in-laws, and your kids' teachers in your educational efforts, if that is appropriate. If there is a problem that won't go away, consider going into family therapy.

It's important that you talk to your kids, but it is even more important that you *listen* to them. Don't allow any child to get stuck in a parenting role. You are still the adult. Enjoy their childhood. Let them know that you plan to have as much fun as is possible—but be realistic. Don't plan things time after time and then disappoint them at the last minute. Be honest with yourself and your family concerning your limitations.

Here are some examples of guidelines you can give to your family before the meeting. This may give them a framework in which to form their own questions. You will probably want to read the guidelines to the younger children as part of the family meeting. These are, of course, only models. They will need to be modified to suit your needs, but they will give you a place to start.

What Your Younger Children Should Know

Dear _____ ,

You know that your (mommy/daddy) has changed, and you may be confused about why. I don't have all the answers, but I wanted to talk to you about this, and I'll let you know as much as I can.

Do you remember when you had a bad cold, and had to stay in bed? You hurt all over, and couldn't do anything you wanted to do. You had to take special medicines, and some of them tasted awfully bad. You didn't sleep well, and you couldn't wait until you got better.

(Mommy/Daddy) has (fibromyalgia and/or Myofascial Pain Syndrome). Those are pretty big names. It means that often I hurt a lot—like you did when you had that bad cold. Some days I don't feel too bad, and some days I feel *really* bad. It's really important for you to understand that *you cannot* "catch" this the way you can catch a cold. This illness is nothing that happened because of anything that you or I did. It just happened.

Sometimes, I can't do all the things I would like to do with you. I may not be able to pick you up anymore, but you can still climb on my lap when I sit down. I might not be able to go to all your school events, but that isn't because I don't want to.

Sometimes, I may get confused, or angry, or mad, and I don't mean it. It's nothing that you did. It is just part of the illness. I sometimes get very tired, and I have to lie down and take a nap. I might need to spend more time taking care of myself. I will have exercises and stretches I need to do to feel the best that I can. Maybe you would like to do some of them with me? It's always more fun if we can do them together.

I will need your help to tell me when I am getting too angry, or too sad. You can help to cheer me up, and we can find more things that we can do together. We may not be able to do as many things as we want to—but we can decide together which things we want to do most.

I won't die from this, so you don't have to worry about that. I won't leave you. We can get through this together. It will be a while before the doctors can come up with a way to cure it. There are a lot of doctors working on that right now. Until they do come up with a cure, I want you to know that you can always ask me any question about this illness. I may not know the answers, but I will try to find them out. We can still have a lot of fun together. Most of all, I want you to know that I love you, and that love will not change. You can help me a lot by giving me a hug whenever you think of it, and I will hug you back. That will help us both feel better.

What Your Older Children Should Know

You may have noticed that your (mom/dad) hasn't been the same lately. This may have caused you some confusion, anger, or fear. I have been feeling these things too, and want to talk to you about it, so that you understand what is going on. I have (fibromyalgia and/or Myofascial Pain Syndrome). You may not know about these condition(s), or have heard or read things that are not true. Fibromyalgia is a neurotransmitter problem. Neurotransmitters are the things that allow the body and mind to talk to each other. My neurotransmitters aren't working properly. That means the communications between my body and mind don't work smoothly, which causes the pain and other symptoms. The pain and other symptoms are very hard to control and they force me to set limits on what I can do at any given time.

Remember how you felt when you had a bad case of the flu? You ached all over, and you didn't want to do much of anything. You were tired all the time. That's how I feel with fibromyalgia. The feeling changes, though. Some days I don't feel too bad, and other days I feel as though I had been run over by a truck. This can be very hard to understand, because I look so healthy. My central nervous system can get so sensitive that I feel noise, odors, and lights and, sometimes, even touch as painful.

I don't get the deep kind of sleep that you get, so when I wake up, I often feel terribly stiff and exhausted, instead of wide awake and refreshed. It can be a challenge to get out of bed. I get tired very easily. Sometimes I get very confused, and have a poor memory—it's called "fibrofog." During those times, I may need your help to keep things straight in my mind. You may have to remind me of things I have promised to do, and in enough time so that I will be able to do them. If I sometimes seem confused or forgetful, that doesn't mean I don't want to do things with you. I just may need some help getting organized.

Myofascial pain syndrome (MPS) is another condition that can occur along with fibromyalgia. MPS is a condition of the myofascia. The myofascia is the covering around muscles and groups of cells that make up the muscles. The myofascia gets tougher, and loses some of its ability to stretch. It's like wearing clothes that are too tight. My muscles can't stretch the way they should. I can develop lumps called trigger points that tighten my muscles and cause pain or weakness. They can also cause dizziness and many other symptoms.

It is important that I keep moving, because if I stay in one place too long, I get stiff and achy. That can make it hard for me to go to meetings or sit through a movie. Sometimes my muscles may give out, and I may fall, so I have to be careful how I walk. I have to spend extra time taking care of myself, so I can be as healthy as possible.

When you have both FMS and MPS, they work together to cause more than double the symptoms. These are chronic conditions. That means that right now, there is no cure for them. I will not die from these conditions, so you don't have to be afraid of that. I want you to understand that some days I will feel a lot better than others. This will change from day to day. I'll try to do what I can to feel as good as possible.

FMS makes other problems, such as MPS, or even symptoms from a cold, feel much worse to me. Fibromyalgia also can cause me to have problems with my feelings. Sometimes I hurt so much I lose my patience with things that I could handle if I wasn't in so much pain. I will need your help with this.

I can be happy one minute and sad the next. I might start crying, or I might get angry very fast, and you won't know why. I might not understand it myself. I may not even be able to find words to explain what is happening, or how I feel. This doesn't mean that you have done something wrong. It is due to the illness, and to the chemicals in my body which aren't working the way they should. Please talk to me about it if it scares you, or if you feel confused about what is happening. Let me know if things are getting out of hand. I will always love you and be here for you. We will find a way to deal with this together.

What Your Significant Other Should Know

I've given you some literature on some of the facts about my chronic illness, but there are other things that you should know to help us get through this together. I want you to know what I need, and I want you to be free to tell me your needs. I don't need a martyr or a hero. Chronic illness is not helped by martyrdom or heroics, but how we both cope with this illness will affect the quality of our lives together.

I do need a companion. I also need a partner. I need you to be understanding, and willing to travel this confusing path with me. Neither of us invited FMS or MPS into our (marriage/partnership), but they're here all the same. They won't go away if we ignore them. I'll try to do everything I can to reduce the pain, fatigue, and other symptoms they have brought.

Things have changed for me. I am not the same person I was before FMS or MPS. That doesn't mean that I am a lesser person. We are still equals, and my identity and life are still important, and so are yours. My values and beliefs are much the same, and the love we share is still there. The passion is there, but the packaging has changed—as the packaging of everyone changes with time and with living. With your help, we can both evolve to have a richer, more meaningful relationship. But I need your help for this, and you need mine.

Change is never easy. I need help to cope with the uncertainties that a variable chronic pain condition brings. I need for you to understand that what I can do one day I may not be able to do the next. Overdoing means I must pay for one day's actions in pain and fatigue on the following day. I will need you to understand that sometimes the risk is worth it, and sometimes it isn't. I need you to help explain to others that this is the way it is.

I need to be able to trust you to be my advocate when my words fail and my steps falter. I need you to be free of guilt and allow me to be the same. I need you to help explain that my condition is real, when neighbors and even family insist that I look just fine.

Don't leave me in isolation. I need your intimacy more than ever. I need to feel desirable, even though sometimes my symptoms aren't very romantic. I need a gentle hug or the soft touch of a compassionate hand to remind me that I am not alone.

I need you to remind me that unaccountable irritability is a symptom of FMS, and that when I'm in pain, my patience runs out too quickly. We both need our space, and we both need to escape sometimes. We can find healthy ways to this.

It's OK if you don't know how I feel, and have to ask. It's good for me to get a reality check sometimes. I know I get moody but please let me know when I do. Please be OK with me warning you when I am having a bad day and need my space. Give me a cheery word—sometimes that is all I need to feel better. It is important we maintain open and easy communication between us.

There may be times when I can't go to events you would like to go to, or do the things you want to do with me. These are not my choices. We can find ways around this without becoming negative. Negativity adds to my illness, and does no one any good.

I know you must get sick of dealing with my illness. So do I. Remember that I am more than my illness, and those other facets of my personality need nurturing and can nurture yours. There are many things we can do together, and many memories of joy we can build. I will need your help to find them, and you will need mine. And that is how it should be.

I may find some types of sexual activity painful at times. At other times I may be just too exhausted. We can talk about this. There may be a way around the problems. It doesn't mean that I don't want or require a sexual relationship with you. We will just have to find a way to make it possible and it may take a little extra effort. It could mean that I need to do some stretching exercises earlier, or use a heating pad, or see a doctor. Maybe we both need to see a counselor. But we can find a way to work things out, because our marriage is important, and sex is a vital part of our marriage.

We need to give each other space, but we need to support each other, too. We will be adjusting our relationship to accommodate FMS and MPS, but we can do it in a way that will bring us closer.

Isolation, Loneliness, and Chronic Pain

We are the square pegs in round holes. We fit, but we don't belong. Chronic pain is hard enough to deal with by itself, but it often brings "side effects," such as isolation and loneliness in its wake. The odds of becoming lonely and isolated are even stronger if your conditions are invisible and not understood. You may be doing the best you can to cope, but you may still feel as if you don't fit in anywhere. Other people don't know how to react to you. You find yourself alone when you don't want to be alone.

Even when you're with someone, you might fail to connect. You may have days when you feel as though your forehead is stamped with "Reject," in big red letters. This attitude may have been reinforced for a long time, before you obtained a correct diagnosis—a time when your doctors and other people—told you that your pain and all your symptoms were "all in your head." That attitude is a recipe for negativity and depression. You don't need that extra grief. You are not a reject and you can create a more positive, life-affirming image of yourself.

Live in the Present—But Take Breaks

Isolation is scary, especially when it becomes comfortable. When you are faced with the daily grind of illness and draining emotions, the sense of loss can be overwhelming. It's easy to get caught in the "might have been" trap. But that's a dead-end. Concentrate on what "is." Try your best to live in the present.

Of course, you will need an occasional escape, a break from reality, especially if you no longer work or get out in the world much, and that's perfectly fine. Your escape could be something as simple as a visit from a friend, an afternoon walk, a few hours with a good book, or a funny video. Also, at times, indulging in a little pure silliness can be a very good thing.

The Dangerous "What Ifs"

You may have many FMS and/or MPS symptoms that cause ordinary interactions with others to become real challenges. For example, you know that you become easily fatigued, and are subject to mood swings, or sometimes clumsy. So a negative dialogue may start up in your head saying, "What might happen if I go out? I might fall asleep or yawn uncontrollably . . . Or I might become very irritable . . . Or I might trip in front of everybody? Then, what would I do? I would look like such a clumsy fool." Once we get into this kind of negativity spiral, we need to take positive action to break out of it. Otherwise, we defeat ourselves before we even begin. We can "What if" ourselves into a box, and then the walls of the box start to close in on us. If any of these imagined events do happen, the world won't end. Why fear them? These things can happen to anybody.

Watch Your Language

Be alert to the use of certain words and phrases in your inner dialogue, terms like "always," "never," "everybody else can," and "nobody else does." The frequent use of these terms indicates distorted thinking, which can be amplified or even caused by FMS neurotransmitter dysfunction. Don't allow yourself to be trapped by your own inner dialogue.

Don't ever call yourself "dumb." At times, you may feel stupid, and you may do things that you think are stupid. With "fibrofog" to contend with, and perhaps even having trigger points affecting your muscles of speech, you may feel that you sound "stupid," even to yourself. That doesn't mean that you *are* stupid!

Give in to Your Animal Nature.

I have an elephant nose, made of soft plastic that I wear some days when I just "need a change." The first time I visited someone in a nursing home while wearing it, I felt a little strange, but the smiles that greeted it were sunshine, and strangers said hello. Victims do not wear plastic elephant noses. You have choices in how you live your life, and a little healthy rebellion on your part can be constructive. When you ask yourself, Why me? sometimes the right answer is, Why not? Life happens. I can still have fun. If I can bring a little joy into others' lives, why not?

This society pays too much attention to packaging, and not enough to substance. Don't fall into that trap. You are under considerable stress, trying to cope with a body and mind that are dysregulated. Many of your internal sensing facilities are out of whack. Life is unpredictable now, at best. *Anything* that you accomplish is deserving of praise. *Respect yourself. You are not stupid. You are not a victim. You can cope. You belong to an ever-growing "FMily" of people with FMS and/or MPS. You are not alone!*

Childhood Negativity

A negativity spiral may have begun in your childhood. As FMS and/or MPS symptoms appeared, you may have become aware that you were somehow different, although you didn't understand why, and you may have started blaming yourself for the difference. This might have been reinforced by your classmates, your relatives, or your teachers. Did you hear any of the following criticisms and admonitions when you were a child?

- Don't be a sissy. Big kids don't cry. It can't hurt that much!

- Why don't you watch where you're going! You stumble over everything. Pay attention!

- You never want to do anything. You're just lazy.

- You would have remembered what I said if you wanted to. You just don't care.

- I got up at 5 A.M. to do a paper route before school. Why can't you?

- Why can't you be as neat as the other children?

If any of these sound familiar, it's time to reevaluate those charges in the light of what you've learned about FMS and MPS. There's no need for you to feel ashamed anymore, because no one understood that you were in a constant struggle. Give yourself permission to accept the fact that you have FMS and/or MPS. Forgive yourself—and them—for not knowing any better. Move on.

Self-Fulfilling Prophecies

Becoming lonely and isolated can become a self-fulfilling prophecy unless you take some positive action to break out of the negativity spiral. This means that you have to start replacing self-defeating thoughts and actions. Develop an attitude of enlightened self-interest. You deserve this. You deserve the respect and support of your doctor, your clergy, your family, and friends—and yourself!

Engage in Activities that Promote Enlightened Self-Interest

When you feel lonely and isolated, consider what *you* can do personally to change these feelings. You may not be able to do the things you once did, or do them in the way you used to, but perhaps you can find substitutes. Take an inventory of what you *like* to do. Make a list of reasons why you haven't been doing them. Then make a list of what you can do to change this.

Have a talk with your librarian, or check out the phone book or newspaper for clubs and organizations that are concerned with your interests. At first, you may be able to attend only a part of a meeting, but that's a start. If you aren't up to meetings, consider contacting a seniors' organization. They might have someone who would love to visit you periodically. Find a contact in your religious organization who could suggest some visitors. If you don't belong to a spiritual group, consider joining one. There may be someone whom you could visit. Having FMS/MPS is not an obstacle to friendship. The true obstacles to friendship are the attitudes that foster dependency, blame, self-sacrifice, conquest, jealousy, or envy.

If you fear that others won't understand your limits because they can't see them, take along some copies of the data sheets from chapter 7. That will avoid long explanations, and you will have the opportunity to spread the word about FMS and MPS. Ignorance is always our greatest enemy. If you have difficulty finding transportation to activities, especially at night, try to find someone at the first meeting you attend who lives near you and might be willing to provide transportation. Or you can call the group's facilitator in advance to help arrange transportation.

Perhaps there is a day group you can join. If there isn't, consider starting one with some friends who share your interests. Explain to them that your symptoms are variable, and that you must pace yourself. Teach others what you need, and what you require. Some people may want to visit you, but are afraid to impose. When you do get visitors, request that they remain as positive as possible, and keep their visits short. Again, you can use others' visits as opportunities to educate. The best way to avoid loneliness and feelings of isolation is to connect with other people. Often, you must make the first move. Do it. It will be worth it. And don't accept negativity from others.

Pets—The Only Love that Money Can Buy

If you are able to care for one, consider adopting a pet. They can provide a world of love and companionship but they require the same of you. As always, to have a friend you must be a friend. My cats have a special interest in FMS, because when they shed, they feel pretty bad if they get hair balls. I call this feeling "Fur-ball Malasia." They are FMily too!

Humor

Find things that make you laugh. We know that anxiety and depression interact with chronic pain and interfere with our ability to function. We need to accentuate positive things. When people ask you how you feel, say "I'm fine." Spell it out. F-I-N-E. Then tell them that stands for Frustrated, Irritated, Nonfunctional, and Everything hurts! It will get your point across, while making a positive statement that you are still able to have some fun in life.

Start a collection of cartoons that "crack you up," or find funny videos and books that you can enjoy and share with others. Read about hobbies you might enjoy, and then follow up on what you discover. Being alone is something that can happen to anyone. Loneliness is a state of mind. With the right attitude and a little planning and effort, loneliness needn't be either *your* state of mind nor your lot in life.

In the Spirit of Things

Many of us get hit with negativity bombs delivered by well-meaning people who try to explain away our conditions, not realizing that they're basically blaming us for having FMS and/or MPS. They say, "If you just forgot about it, you'd feel better." Clearly they need to be educated. So, educate them. Well-meaning religious representatives can also deliver mighty blows, kicking us when we are down. When we are told that sickness is the way we are "paying for our sins," that constitutes "cruel and unusual punishment." Try to educate them. Don't accept the guilt.

I have spoken with religious leaders and others, and with few exceptions, I've been told to explain clearly that illness is not our fault. God doesn't want people to suffer. Unconditional love seems to be the Golden Rule here. So why do we fall ill?

Native American healers and leaders believe that sickness is a way to learn—a process by which we can evolve to a clearer, deeper understanding of what it means to be a human being. Sometimes an unusual illness is the first sign that a person has been chosen to become a shaman, or healer. Perhaps we have all been chosen to be healers in some way. Perhaps we are teaching others—and ourselves—patience and compassion. Many great souls in history have had difficult, painful lives.

Many FMS and/or MPS patients who believe in reincarnation have written to me asking if they were horrible people in their previous lives. Why else would they have FMS/ MPS Complex? I spoke to Gordon-Michael Scallion, an internationally known psychic and friend, about this. He said that we may simply have wanted to understand the essence of life more thoroughly.

My friend, Paul Gallagher, the director of the Deer Mountain Taoist Academy, agrees. He said that an illness such as this can be a path to spiritual enlightenment. Your spiritual belief system can be a great emotional support to you, and a positive influence in your life and the lives of those around you. What are your spiritual beliefs? How do they help you cope with chronic illness?

Take Care of Yourself

Do you enjoy life? When was the last time you really had fun? When did you last laugh? Can you remember? Does pain interfere with your home life? With your job? Your social life? Are you hampered by negatives like self-hate? That may seem like an absurd question, but sometimes we hate ourselves for getting ill. As if we had a choice! That kind of self-hatred is a form of surrendering to the illness. Sometime we hide this feeling by allowing ourselves to be abused, or by forms of self-abuse. This can come in the guise of denying yourself appropriate medication or food, or as destructive habits, or otherwise not taking good care of yourself.

Part of taking good care of yourself is keeping accurate files with whatever data you need. You may decide to get a medic-alert bracelet, or other health aids. Check out your insurance and find out what it does and does not cover. Have an easily accessible list of your doctors' and therapists' names, addresses, and phone numbers. Write their job titles alongside their names in case someone else has to contact them for you. Keep a record of your bills and your medications. Help others to help you.

In every family, the partners bring different habits and ways of viewing the world to the relationships. Even the meanings of common words can differ enormously between partners from different cultures. When one member of the family has a long-standing health issue, it has a profound effect on the entire family. Because of the illness, a lot of time, money, and emotional energy is expended, bringing more stress to family dynamics. It is almost a form of culture shock, thrust on the entire family without any choice in the matter. You need time to adjust. You look just like everyone else, but you have special needs. You need time to establish new routines—routines that respect the realities of your situation, not that go against them.

Be Glad Now

One of my friends, a counselor, tells people not to "should" themselves. "Should" signifies expectations. Beware of implied "shoulds." "Life isn't fair." Should it be? Who said it should? How would we learn if life was always fair? The "why" of life is not always ours to control. The "how" of life is. The "how" of life often depends on the "now" of life. Learn to live in the now.

Catch yourself when you say "I will be glad when such and such happens." Will you really? For how long? Then what will you be? Would gladness now eliminate the joy when the thing that will make you happy in the future finally happens? Why not be glad now? It's more fun, and it'll take some of the pressure off tomorrow.

15

Crisis, Conflict, Communication, and Survival Skills

Letter to Those Who Do Not Have FMS and/or MPS

Having fibromyalgia (FMS) and/or Myofascial Pain Syndrome (MPS) means that many aspects of life change. Unlike the effects of cancer or accident injuries, the effects of FMS and/or MPS are invisible. Most people do not understand anything about FMS/MPS, and of those who think they do, many are actually misinformed.

In the spirit of informing those who wish to understand, these are the things that I would like you to understand about me before you judge me.

- Please understand that being sick doesn't mean I'm not still a human being. I have to spend most of my day dealing with lots of pain and considerable exhaustion, and if you visit, I probably won't seem like much fun to be with, but I'm still me stuck inside this body. I still worry about school and work and my family and friends, and most of the time I'd still like to hear you talk about your concerns, too.

- Please understand the difference between "happy" and "healthy." When you've got the flu, you probably feel miserable for a week or two, but I've been sick for years. I can't be miserable all the time; in fact, I work hard at not being miserable. So if you're talking to me and I sound happy, it means I'm happy. That's all. It doesn't mean that I'm not in a lot of pain, or extremely tired, or that I'm getting better, or any of those things. Please, don't say, "Oh, you're sounding better!" I am not sounding better, I am sounding happy. If you want to comment on that, you're welcome.

- Please understand that being able to stand up for ten minutes doesn't necessarily mean that I can stand up for twenty minutes, or an hour. Just because I managed to stand up for thirty minutes yesterday doesn't mean that I can do the same today. With a lot of diseases you're either paralyzed, or you can move. With FMS and/or MPS the issue of being able to move becomes more confusing.

- Please reread the last sentence in the paragraph above substituting "sit," "walk," "think," and "be sociable" for "move." That's what FMS and/or MPS does to you. It changes everything.

- Please understand that the effects of FMS/MPS are variable. It's quite possible that one day I may be able to walk to the park and back, and the next day I will have trouble getting to my own kitchen. Please don't attack me when I'm ill by saying, "But you did it before!" If you want me to do something, then ask me whether I can do it. For the same reason, I may need to cancel an invitation at the last minute. If this happens, please do not take it personally.

- Please understand that "getting out and doing things" does not make me feel better, and can often make me seriously worse. Telling me that I need a treadmill, or that I just need to lose (or gain) weight, get this exercise machine, join that gym, try these classes, and so forth, is not correct and may frustrate me to the point of reducing me to tears. If I was capable of doing these things, don't you know that I would? I am working with my doctor and physical therapist and I am already doing the exercise and diet that I am suppose to do.

- Another statement that hurts a lot is, "You just need to push yourself more, exercise harder." Obviously FMS and/or MPS are directly concerned with muscles, and because my muscles don't repair themselves the way your muscles do, this does far more damage than good. It could result in a single activity costing me days or weeks or months in recovery time. Also, be aware that although FMS and/or MPS may cause secondary depression, they are not caused by depression. (Wouldn't you get depressed if you were hurting and exhausted for years on end?)

- Please understand that if I say I have to sit down/lie down/take these pills now, that I do have to do that immediately. It can't be put off or forgotten just because I'm out for the day (or whatever).

- FMS/MPS does not forgive me if I don't do what I need to for my health. I pay the price in the quality of my life. At times that price may be very steep.

- If you want to suggest a cure to me, don't. It's not because I don't appreciate the thought, and it's not because I don't want to get well. It's because almost every one of my friends has suggested a "possible cure" at some point or another. At first, I tried them all but then I realized that I was using up so much energy trying things that I was making myself sicker, not better. If there was something that cured or even helped those of us with FMS and/or MPS, we'd know about it. This is not a drug-company conspiracy. There is worldwide networking (both on and off the Internet) among people with FMS/MPS. We keep up with the medical literature. If something worked we would *know* it. If, after reading that, you still want to suggest a cure, then do it, but don't expect me to rush out and try it. I'll take what you said and discuss it with my doctor.

In many ways I depend on people who are not sick. I need you to visit me when I am too sick to go out. Sometimes I may need you help me with the shopping, cooking, or cleaning. I may need you to take me to the doctor, or to the physical therapist. I need you on a different level too . . . you're my link to the outside world . . . if you don't come to visit me, then I might not get to see you at all. And, as much as it's possible, I need you to understand me.

(This letter is based on an open letter that was written by Bek Oberin. It has been modified for FMS and/or MPS and adapted from "Living with FMS" from Paula Payne's website: http://www.tidalweb.com/fms/)

Life on the Edge

People with FMS and/or MPS are often pushed to the edge by their medical conditions, and any additional factors, even "good stressors," can drive us over the brink. Anything that interrupts or disrupts sleep—injury, a new baby, illness, visitors, holidays, time changes, travel and vacations, shift work—can cause a major flare. We have this tendency to push ourselves a little too far, and then someone else comes along (either unaware or purposefully), and gives us a shove!

Dealing with Change

No matter how much you try, you can minimize change, but you can't avoid it. Change is essential to life. After any change to your schedule, resumption of adequate restorative sleep is essential as soon as possible. Don't overdo anything during times of stress. Menstruation, sudden temperature changes, and emotional strains can overload your already overloaded system. Something as minimal as the pain of having your teeth cleaned (even if topical anesthetics are used) can be enough to send you over the edge if you're already tottering.

Sometimes you can modify a change to make it less disruptive. For example, an increased immune response, which may happen during allergy season, usually means increased myofascial pain. Antihistamines will help this, so you can often minimize the impact by using them. Start adjusting to a time change (including travel times) early, a little at a time, and ease into it. Do what you can to modify all of your perpetuating factors so that the total stress impact on your life becomes as minimal as possible.

Dealing with Flares

An increase in the jerks and spasms your body produces is often a warning that your muscles are not getting sufficient oxygen, and that a flare is on the horizon. At that time,

Riding Skyhook One

When things seem out of control, it is a great relief to me to cheerfully give up whatever remnants of control I have. I call it "riding Skyhook One, with the Master at the controls." As I give up the need to be "controlling," I find I am more "in control" than ever. Dealing with a book deadline and an ever-increasing stream of correspondence has constantly threatened to put me under. I had to take a good look at my limits and my needs. No amount of "positive thinking" can enable you to handle too much input.

your muscle strength often becomes more unreliable, and objects will drop unexpectedly from your grasp. When this happens, don't panic. That will only further add to the stress on your system. Your body is talking to you. It's time for a "time-out."

Keep a journal, so that you will have a record to consult and know what to look for when flare is threatening. Get your family and friends to help you with this. If they inform you that you've put laundry detergent in the freezer, or that the chocolate drink you placed on the shelf some time ago has turned a poisonous green, then you will know that you've been operating in a fibrofog, and that a flare may be imminent.

There are times when flare can be headed off by accomplishing something simple. Cleaning out a closet or organizing something may give you a feeling of control if you have the time to devote to it. You may decide to take a virtual vacation, by meditating on a picture you have of a pleasant location. I keep a folder of interesting pictures handy for this type of mind journey. You may want to keep a small picture of your escape route on the refrigerator or some other convenient place. Just looking at it will remind you that you can escape if you but take the time.

People with FMS and/or MPS are many things, but we are never dull. I have found most of us tend to be exceptionally creative. It's a survival mechanism. We don't have the luxury of falling back on "Plan B"; we are usually halfway down the alphabet before we realize it. Use your creativity to get out of difficult situations. Don't accept the blame for your condition. Do take responsibility for optimizing it. Use "either/or" choices when confronted with too much to do.

The Art of Triage

When life becomes overwhelming, take a moment to inspect your chest carefully. Do you see a big red "S" there? Is there a red cape furling around your shoulders? No? Well, there are some things you just won't be able to do today. It's time for a reality check. Stop trying to leap tall buildings with a single bound. Be content with just "being" for a while. Give your body and mind a chance to catch up. Each of us has limited energy and time. We must each become expert in the art of "triage."

Triage is a word that came into use in emergency room settings, where patient care is prioritized by need. Learn to do this with your job list, your mail, and anything else that is piling up. Streamline your life, and educate your companions. Decide right now to simplify, delegate tasks, set limits, and pace yourself. When you are exhausted and in pain, you have less patience with the needs and desires of others. Get your own needs met, so that you can help meet the needs of the important others in your life.

Conflict

Life is not only change, it is also conflict. There are times you will be in disagreement with others. This will further heighten your already overactive "flight or fight" response. See whether you can back off from the conflict and observe what is happening. Make an assessment. There will be times when you can't win. Learn to pick your battles, and avoid wasting your energy. Try to use humor to get through difficult times. Anger is part of the stress response, and our neurotransmitters—and our stress response—can be dysfunctional and/or disproportionate to the cause. You may experience uncontrollable and even violent rages. This can be dangerous both to yourself and to those around you. If you are one of these people, you may need some medical support to help control your raging neurotransmitters.

One of the biggest sources of conflict in my life occurs when I hear or read something misleading about FMS or MPS. I am fully aware of the damage an incorrect, misleading article can do, and the pain and misery it can cause, and my first instinct is to attack any article that presents itself. I am learning how to deal with these events more constructively, however.

For example, I recently read an article that disturbed me greatly. It did have some true facts, but the rheumatologist (Bluestone 1998) who wrote it spoke as an authority, and kept mentioning "fibromyalgia trigger points." He didn't even know the difference between FMS and MPS. There were contradictory statements in the article, and the entire tone was to blame FMS and MPS on depression, stress, and downright malingering.

The article contained such quotable (by insurance lawyers) statements as "If the patient has been suffering from fibromyalgia for any length of time, there is *often* (italics added) an overlay of anxiety, depression, inappropriate drug use, and even drug-dependent problems, including distinct drug toxicity"(1998, 7). Incorrect, biased statements such as "Interestingly, cumulative physical trauma or acute sprains to the spine are *rarely seen to result in the development of fibromyalgia outside of the workers' compensation or personal injury arena*" (italics added) (1998, 11). And "Interestingly, once society rejects all such claims as valid for workmen's compensation award, the claims of such forms of chronic pain almost disappear!" (1998, 12).

The author several times indicates that he believes both fibromyalgia and chronic fatigue syndrome to be psychological, and that powerful painkillers are to be scrupulously avoided. These statements will show up in courtrooms, even though they are erroneous and biased. What will be missing is that the article appeared in *The Workers' Compensation Quarterly*.

It is almost a given that you will at some time be confronted with this sort of misleading claptrap. Remember, it is in the interests of many to keep us down. Arm yourself with information and know that there are others helping you. Think of such attacks—and they are attacks upon our credibility—as tests. Try to educate these people, and inform their employers with properly documented information that they won't get away with printing this kind of degrading article for much longer.

It has been said that the smallest support group in the world is called the "Children of Functional Families." Many of us have never learned how to communicate our feelings effectively. Lack of adequate communication is a threat to health and well-being, and it blocks our attempts to achieve harmony with those around us. There are many books that can help you communicate more effectively and can teach you conflict resolution skills. They are not a substitute for professional counseling or medical help if that is what you need, but they may help you to understand what you do need. It is necessary to *practice* these skills. They take time, perseverance, and dedication. But it is worth the effort. Learning how to communicate effectively brings wonderful rewards in its wake. (See the Advocate's Reading List after the Bibliography.)

Do You Need Counseling?

Some of us have developed the habit of using anger to block pain, frustration, loss, guilt, and other negative emotions that threatens us. This can get worse when we are faced with an overwhelming workload, overstimulation, or an excess of muscle tension. If you find this is happening to you, or if members of your family tell you this is happening to you, look into marriage and family counseling. Until you can get help, it may be wise to distance yourself from anyone you can hurt. There is help for you out there, but it's up to you to accept it. This may not be easy.

If you are constantly running into family conflicts, there is a simple exercise below that may help you get a clear picture of what is actually happening. Fill in the blanks as accurately and completely as you can, and then think about your answers. You may come to a much clearer understanding of what is really going on during these conflicts.

Exercise: Finding Out What's Really Bothering You

I. Situation: Describe the situation in one paragraph.

_____

_____

_____

_____

_____

Who is involved? Name the other people.

_____

_____

_____

What happens? What is done or not done that bothers you?

_____

_____

_____

Where does it happen? Describe the location.

_____

When does it happen? What time of day, how often, how long does it go on?

How does it happen? What are the rules it seems to follow? What are the moods involved?

Why does it happen? What are the reasons you or others give for the problem at the time it is taking place?

II. Response: Summarize what you do or don't do after the problem has subsided.

Where do I respond (or not response)?

When do I respond? What is my reaction time, what is the duration of my response?

How do I respond? What is my style, mood, degree of force or restraint?

_____

_____

How do I feel? What are my dominant emotions? Are they anger, depression, confusion, sadness, or grief?

_____

_____

_____

Why I do respond that way? What do I really think about it? What are my thoughts, theories, explanations, rationalizations?

_____

_____

_____

What do I want? What are my goals that, if accomplished, would mean that the problem is solved?

_____

_____

_____

Try to complete this exercise honestly. You don't have to show it to anyone, but it may help you to communicate with them better if you do. What have you learned by answering these questions?

Communication Skills

I wish more schools taught communication skills as formal courses. They need to be taught somewhere. Just reading a daily newspaper makes it painfully obvious that many people need to learn to communicate more effectively. Sometimes we are unaware that we aren't saying what we mean. At other times, we are not aware that we haven't listened to the other person carefully enough to truly have heard what was said. Too often, we don't know how to express our feelings and needs in a way that is nonthreatening to others. All this leads to poor communication and to a lot of unnecessary stress, which, in turn, leads to a stressful, unhealthy mode of living.

You must learn to accept that it is OK to disagree with others, and it is OK for others to disagree with you. We all need to learn how to disagree in a mature manner. Very few issues in life are "all right" or "all wrong," and differences of opinion need not mean that one person "wins" and another "loses." We can agree to disagree. If there is no "all right" and no "all wrong," there is no need to argue—or if there is still a desire to argue, it need not be a bitter fight that leaves everyone feeling bruised and ill-used.

Giving up the need to win, and learning how to think in a nondualistic mode are probably the most difficult mental tasks we can set ourselves, and they might take a lifetime to achieve. If you can learn and practice these arts, you may find that at least some of your conflicts have a way of resolving themselves. If you can learn to find ways to cooperate, and find solutions in which both parties win, everyone's life becomes much more pleasant, and much less stressful.

In *The Tao of Conversation* (Kahn 1995) the author proposes a "barn raising" method of solution-building. When my husband and I built our post-and-beam house on a hill in New Hampshire, we spent some time preparing the grounds. Once the site development and foundation were ready, our neighbors and friends gathered together and we had a house raising. The timber frames had been cut, and we manually assembled them and raised them by working together with the proper tools. We all taught, and we all learned. By the end of the day, we had the frame raised, and the roof was on and shingled. Our home will always be the better for the part that friendship played in its construction.

In the same way, you can learn to build a solution to a problem. You can't learn much if everyone around you agrees with everything you say (except perhaps that some of the people around you aren't truthful). Differences are healthy, and allow room for growth. The solution that you build with others is often more substantial than one you could build by yourself. Once you forget about "scoring points," or "winning," you can accomplish a great deal. With the single goal of "solving the problem," everyone works together. Starting with a solid foundation of a mutual goal, everyone contributes ideas until the structure of the solution takes form. The structure of debate and defensiveness gives way to collaboration, and one more problem falls before the power of collaboration.

Survival Skills

It's frustrating to have to change your clothes fifteen minutes after you put them on, because you spilled something all over them. Eating can be painful when you have bitten the inside of your cheek or your tongue since you don't always know exactly where your teeth are in relation to the rest of your mouth, due to the proprioceptor problems of MPS. It's infuriating to have to do your wash twice because you put the detergent in the rinse dispenser the first time because of fibrofog. Those of us with FMS and/or MPS go through so much grief

---

Fish Meditation

When you're in flare, or facing any stressful situation, you might find this meditation helpful. It came to me when I was snorkeling over a Grand Cayman island reef. Sometimes the greatest teachers come in the most unexpected places, and from the most unassuming sources. This meditation helped me while writing this book, and I use it when I need to go into what I call "survival mode." I enter this mode when I note that my symptoms are getting worse, and I start doing things like throwing my bath towel instead of the face cloth into the bath water. This is a clue that I am overloaded, and have to slow down and attune myself to the life force. It's time to regain the inner harmony I need to once again become an effective teacher and student in the school of life.

While snorkeling, I observed a small wrasse hovering over a coral outcropping. A wrasse is a tiny but beautiful fish; a very unassuming creature. This wrasse became

(Continued on next page)

my "Roshi," or Zen teacher. I hovered over the fish, observing. It remained nearly motionless. Every now and then a corner of a fin would flip a little, and it would return from where it had drifted. It expended the smallest amount of energy necessary to get it back over the relatively easy pickings of the reef outcrop. It ate anything edible that came its way, and took life as easy as possible.

I floated over the wrasse, essentially weightless. Every now and then I moved my hands an infinitesimal space, or angled one of my fins enough to keep me hovering over the fish and the coral reef, my arms outspread. Watching. Learning. The fish was expending the minimum amount of energy to survive. Keeping in place. Not worrying about going anywhere, not trying to be anyplace but here. The feeding was fine.

I think of that wrasse Roshi often. When I am focused on a task, I try to do my job. If I must depend on others, I try to see that their jobs get done

(Continued on next page)

and frustration that can't be categorized under ordinary, everyday "pain and fatigue." Yes, I know. You're nodding your heads as you read this. You *know* what I mean, because you've been there. But how can we get people outside the FMily to understand? How do we deal with these endless frustrations?

There are coping strategies that can dramatically improve the quality of your life. The following are the most important:

- You must deal vigorously with your perpetuating factors.

- You must get sufficient restorative sleep, adequate medication, and relaxation.

- You must understand that people with chronic pain syndromes are not victims.

- You can alter your response to pain to some degree. This takes mindwork (see Starlanyl and Copeland 1996).

- You can also minimize the frustrations of your day-to-day life.

Cultivate the art of creative problem solving. Customize tasks to your needs and style. Create no-lose situations. You may need the help of an occupational therapist to help redesign your tasks. Ask yourself these questions: What do I want? What do I need? What do I have available to help make this task easier or more enjoyable? What must I overcome to reach my goals?

Make your chores as pleasant as possible. Cultivate the healing use of music, and dance through your work. Pick the tempo to suit your needs. Lighten up. Don't become obsessive about your chores lists. The sooner you fall behind, the more time you have to catch up. Save some time by combining chores. For example, if you reuse freshly washed sheets immediately, you don't have to fold them.

Reduce clutter in your house. Give freely to the local tag and garage sales. Simplify your clothing as much as possible. Get rid of those items you no longer wear. If clothing labels irritate your skin, cut them off. Dress for comfort.

Friends: The Family You Choose

Educate your friends about FMS and MPS. Remind them that you are much more than your illness. You may find out the quality of your friendship. At first, your illness may scare your friends. They might not know what to do or say to help you. It's bad enough that we have a chronic illness, or two, or more, but to have conditions that are not well known, and with such clumsy, unwieldy names to boot! There has been more information in the popular press about fibromyalgia lately, but much of it is incorrect or incomplete. Myofascial Pain Syndrome has been completely ignored. We must change this.

Talk to Your Friends

Talk to your friends about your condition. Explain your limits quietly and carefully, but let them know that there are a lot of things you can still do. Explain that your symptoms vary, and that, on some days, you can do things that on other days you can't. Let them know early on that you may have to withdraw from planned events at the last minute due to flare.

It's OK to ask for help, and it's OK for you to say that most of the time, you don't want to talk about FMS or MPS. Have a few replies ready for the expected "But you look so good!" The director of the Portuguese FMS Association, Jaime De Lemos Revolo Pinto, has a good response to that one. He tells people, "I am not complaining about my looks!" A sense of humor can get your point across.

without my worrying or micro-managing. As long as my needs are met, I can get through the stressful times of life by doing the minimum possible to survive. You may lose a little ground when the going gets rough, but you'll get back to where you were eventually. Let yesterday, and tomorrow, take care of themselves. For now, just be.

Don't burn out your friends. You need a large support structure. Be a support for them, too. You may not be able to do a lot, but you can listen. You can be an attentive listener, and try to support and understand them when they are in need. Let them know that things have changed for you, but that you still care about them and can be a good friend. Maybe you can't go mountain biking anymore, but you can still have a good chat or take a walk together.

Accept Your Limits

Understanding and accepting your limits means not taking on too many responsibilities and knowing how to set your priorities. Let your friends know what they can do to help. Then learn to accept offered help, and to give thanks graciously.

The word "can't" has its place. But change is always possible. Be reasonable and evaluate your options. For example, I know that I can't fly, since I don't have wings. But if I purchase an airline ticket, or get on a hang glider, that changes—temporarily. With a little bit of help, many things are possible. Whenever you catch yourself saying "can't," investigate what goes around it. Place a "but" at the end of the sentence, and see how you can modify whatever it is that you "can't" do to make it possible. Optimize your options.

Don't Hold On to Resentments

Investigate forgiveness. Then invest in it. This doesn't mean you should let anyone get away with wrongdoing. It's part of our responsibility as nonvictims to take assertive control of our destiny, as much as we can, and to prevent victimization from happening to others. Having FMS and/or MPS can teach us a lot about compassion.

Understand that resentments can keep you from living your life in full color, they can keep you mired in shades of gray. You can't carry on with life when you are busy carrying a grudge. Allow your lightened and enlightened self to emerge.

Don't Spend Your Valuable Time on Negativity

You may have to drop some people from your life. Each of us has negative moments, but there are some people who make a practice of negativity, and who can never be enticed into a good humor. You can't afford to have constantly negative people draining your energy and time. You need to spend quality time with people who will nourish you and help you to feel good. This may mean some painful choices. You may decide not to spend any more time with certain friends—or relatives. Give yourself permission to do this. As the manager of your own health care team, you know what you need. And you know what you don't need.

We can move more effortlessly through life if we eliminate packaging as much as possible. Most of us can't do packaging, and much of the clutter that complicates our life is "packaging"—things that we hold on to because we or someone else feels that we should have them. We need to strip down to the essentials. Clean out the closets. Hold fast to what we really use and enjoy, and get rid of those things we believe we "should" keep but that add nothing to our lives. That size 8 dress that never fit, or the calligraphy set your aunt gave you that you don't want and can't use—send it to the tag sales, and send along any guilt that goes with them. Lighten your burdens as you travel through life.

We need to accent function. For example, most women with FMS and/or MPS need handbags that are soft and flexible, with several compartments. The strap must also be soft and flexible, or it won't stay on the shoulder. In general, we aren't going to use uncomfortable, awkward handbags. Some of us even use fanny packs instead. Ditch the ones that you don't use.

Create Winning Scenarios

Learn to give yourself choices to create winning situations. For example:

- I can't handle a big garden this year, but . . . I'd like to try some herbs and a few container plants.

- I can't stay up for a New Years' Eve party, but maybe I can get some neighborhood friends together. If we do a potluck, we can have a nice gathering without fuss.

- It's late and I can't sleep, but if I write that letter now, I'll be able to relax a little.

- I can't do everything on my job list, but if I prioritize what needs to be done, I'll be able to do the most important. The less important tasks can be put off for a while, or modified so that I can accomplish some of them sooner.

Relief from Stressors

Take a brief inventory of what you do with your time. Are you spending all of your "leisure" time doing physical therapy and otherwise coping with your illness? It takes us longer to do many tasks due to the added burden of FMS and MPS. That leaves less time for activities that make life rich and worthwhile. This is not healthy. It isn't sufficient that you can function. You must be able to maintain an adequately satisfying quality of life. You must make some time to enjoy life.

Keep resources handy that will help you to prevent stress overload. *The Daily Relaxer* is a handy book that will give you lots of good ideas to reduce stress (McKay and Fanning 1997). Learn the art of meditation. Get outside and expand your soul by spending some time in nature. If you can't get out, take nature walks in virtual reality by mentally visiting "inside" a photograph or painting. Create a "sacred space," or several spaces, where you can be mindful without distraction. Create such a space indoors, outdoors, and one within. Recognize others as people with their own problems and obstacles to overcome, and give them the benefit of the doubt. Lived mindfully, your life, or at least parts of it, can become a meditation. Don't take life for granted.

The Notion of "Ness"

One idea that helps me adapt to difficulties and to think creatively is being aware of "ness." The principle of ness is all about problem solving. People with FMS and/or MPS need creative solutions. All objects have "ness." Chairs have "chair-ness," of course, but if you stand on them to reach something, they can have "ladder-ness." If you sit on a table, then it can have "chair-ness." Function is what "ness" is all about. It's important for us to realize that many objects have many possibilities—many types of "ness." For example, one of our local group members asks for a booster chair whenever she goes to a restaurant. She uses it to prop her feet up, so that her hamstring muscles won't be compressed. She has recognized the inherent "footstool-ness" of the booster seat. Use "ness" creatively and it can make your life easier.

Pamper Yourself

Learn to pamper yourself. When something disrupts your routine, such as a storm front moving in, you may have to surrender to the disruption and not do the things you had planned to do. In such a case, don't fret about what is not getting done, use the time that has been "freed up" to take a hot bath and a nap. Keep a list of things that help you to block or detach from pain. Become aware of body movements and positions. Learn to avoid immobility, and respect pain and its consequences.

Take a Deep Breath, Settle Your Body, and Meditate

Throughout the day, be mindful of your breathing. Breathing is an automatic function, so we take it for granted. You are breathing well enough to stay alive, but that doesn't mean you are breathing *well*. Most adults use only a small portion of their lung capacity. Is your breathing deep, rhythmic, and relaxed? If it is shallow, jerky, or constricted, you need to learn better breathing habits (see Starlanyl and Copeland 1996). You need to breathe properly to get the most out of exercise, and out of life.

As you move through the day, take periodic pauses to check your body alignment (see Starlanyl and Copeland 1996). Have your shoulders crept up toward your ears? Is your head thrust forward from center? Adjust your posture during the day to give your body a chance to return to its proper alignment. Then take a meditation break.

Cloud Meditation

If clouds were seen only in specific areas, and only for a limited time, people would be willing to spend a great deal of money and effort just to catch a glimpse of this ever-changing phenomenon. Clouds are a masterpiece on the canvas of the sky. I am a scientist. I know why there are clouds. I don't understand why they are so magnificent and inspiring in their diversity and beauty. I am thankful that they go about their work with such grace and beauty that they can bring pleasure to anyone who takes the trouble to watch them.

Sometimes, when the clouds get gray and heavy, if you look far enough, there will be a patch of clear sky. A similar opening occurs on ice sheets in the far north. A little patch of clear water forms, called a polynya, that allows seals and other mammals to come up for air. The contrast of a bit of blue sky allows us to come up for air, too, sort of like God is reminding us that no matter how dark and heavy things get, the blue sky is there all the time, waiting for the clouds to do their thing and then break up. There are times when the entire sky is overcast, but once the clouds get busy and give the thirsty earth what it needs, there will be blue sky once again. We need to hang on and appreciate the beauty in the shades and shadows while we have them.

Holidays

Holidays can be the most stressful times of the year. These times may be when you discover how well you've learned to take care of yourself without feeling guilty. Too often, a time that should be joyful is heavy with stress and guilt. Be reasonable in your demands on yourself. Try to keep to your normal schedule as much as possible when it comes to eating, sleeping, and exercising. Stay within your budget.

As holidays approach, plan ahead. Whenever possible, shop by catalog, or gather or make things all year. Consider IOU presents, and gifts of nonmaterial things. Determine what causes extra stress, and be specific. Make a written list. Delete or diffuse holiday stressors. Don't take on responsibility without authority. It only leads to loss of control. Avoid late nights.

At the end of the day, make a list of what you hope to accomplish the next day. That way, you can start right in, even if you're not quite "together." It's empowering to decide that some chores can be put off until after the holidays, delegated to others, or not done at all. Think of your work list as a tool that helps you to achieve your goals. Dress for comfort when you go to holiday parties.

Take time for self-massage and mini-meditations. Ask for a massage for a present. Survive holiday "one-upsmanship," which is a major stress, *by letting them "win."* That's how you win. Just say *"No"* when necessary—and tell everybody, "Please don't visit if you have a cold." Holidays are supposed to be times of joy. Don't allow them to be times of stress. Take control. Have some fun. Fibromyalgia and/or MPS adds enough stress and frustration to our lives. It's time to slow down, look around, and enjoy the wonders of the holiday season.

Modify or combine the data sheets from chapter 7 to create "What Your Guests Should Know" and "What Your Hosts Should Know." Include specifics about meals, the importance of sleep, and information about anything that you must avoid. It is difficult to act ecstatic about a gift of perfume when you can't even tolerate the scent that is emitted from the gift box. Remember your limits. Be realistic. Eagles may soar in majestic grandeur, but house cats are seldom sucked into jet engines.

The Support Group

See if you can find a local FMS support group. If necessary, educate them about MPS. Too often, FMS support groups are places where people come to discuss how to deal with MPS—only they don't know it. Knowledge is power—and healing. Your support group can be a lifeline. As soon as you enter the room, you know that you have more in common with the strangers there than you have with many members of your own family. There is an instant understanding, and a great relief that comes with the lack of the need to explain. They *know* where you're coming from, they understand the language that you speak.

Support groups should be places of *positive* energy. Support holds you up, it doesn't drag you down. A little venting is fine, but it shouldn't be the reason for the meeting. Acceptance, information exchange, and kindness should rule. There should be ground rules of confidentiality and trust. Everyone should feel welcome, and the atmosphere should be nonjudgmental.

Find a group that is open to new ideas with compassionate people who share love and laughter. The group should reflect the members' needs and desires. In our local group, anyone can "pass" on any topic. That means that no one is under any pressure to discuss anything that he/she doesn't want to talk about. Anyone can get up and move around at any time, or even leave. Family and friends are welcome.

Avoid moan and groan clubs. There are too many of these negative groups around. Some doctors even tell their patients to stay away from support groups for this reason, but a support group does not have to be permeated with negativity. Educate them. A good support group can add a new dimension to your healing.

Also avoid groups where there is a guru with *one* idea that is the "only path" to better health. Avoid groups that won't even talk about the benefits of supportive care such as physical therapy, massage, good nutrition, and meditation.

If you can't find such a support group near your home, consider forming a self-help group with others. You may have to place an ad in the newspaper to inquire about local interest in such a group. Talk to an editor of your local newspaper. They might want to do a story on you, and on FMS and MPS. There is true joy in taking action to help others, and getting your story out.

16

Special Issues

Save us from troubled, restless sleep,
From all ill dreams your children keep;
So calm our minds that fears may cease
And rested bodies wake in peace.

—"To You Before the Close of Day"
(Sixth-century hymn)

Sleep

Often, unrestorative sleep is the first obvious manifestation of fibromyalgia (FMS), but refreshing sleep is an essential, vital part of human life. In my first book (Starlanyl and Copeland 1996), I discussed the alpha-delta sleep anomaly and described how it disrupts the deep-level sleep of those of us with FMS. The issue also has been touched upon in several chapters in this book (see chapters 1 and 3, particularly).

Disrupted sleep also can be one of the first side effects of Myofascial Pain Syndrome (MPS), when during the night, movement from changing the body's position brings pain. In addition to suffering from sleep-destroying pain, our neurotransmitters are working against us, so we must take care to avoid any preventable sleep interruptions and we must be vigilant in our efforts to get sufficient restorative sleep.

Too many doctors hold the notion that if you're in bed with your eyes closed for eight hours, that's sufficient. Not so. You need that delta sleep—that deep, *restorative* sleep—and until you get it, you are not resting properly, and as a result, you are not healing. During deep-level sleep, the neurotransmitters are regulated, and the body is repaired at a cellular level. To achieve this kind of sleep, you may need to take Benedryl, that over-the-counter sedative antihistamine that is often used for its slumber-inducing side effect.

Unfortunately, for about 25 percent of those of us with FMS, Benedryl doesn't knock us out—it gets us wired. If we take it, we are kept *awake,* with "Little Orphan Annie Eyes," all night long. If this is the case, we need to keep searching for a medication that works for us.

There are other sleep disrupting mechanisms that plague us. Some of us experience visual sensations of lights and explosions, falling sensations, and even vocalizations as we are about to fall asleep, although they can also take place when fully awake. I turned to our Internet Fibrom-l resident neurologist, David Nye, for an explanation of this. He says that these are all part of a phenomenon called "sleep starts," and can happen to anyone, especially if s/he is stressed, over-tired, or physically exhausted. People with FMS fit right into these categories, and some of us seem to experience them fairly regularly. These disturbances can be terrifying if you don't understand what they are. This also has been called "the exploding head syndrome," and one study indicates that it can be relieved by Anafranil (clomipramine) (Sachs and Svanborg 1991). You also may have night sweats, which may be worsened by some medications.

There is also the "burning feet" syndrome. This is a burning sensation that occurs on the feet, especially the bottom, and is most often noticed at night. According to Birkmayer and Riederer (1989) it may be due to a parasympathetic activation by the limbic system. As usual, FMS amplifies the sensation. Sometimes, this can be avoided by soaking your feet in cool water before going to bed. Otherwise, you may have to kick the covers off your feet to cool them down during the night.

The Cost of Shallow Sleep

Lack of restorative sleep is a major perpetuating factor that must be addressed as soon as possible, because the lack itself brings more muscular aches and even more symptoms to compound our miseries. It can get so bad that we sometimes get to the point where we are afraid to go to bed. We know that we might be facing a restless, painful night of tossing and turning with no relief in sight. We also know that, if we do fall asleep, we might be subject to bizarre and frightening dreams when our REM sleep is disrupted. We may fear that when we wake up, we will hurt more than we did when we went to bed.

In the morning, we may find that our fears were justified, when we feel as if our every muscle is rigid, and our every cell is crying out for relief. In such a state, it is sheer misery to force ourselves out of bed. The line," I feel as if I've been run over by a truck," is a typical comment on the kind of sleep those of us with FMS commonly experience.

Not only does interrupted or shallow sleep cause more muscular pain, it also hampers thinking processes. We can't afford to lose any more brain power. It is all too easy to get caught in a descending spiral. The lack of sleep worsens symptoms which then cause further lack of sleep, and so on. Too many of us spend too many waking hours in the horizontal state, because of fatigue and inadequate pain control.

It's vital that our chronic pain be addressed at once, as well as the lack of restorative sleep. Only then can we use the feeling of well-being that comes from *adequate* pain control and *adequate* restorative sleep to begin to build endurance and physical fitness. There again, we have to proceed carefully, ensuring that our trigger points are being *adequately* treated. Recovery isn't like piece work—we must treat the whole person. That's why I like the spelling "wholistic" rather than "holistic." Words are important. We've been in the "hole" long enough. Let's emphasize the "whole."

Reactive Hypoglycemia

If we start feeling sleepy at an inappropriate time, say, a few hours after a meal, reactive hypoglycemia may be the culprit, and we need to look to our diet for solutions (see the section "Reactive Hypoglycemia" in chapter 3). External sleep disrupters, such as light or noise, may prompt us to buy blackout curtains, a sleep mask, or ear plugs. We may have to bar the cats and/or dogs from the bedroom. (I admit I haven't been able to bring myself to keep my "catkids" off the bed, but it costs me.) Fibromyalgia amplifies the effects of these disrupters, and then we "work ourselves up" emotionally because we can't get back to sleep. We must remember that it is also in our power to "work ourselves down" as well, like turning a volume control on the radio. We need to do whatever it takes to help us get uninterrupted sleep.

Virtual Dreaming and Other Aids to Sleep

If you can't sleep, try virtual dreaming. What have you always wanted to do? Go to bed and "daydream" that you're doing it! You can fly, relax on an island, walk in a forest, or visit places you have always wanted to see. Sometimes the "daydreams" meld into night dreams. Read about your planned dream vacation just as though you were going there. That adds a realistic feel to your dream setting. I am often able to escape into a science fiction universe where I feel comfortable.

> **Oh to Sleep, Perchance to Dream!**
>
> Sometimes if I can't sleep I get up and take extra medication and decide to work or read until it takes effect. More often, I use meditation and prayer. I have also found imagery very beneficial. Often I will do a body scan, and see if there is an area that is painful and keeping me awake. Then I will use mindwork to ease the pain. Doing the fish meditation or visualizing myself in a space ship (two different weightless states) can be very helpful. The weightless state often feels quite realistic to me. Of course, one of these days I may wake up and find my nose rubbing against the ceiling. Anything is possible to a mystic!

There are other actions you can take to help in your quest for sleep. Avoid excessive fluids after 6 P.M. This will lessen the urinary urgency that may have you leaping up to visit the "facilities" during the night. Also, avoid stimulating activity just before bed, and don't use stimulants such as caffeine and chocolate. You may want to cut down on noise and bright lights during the hours before bedtime as well. If periodic leg movements or snoring are disrupting your sleep, do something about them. Talk with your doctor, and explain your concerns.

Try a cervical pillow, although it may be difficult to find one that fits your neck. You may have to try several to find one that fits just right. The shape you need varies with how tight the scaleni and sternocleidomastoid muscles are at any given time. Your chiropractor or physical therapist might lend you a (plastic covered) cervical pillow to try out before you buy your own. You also may want to try a water pillow. It's great to have a few choices that work for you.

Legal Evils

There are many drugs we consume in our daily lives that have all sorts of adverse effects on our health. We are not accustomed to thinking of them as drugs because they are so much a part of ordinary life. Nevertheless, caffeine, alcohol, and tobacco are drugs that come with the same kinds of side effects that heroin and crack cocaine do: tolerance, physical dependency, and unpleasant withdrawal symptoms.

Caffeine

Caffeine acts strongly on neurotransmitters. It can increase repetitive involuntary muscle twitches and restless jumpy legs. It increases acetylcholine, a neurotransmitter that can cause heart palpitations. Caffeine stimulates both urination and defecation. It can also cause the cerebral blood vessels to dilate, causing a headache. Some people have found that a small amount of caffeine helps their headaches, if their cerebral blood vessels are constricted. But, unfortunately, the body builds a tolerance to caffeine very quickly. A rebound headache frequently develops when you try to quit drinking caffeinated beverages. You have to taper off gradually to avoid or at least to minimize these headaches.

Alcohol

Alcohol can be a clear and present danger. Alcohol inhibits the N-methyl-D-aspartate (NMDA) receptor. NMDA is responsible for mediating the effects of the amino acid glutamate, the brain's most common excitatory neurotransmitter (Tsai and Coyle 1998). The net result is a slowing of activity in parts of the brain. Glutamate in large doses can even kill neurons containing glutamate receptors. If this slowdown affects the neurons controlling your muscles, the resulting physical incoordination may become unmanageable. If it affects a speech area of the brain, you will have more trouble getting out your words. If the neurons that govern the autonomic nervous system are affected, your heartbeat and breathing may be changed.

Alcohol damages the NMDA receptors in healthy people. These receptors may already be hurting due to FMS. Do you need the extra grief? I'm not saying that you should never take a drink. The risk is up to you. Just *know* what you are risking. The molecules that normally would be hard at work trying to clear your muscles of excess lactic acid (the clearance is already impaired by FMS) will be sidetracked to detoxify the alcohol instead. This will allow the lactic acid to build up, causing more muscle aches and mandatory overtime for your liver. In addition, as alcohol metabolizes, its main waste product is acetic acid. We don't need more acid. Think of the symptoms of a hangover, and remember that FMS amplifies sensations. This is a part of your life that is under your control. If it isn't, it is time to seek help.

There is a study that indicates that sensitivity to ethanol may be at least partly dependent on neurotransmitters (Masood, Wu, Brauneis, et al. 1994). This may explain why many people with FMS are so sensitive to the effects of ethanol.

Tobacco

Smoking is part of the lives of too many people with FMS and MPS. Some patients claim it helps their symptoms. There is a logical reason why this may seem so. The neurotransmitter acetylcholine has two different types of receptors. One is called a *muscarinic receptor* because the chemical muscarine has the same effect as stimulation of the parasympathetic nerves. The other type of receptor is called a *nicotinic receptor.* Nicotinic receptors are found where skeletal muscles and voluntary nerves come together. The effects of nerve stimulation on these muscles and nerves are duplicated by the potent chemical nicotine. Most cholinergic receptors at the autonomic nervous system ganglia are nicotinic receptors (the autonomic nervous system is profoundly affected in FMS). These receptors are excited and later blocked by nicotine. What this interaction causes depends on where the ganglion is located and what its function is.

Smoking is not healthy for anyone. It is logical, however, that smoking, and also the abrupt cessation thereof, will have profound effects on anyone with a neurotransmitter dysfunction such as FMS. It is a courageous and positive step to quit smoking. Take it slow and easy when you quit. Abrupt nicotine withdrawal can shock your system into FMS flare.

It makes no sense if we are using air and water filters to cut down the chemical irritants in our lives, and then deliberately suck in the concentrated pollution of cigarettes. Most of us should even avoid smoke-filled rooms. The risks, and the choices, are yours.

On the Job

Those of us who work in spite of chronic pain conditions often have to live with many job-related fears. Among these are the fear of failure, the fear of getting fired, the fear of being misunderstood by co-workers, and the fear of ridicule or pity. These fears can weigh us down. You can't change the personalities of your boss or co-workers, although you may be able to educate them. It is vital that you understand this. Don't compare yourself with other people, or focus on your failures. Instead, consider how much you've accomplished. The power of positive thinking can give you added energy. Frustration and lack of control can be destructive.

If you dread going to work, and can't "be all that you can be" on the job, it's time to assess your work and work environment. Below is a checklist from *Wellness at Work* (O'Hara 1995), which will help you to identify your workplace stressors. The author has kindly given permission to adapt it for use here.

Checklist for Work Site Stressors

Rate each of the ten stressors listed below on a scale of one to ten, one for a low-impact score, ten for a high-impact score. There are some possible variations listed under each stressor. Check those that apply to you. You may have some of your own unique variations. You can add these to the list. The purpose is to assess accurately what causes you the most stress at work. Rate stressors that have occurred anytime during the past year. Then total your score.

1. I have inharmonious work relationships, because of:
   - uncommunicative co-workers or supervisors _____
   - aggressive colleagues or customers _____
   - discordant relationship with boss _____
   - incompatibility with boss or co-workers _____

2. I have little say in the decision-making process, including such examples as:
   - responsibility without much authority _____
   - to voice my opinions or feelings would jeopardize my job _____
   - not being included in important planning meetings/decisions _____
   - my decisions are often challenged or contradicted _____

3. My job conflicts with social/family obligations because of:
   - incompatible working hours with spouse/family members _____
   - constant shift changes _____
   - change in working hours _____
   - transfer to new office/location _____

4. I have an unpleasant, relatively unsafe work environment or commute, such as:
   - work conditions with little privacy _____
   - long commute with lots of traffic _____
   - noisy or hazardous environment _____
   - uncomfortable environment; poor lighting, recycled air, no windows _____
   - physical discomfort: long hours sitting or standing _____

5. There are uncomfortable aspects about my workload such as:
   - deadline pressures _____
   - information overload _____
   - decrease in hours and/or income _____
   - too much or too little work _____

6. I am hassled or discriminated against at work due to:
   - sex, race, or age _____
   - religion, politics, or fashion _____
   - appearance, lifestyle, or values _____

7. I don't feel adequately appreciated for the work I do because of:
   - inadequate pay for amount of work _____
   - others take credit for my ideas _____
   - boss is highly critical and rarely says thank you _____

8. I do not have job security because of:

   - business reorganization—layoffs, mergers, bankruptcy _____

   - ambiguity of job description _____

   - my overqualification or underqualification for the job _____

   - highly competitive and shrinking job market _____

9. My job, or job description, has changed or is changing due to:

   - promotion _____

   - demotion _____

   - retirement _____

   - change to a different line of work _____

10. I do not feel proud or rewarded by my work because:

   - it is tedious and treated as trivial by other employees _____

   - it isn't the type of work I most want to do or isn't in my field of interest _____

   - there are conflicts with my values and beliefs _____

   - my friends/family don't respect what I do _____

Job Stress Score Rating
10–29 = Low   30–59 = Moderate   60–80 = High   81–100 = Intense

Choosing Your Battles

Review the list and categorize the stressors according to those you can change and those that you can't. Focus your time and creativity on those stressors you can change. For example, what is your contribution to a discordant relationship with the boss or incompatibility with a co-worker? Or, for another example, do you need to learn to be more assertive regarding deadline pressures or unpaid overtime work?

Under the following columns categorize these stressors as those you think you can change and those you think (or feel) you can't change.

Stressors I Can Change   **Stressors I Cannot Change**

_____   _____

_____   _____

_____   _____

_____   _____

_____   _____

Are some of your stressors ones that you cannot realistically change? For example, a long commute with lots of traffic, working hours incompatible with your spouse's, or a hazardous work environment may be beyond your ability to change. Acknowledge those stressors you can't do anything about and "let go" or reconcile yourself to this lack of control. This is a challenging task, and perhaps a lifelong project, but there are skills you can learn in order to let go more easily.

Fear of Being Known as Having FMS and/or MPS

You may be afraid to talk to your employer about FMS and/or MPS. Those people who are maintaining regular jobs in spite of having FMS and MPS rarely make the news. Many employers, if they have heard of FMS or MPS at all, view these conditions only in terms of costs. If you love your job and the challenges it presents, and don't come home at the end of the day too tired to eat (or even to make dinner), there are ways to relieve your worries about job security. Even if you're totally tired and exhausted after work, but you still love your job, perhaps you will be able to work part-time with the same employer. Perhaps you can find a less demanding job.

In most states it is illegal for an employer to fire a person because of illness or disability. Personal issues such as lateness, lack of productivity, attitude, or time off, however, are legitimate causes for dismissal. It can be difficult to prove that your frequent absenteeism is due to a chronic disability. You may want to take the following precautions.

Explain your illness to your employer. Talk about what changes it might make in your job, and what you both can do to make work a healthier and happier place. Follow this up with a written agreement or memo signed by the two of you. Be honest and realistic about your limits, and about the variability of your symptoms. Specify any needed modifications. Explain the dangers of immobility and other perpetuating factors. Some work changes that you need may be relatively easy, such as substituting a track ball or similar user-friendly apparatus for a computer mouse. Be sure that what you ask for will actually help. I tried a touch pad instead of a mouse, and found that I lacked the fine motor control it required. It only added frustration to my work procedures. You want changes that will work *for* you.

Many companies have Employee Assistance Programs. These include counseling and help with handling stress, including marriage and family counseling. The fitness and wellness programs some companies have may not be suitable for people with FMS and MPS. See what's available in your company disability plan.

A lot depends on the work relationships you already have. It's up to you to decide what to tell co-workers. They may resent it if you aren't carrying "your share" of the work load. On the other hand, you might view this disclosure as an opportunity to educate them about FMS and MPS. Be sure to stress the variability of your symptoms.

The Americans with Disabilities Act

If your employer has at least fifteen employees, you are covered by the Americans with Disabilities Act. The ADA prohibits discrimination in all employment practices, including job application procedures, training, hiring, firing, advancement, compensation, and other terms, conditions, and privileges of employment. The ADA applies to persons with substantial, as distinct from minor, impairments. These include impairments that limit major life activities such as seeing, hearing, speaking, walking, breathing, performing manual tasks, learning, caring for oneself, and working. The ADA also covers institutions of higher learning, and includes your right to a convenient parking space (see chapter 11 for a more extended discussion of the ADA).

A qualified individual has the skill, experience, education or other requirements of a position that he or she holds or seeks, and who can perform the "essential functions" of the position *with* or *without* reasonable accommodations. Do you fit this category? You may wish to consult an occupational therapist to verify this.

Pregnancy

Pregnancy is a challenge for women in the best of health. For women with FMS and MPS, there are many added stressors. Some women have told me that their FMS symptoms got better with pregnancy, but their MPS symptoms got worse, especially during the last trimester and after delivery. Other women have reported that their FMS went into remission for most of the pregnancy, but returned in the last few months with headaches, depression, and pain.

Recent studies have shown that trigger point injections during delivery (even with epidural anesthesia) can prevent a lot of pain later (Tsen and Camann 1997). These injections are similar to the trigger point injections that can be made in surgical incision areas.

In FMS, hormone fluctuations may increase in women, due to another imbalance in the body, called the HPA-gonadal axis. Some pregnant women developed toxemia and diabetes, and had to be put on strict bed rest, which worsened their MPS. One woman with FMS, carried her babies for ten months—in two separate pregnancies. I have heard reports of five other women who experienced ten-month pregnancies. Some women have told me that they craved protein during their pregnancies, but their protein levels always remained low in spite of their increased intake of protein.

Worsening reflux can be an aggravation during pregnancy, especially when coupled with morning sickness. Pregnant women have reported more joint pains when sleeping, mostly in the shoulders, hips, and knees. Some have reported worsened insomnia and nighttime leg cramps. Benedryl is one of the few sleep medications available for pregnant women, and the normal pain relievers may not be advisable during pregnancy. Flexeril may be helpful. Discuss the options with your doctor. It is also vital to ensure adequate vitamin and mineral intake.

Sleeping in the fetal position, with the legs drawn up, can perpetuate the iliopsoas trigger points. Back pain caused by the psoas muscles is common in pregnancy. A small pillow under the knees when sleeping on your back, or between the knees when lying on your side, will help.

Change Is Inevitable—Except from a Vending Machine

It's hard for anyone to accept change. It took a long time, but I've finally accepted that I cannot function as an Emergency Room physician. Many days I can't keep my shoes tied, and I usually have difficulty managing buttons. Even though my ER days are over, God has provided a chance for me to touch many hearts. I feel blessed. There is always a path for you. If you are in the job market, I recommend *Job-Hunting Tips for the So-Called Handicapped or People Who Have Disabilities* (Bolles 1992).

If you are pregnant, you may find that you have less endurance and more heart palpitations. To exercise, walk on level surfaces, avoid hills and stairs, and take frequent rests. Check out those trigger points. I've had two reports of immune problems during the first four months of pregnancy, with one sickness after the other. I've also heard about supersensitivity to odors, noises, and heat. A few women have reported trigger points that seemed to result after episodes of strong kicking by the fetus they held within.

One woman had a complication with prolonged pushing while squatting during labor. She developed cramps in her leg, and after delivery, when the epidural wore off, her shin was painful and she couldn't wiggle her toes. She developed a visible, painful knot on her shin. Tests for blood clots or bone damage were negative, but her doctor didn't treat her for trigger points. She developed a profound limp and foot-drop. Eleven days later, she was sent to the Emergency Room and had three muscles removed and a tendon transfer due to anterior compartment syndrome. Her recovery will take months. Her story might have been different if she had had prompt treatment for tibialis anterior trigger points. We must demand that doctors become educated about FMS and MPS.

In every case of a pregnant woman with FMS and/or MPS that I know about, the mothers delivered healthy babies. They do need as much help as they can get to cope with their infants, however. Any new baby provides a study in sleep deprivation for its mother. Furthermore, all the usual FMS/MPS medications get into breast milk, so it's very difficult for the new mother to breast-feed.

Recent studies (Thomas and Palmiter 1997b) with mice indicate that the lack of the neurotransmitters norepinephrine and epinephrine causes deficits in the maternal nurturing instinct. This, coupled with mood swings and uncontrolled irritability, could lead to disaster. *If you are a new mother and feel that you lack the desire and patience needed to adequately tend your infant, please talk to your doctor without delay.*

Menopause

Some women find that menopause makes FMS much worse. Further sleep disruption seems to be one of the worst side effects. Before menopause, the hormonal balances of a woman with FMS wobble the way a top does before it stops. When menopause arrives, it can play havoc with the already dysregulated HPA-gonadal axis, and put a woman with FMS on an emotional roller coaster that is no fun at all. FMS menopausal women tend to get *intense* hot flashes, which may be resolved with hormone replacement therapy. Remind your doctor that sensations are often amplified by FMS. The heat is severe and sudden, and sometimes may be modified with ice. I had killer hot flashes that woke me up about twenty times a night.

Here, I want to clear up a misconception. Guaifenesin therapy will not worsen menopausal hot flashes—but FMS will, dramatically. The hypothalamus "thermostat" is already off, and the FMS pain amplification and hypersensitized central nervous system can cause extreme symptoms. Menopause can even serve as a trigger for the FMS neurotransmitter cascade.

Excess sweating may be somewhat helped by soaking in Epsom salts baths. The sweat may turn your sheets dark. It is important to get the sweat off your skin, because it can promote severe itching. I believe this to be a result of hyperacidity and the toxic FMS state. (See

"New and Experimental Treatments" and "Guaifenesin" in chapter 9; and "The Alternate Tryptophan Pathway" in chapter 5.)

The Elderly

As the years go by, we tend to develop more trigger points, so as elderly folks we often restrict our movements to avoid pain. I believe that a lot of symptoms we call "old age" might be from tightened constricted myofascia caused by trigger points.

If we treated trigger points and FMS, some of the symptoms of some of our senior citizens might be eased. Circulation could be improved and cognitive impairments diminished. Many of our elderly are polydrug users. With appropriate attention to perpetuating factors, we might be able to lessen the amounts of medication needed to control their symptoms. It is important to evaluate thoroughly all medications and their side effects periodically.

Many of the elderly experience chronic pain that impairs their functioning, and yet they receive inadequate pain management (Gagliese and Melzack 1997; Nikolaus 1997). This pain often lessens their activity level, which encourages the downward spiral of their health. Pain is not a normal sign of aging. You don't "have to live with it"! Doctors must be educated in the methodology of prescribing for the elderly, because many metabolic changes take place as we age (Gloth 1996). It is your *right* to have a doctor who understand your needs.

Children with FMS and MPS

All the indications are the sooner emerging FMS and/or MPS are identified and properly treated, the less likely it is that a full-blown case will develop (Buskila, Neuman, Herschman, et al. 1995). It is often easy to head off sleep disruption as it first begins, if you recognize it promptly. You can look for perpetuating factors. If you find an early sleep disturbance, for example, you can talk to your pediatrician about Benedryl, and encourage your child to develop regular bedtime habits. Children often don't know what is happening to them if they have FMS and/or MPS, however, and it is important that you encourage them to talk to you about how they feel, especially if FMS and MPS are in the family.

MPS is caused by mechanical breakdowns, but physical traits that perpetuate trigger points, such as short upper arms, run in families. There are studies that indicate that the tendency to develop FMS is genetic (Pellegrino, Waylonis and Sommer 1989).

FMS and MPS can occur at any age. There are specific trigger points that Travell and Simons found to be common in children. I've identified these in my video (see Resources). There are preventative measures that can be taken. For example, you can ensure that a child's legs are supported by a footrest on a highchair, rather than allowing the child's legs to dangle.

Children, even infants, can feel pain. Because young children can't advocate for themselves, you must advocate for them. "Growing pains" are not normal. If your child has achy muscles, try a gentle massage. Check for trigger points. Don't stop your efforts until your child receives adequate pain relief and restorative sleep.

You may want to write a specific data sheet for your child's teacher, babysitter, or daycare worker. Of necessity, this must be specific to your child. Emphasize your availability to answer questions. Include your phone number and the times you can be reached. Let them know that your child's hesitance may be due to pain, confusion, or other FMS or MPS symptoms. Take your child's symptoms one at a time, and consider how each symptom might have an impact on your child in the setting for which you are preparing the data sheet.

Go through the self-diagnostic test (Appendix A), and use it as a guide to explain in simple terms what your child's caretaker needs to know. It's important that s/he knows what works best for your child when there is pain. It's also important that your child not be classified as a behavior problem, or as a "slow student," simply because of FMS or MPS symptoms.

Your pediatrician should be familiar with the concepts of FMS and MPS. S/he should not dismiss your child's aches as "growing pains," but should actively be searching for and eliminating perpetuating factors. Use the data sheet and pick out the relevant titles from the Reference and Bibliography sections for everyone on the child's medical team.

Post-Traumatic Hyperirritability Syndrome (PTHS)

In a very small section of my last book (Starlanyl and Copeland 1996), I mentioned what Travell and Simons call Post-Traumatic Hyperirritability Syndrome (PTHS). They gave it less than a page in Volume II of their *Trigger Point Manuals* (1992, 545). What a world of pain and despair lies within those few lines. I have received phone calls from people who had become isolated from their families because they had become supersensitive to nearly everything. Often their condition started with simple FMS or MPS, but due to lack of proper treatment/ diagnosis or attention to perpetuating factors, they developed sensitivity after sensitivity until their hypersensitive nervous systems rejected almost everything in their environment. Frequently, there were very few foods that they could tolerate. Their restricted diet furthered their metabolic imbalances. They were often unable to take any medications, which made their pain and sleep problems worsen.

These people not only have severe hyperalgesia, or enhanced pain, but they often have severe allodynia (see chapter 5). This means that stimuli that normally would be nonpainful, such as a breeze or an odor, will cause pain. The slightest fall or minor bump can worsen the condition for a long time. Even moderate stress or exercise can intensify the pain.

It is no easy task to unravel PTHS perpetuating factors, and great care must be taken to gently defuse the trigger points. There are doctors who specialize in multiple chemical sensitivity, and often they must do their best to minimize irritants and gently lead these sorely tried individuals onto a path of healing. I have no easy answers for PTHS. I do urge people with PTHS to deal with individual symptoms and perpetuating factors, and to seek compassionate and educated medical guidance.

In Conclusion

At first, trying to develop a healing program as well as advocating for yourself may seem like a twenty-four-hour-a-day job. It may seem as if there is not enough time left to work, let alone to have a life! But, as you gain exercise skills, stretching will become second nature, as will balancing your diet. As you regain harmony, you will get more energy, and the fibrofog will lift. Life will brighten.

Take heart when reading the Reference and Bibliography sections. Use those articles, and the data sheets in chapter 7, to convince your medical team that your symptoms are real. Today, medical teams are doing research on FMS and/or MPS all over the world. Every day brings new discoveries. Each time we help to educate a doctor, scientist, or nurse we are enlisting one more mind that may contribute answers we need. We know more than we did yesterday, and much less than we will tomorrow. We still don't have a cure for FMS or MPS, but we have come very far. The view is getting better with every step!

PART V

Arm Yourself with Documented Information

Part V is a vital and important part of this book. Appendix A provides a self-diagnostic test for trigger points. Appendix B is offered in the hope that this AMA-approved policy statement on the use of opioids will help you to obtain adequate pain medication. Appendix C gives you the opportunity to advocate for all of us with FMS/MPS without having to leave the comfort of your home. And Appendix D is intended to aid in your efforts to obtain disability benefits.

The References, Bibliography, and Advocate's Reading List are the basic tools you need to enhance the quality of your interactions with the medical profession. If you should meet someone who tells you that either FMS and/or MPS "Is All In Your Head," here are the documents to refute that statement. Here, too, is information that will help you find the newest and best treatments. The names of some of the medical journals may seem formidable at first, but if you take the time to read the titles of the journal articles, the chances are good that you will find information that will really help you in your quest for better health and a happier life.

APPENDIX A

Self-Diagnostic Guide to Trigger Points

The following list is a self-diagnostic guide to help you isolate those of your symptoms that may be coming from fibromyalgia (FMS) or coexisting with it, those that could be caused by Myofascial Pain Syndrome (MPS) trigger points, and those that may be due to reactive hypoglycemia. This list is by no means complete, nor does it indicate that these symptoms are caused by these conditions.

It isn't unusual to have both trigger points (TrPs) and FMS contributing to one symptom—sometimes with the addition of reactive hypoglycemia (RHG). Furthermore, some of your symptoms may be caused by the side effects of medications. There are other medical conditions that can cause some of these symptoms as well. This guide will, however, indicate whether there is a pattern. For example, if you have ten symptoms indicating possible TrPs, you have a greater likelihood of having other symptoms also caused by TrPs, and a good possibility of having MPS. Visual locations of TrPs and their reference zones can be seen in the video "Chronic Myofascial Pain Syndrome: The Trigger Point Guide" (see Resources).

Key to Understanding the Self-Diagnostic Guide

"(FMS)" indicates that the preceding symptom often accompanies fibromyalgia. "(H)" indicates that reactive hypoglycemia may contribute to the symptom. The Latin-derived names of the muscles in brackets [ ] indicate the *most likely sites* for myofascial trigger points (TrPs) that could cause the symptom. The symptoms are listed in boldface type, but by design, they are not in any particular order. There may be a variety of causes for every symptom, and there are many ways of categorizing the symptoms. I do not wish to imply connections where there may not be any, nor, by separating symptoms, to exclude them where they may exist. Each of us is different and our patterns of symptoms may be different.

Symptom List and Possible Causes

childhood growing pains: [early TrPs]

FMS/MPS sinus syndrome: ("traveling" nocturnal stuffiness) [pterygoid, sternocleidomastoid, posterior digastric]

allergies: (FMS)

post nasal drip: (FMS), [pterygoid, sternocleidomastoid]

drooling in sleep: [internal medial pterygoid]

swollen glands: [digastric]

difficulty swallowing: [digastric, pterygoid]

dry cough: [lower end sternal sternocleidomastoid]

TMJ symptoms: [masseter, trapezius, temporalis, pterygoid]

dizziness when turning head fast or changing field of view: [sternocleidomastoid], (H), Medications

runny nose: (FMS), [sternocleidomastoid, pterygoid]

sore throat: [sternocleidomastoid, digastric, pterygoid]

stiff neck: [levator scapulae]

mold/yeast sensitivity: (FMS), (H)

reflux esophagitis: [external oblique], (H)

headaches/migraines: (FMS), [trapezius, sternocleidomastoid, temporalis, splenii, suboccipital, semispinalis capitis, frontalis, zygomaticus major, cutaneous facial, posterior cervical], (H)

light and/or broken sleep pattern with unrefreshing sleep (possible alpha-delta sleep anomaly): (FMS)

sweats: (FMS), (H), Medications

morning stiffness: (FMS), [multiple TrPs]

fatigue: (FMS), [multiple TrPs], (H), Medications

shortness of breath: (FMS), [serratus anterior, diaphragm, other respiratory muscle TrPs], (H)

painful weak grip that sometimes lets go: [infraspinatus, scaleni, hand extensors, brachioradialis]

hypoglycemic symptoms: (FMS), (H)

menstrual problems and/or pelvic pain: (FMS), [coccygeus, levator ani, obturator internus, high adductor magnus, abdominal obliques]

PMS: (FMS)

loss of libido: (FMS), Medications

low back pain: [quadratus lumborum, thoracolumbar paraspinals, longissimus, ilicostalis, multifidi, rectis abdominis]

nail ridges and/or nails that curve under: (FMS)

difficulty speaking known words: (FMS), (H)

directional disorientation: (FMS), (H)

visual perception problems: [sternocleidomastoid], (H)

tearing/reddening of eye, drooping of eyelid: [upper sternal sternocleidomastoid]

loss of ability to distinguish some shades of colors: (FMS)

short-term memory impairment: (FMS), (H)

weight gain/loss: (FMS), (H), Medications

sensitivity to odors: (FMS)

mitral valve prolapse: (FMS)

double/blurry/changing vision: [internal eye muscles, temporalis, sternocleidomastoid, trapezius, cutaneous facial, splenius cervicis]

visual and audio effects/falling sensations before sleep (called "sleep starts"): (FMS)

earaches/ringing/itch: (FMS), [SCM, masseter, pterygoid], Medications

unexplained toothaches: [temporalis, masseter, digastric]

rapid/fluttery/irregular heartbeat/heart attack-like pain: (FMS), [sternalis, pectoralis], (H)

bloating/nausea/abdominal cramps: (FMS), [abdominals, multifidi, iliocostalis, paraxiphoid rectus abdominus, quadratus lumborum, upper thoracic paraspinals], (H) [Note: for excessive gas and belching, check for TrP at angle of 12th rib, either side.]

appendicitis-like pains: [iliopsoas, rectus abdominis, piriformis, iliocostalis]

carbohydrate/chocolate cravings: (FMS), (H)

sensitivity to cold/heat/humidity/pressure changes/light/wind: (FMS)

abdominal cramps, colic: [periumbilical rectus abdominus]

panic attacks: (FMS), (H)

mottled skin: (FMS)

depression: (FMS), (H), Medications

confusional states: (FMS), (H), Medications

thumb pain and tingling numbness: [brachialis entrapment of radial nerve, adductor pollicus]

urine retention: [upper public, inguinal ligament, lower internal oblique and lower rectus abdominus TrPs]

tendency to cry easily: (FMS), (H)

night driving difficulty: (FMS)

weak ankles: [peroneus, tibialis]

lax, pendulus abdomen: [abdominal TrPs, especially rectus abdominus]

upper/lower leg cramps: [sartorius, gastrocnemius]

tight Achilles tendons: [tibialis posterior]

groin pain: [adductores longus and brevis, iliopsoas]

irritable bowel: (FMS), [pelvic TrPs, multifidi, high adductor magnus, abdominal obliques], (H)

sciatica: [thoracolumbar paraspinals, gluteus minimus, hamstrings, piriformis, iliopsoas]

urinary frequency: (FMS), [cutaneous and myofascial lower abdominal TrPs]

impotence: (FMS), [piriformis pudendal nerve entrapment]

stress incontinence, anal/genital/perineal pain: [pelvic floor TrPs, high adductor magnus, piriformis, paraspinals]

painful intercourse: [vaginal TrPs, pelvic floor TrPs, piriformis pudendal nerve entrapment]

muscle twitching: (FMS), [local TrPs]

numbness and tingling: [nerve entrapment by TrPs]

diffuse swelling: (FMS), [vascular entrapment by TrPs]

hypersensitive nipples/breast pain: [pectoralis]

fibrocystic breasts: (FMS), [possible ductile entrapments by TrPs]

buckling knee: [vastus medialis, quadriceps, adductor longus]

problems climbing stairs: [sartorius, quadriceps femoris, vastus medialis]

problems going down stairs: [popliteus]

free-floating anxiety: (FMS), (H), Medications

mood swings: (FMS), (H), Medications

unaccountable irritability: (FMS), (H)

trouble concentrating: (FMS), (H), Medications

shin splint-type pain: [peroneus, tibialis]

heel pain: [soleus, quadratus plantae, abductor hallucis, tibialis posterior]

sensory overload: (FMS), (H)

handwriting difficulties: [adductor/opponens pollicis]

sore spot on top of head: [splenius capitis, sternocleidomastoid]

problems holding arms up (as when folding sheets): [subscapularis, infraspinatus, supraspinatus, upper trapezius, levator scapulae]

"fugue"-type states (staring into space before brain can function): (FMS), (H)

tight hamstrings: [hamstring complex, adductor magnus, quadriceps femoris, iliopsoas, gastrocnemius]

numbness/tingling on the outer thigh (meralgia paresthetica): [quadriceps femoris, vastus lateralis, sartorius, tensor fascia latae entrapment]

carpal tunnel-like pain in wrist (watchband area): [subscapularis]

balance problems/staggering gait: [sternocleidomastoid, gluteus minimus], (H), Medications

restless leg syndrome: [gastrocnemius, soleus]

myoclonus (muscle movements and jerks at night): (FMS), [local TrPs]

feeling continued movement in car after stopping: [sternocleidomastoid]

feeling tilted when cornering in car: [sternocleidomastoid]

first steps in the morning feel as if walking on nails: [long flexors of toes, tibialis posterior]

pressure of eyeglasses or headbands is painful: [head, neck, and shoulder TrPs]

thick secretions: (FMS)

bruise/scar easily: (FMS)

some stripes and checks cause dizziness: [sternocleidomastoid]

bruxism (teeth grinding): (FMS), [digastric, masseter, soleus]

inability to recognize familiar surroundings: (FMS), (H)

delayed reactions to "overdoing it": (FMS)

family clustering (other members of the family have FMS): (FMS)

tissue overgrowth (fibroids, ingrown hairs, heavy and splitting cuticles, adhesions): (FMS)

Suggestions for Dealing with FMS and MPS

You must first deal with any perpetuating factors.

For reactive hypoglycemia, each snack and meal must be balanced with protein, carbohydrates and fat in a 30/40/30 ratio as per *Mastering the Zone* (Sears 1997b).

For specific trigger points find what combination of therapies works for you.

Gentle stretch, "Spray and Stretch," tennis-ball compression, acupressure massage, gentle nonrepetitive exercise such as Qi gong (Chi kung) are among your choices.

- Use ice if there is nerve entrapment pain/muscle tightness.

- Use galvanic muscle stimulation and/or craniosacral or myofascial release to break up TrPs. Consider TrP injections if available.

- Use heat to ease muscle pain and pay attention to body mechanics.

- Use warm saltwater as nose drops before bed if needed to ease throat and neck TrPs.

- Climb steps at 45 degree angle if needed to avoid loading the TrPs on the front of the thigh.

- Use a triple-folded hand towel pinned as a collar splint before riding over bumpy roads if sternocleidomastoid TrPs are a problem.

- Use pillows under knees (or between knees if you sleep on your side) during the night to ease strain on hips in cases of sciatica.

- Eye exercises are beneficial when the muscles around the eye are suspected of holding TrPs.

- Use a wrist rest for computer work, and Hand-eze supports (Starlanyl and Copeland 1996) for handwriting pain and keyboarding strain.

- Use Travell modified shoe insert as per the *Trigger Point Manual, Vol. II* (1992) or *The Survival Manual* (Starlanyl and Copeland 1996).

- The use of flexible shoes with good support will aid balancing problems.

- Avoid restrictive clothing.

APPENDIX B

Public Policy Statements from the American Society of Addiction Medicine

Adopted by the ASAM Board of Directors, April 1997

I. Public Policy Statement on Definitions Related to the Use of Opioids in Pain Treatment

Background

Opioid medications have an important role in the treatment of acute pain and cancer-related pain, and they are sometimes helpful as a component of the management of intractable pain of noncancer origin. However, a number of issues of clinical concern may arise in the course of opioid therapy of pain. Physical dependence on opioids may occur under certain circumstances. Some individuals may develop addiction in association with the prolonged use of opioids.

The clinical implications and appropriate management of physical dependence, tolerance, and addiction differ. It is therefore important that clear definitions be established to facilitate identification and appropriate management of these occurrences.

The standard DSM IV criteria for diagnosis of psychoactive substance use disorder cannot be used reliably to diagnose addiction in the presence of opioids prescribed for the treatment of pain. Many of the DSM IV criteria defining addiction refer either to physical dependency or tolerance which are physiological and expected with the long-term opioid use (criteria 1 and 2), or to other occurrences which may be normal and expected in the course of opioid therapy of chronic pain (criteria 3 and 4). If DSM IV criteria are considered in diagnosing addiction in the context of pain treatment, only those criteria which reflect addictive behaviors (criteria 5, 6, and 7), rather than the physiologic phenomena of physical dependency and tolerance, should be used in formulating the diagnosis.

Recommendations

The American Society of Addiction Medicine recognizes the following definitions as appropriate and clinically useful definitions and recommends their use when assessing the use of opioids in the context of pain treatment.

Physical Dependence

Physical dependence on an opioid is a physiologic state in which abrupt cessation of the opioid, or administration of an opioid antagonist, results in a withdrawal syndrome. Physical dependency on opioids is an expected occurrence in all individuals in the presence of continuous use of opioids for therapeutic or for nontherapeutic purposes. It does not, in and of itself, imply addiction.

Tolerance

Tolerance is a form of neuroadaptation to the effects of chronically administered opioids (or other medications), which is indicated by the need for increasing or more frequent doses of the medication to achieve the initial effects of the drug. Tolerance may occur both to the analgesic effects of opioids and to some of the unwanted side effects, such as respiratory depression, sedation, or nausea. The occurrence of tolerance is variable, but it does not, in and of itself, imply addiction.

Addiction

Addiction in the context of pain treatment with opioids is characterized by a persistent pattern of dysfunctional opioid use that may involve any or all of the following:

- adverse consequences associated with the use of opioids
- loss of control over the use of opioids
- preoccupation with obtaining opioids, despite the presence of adequate analgesia

These consequences may be accompanied by distortions in thought, chiefly denial, and a tendency to relapse, once in recovery.

Adverse consequences suggestive of addiction in the context of pain treatment with opioids may include persistent oversedation or euphoria, deteriorating level of function despite relief of pain, or increase in pain-associated distresses such as anxiety, sleep disturbances, or depressive symptoms. Common and expected side effects of the medications, such as constipation, should not be interpreted as adverse consequences in this context. Loss of control over use might be reflected in prescriptions used up before the expected renewal time, obtaining multiple prescriptions, or using street sources of opioids or other drugs. Preoccupation with opioid use may be reflected in noncompliance with nonopioid components of pain treatment, inability to recognize nonphysical components of pain, and the perception that no interventions other than opioids have any impact on pain whatsoever.

Individuals who have severe, unrelieved pain may become intensely focused on finding relief for their pain. Sometimes such patients may appear to observers to be preoccupied with obtaining opioids, but the preoccupation is with finding relief of pain, rather than with using opioids per se. This phenomenon has been termed "pseudoaddiction" in the pain literature. Such therapeutic preoccupation can be distinguished from true addiction by observing that when effective analgesia is obtained, using either opioids or other pain treatment interventions, the previous behavior, which might have suggested addiction, resolves. If opioids are used for pain treatment, the patient does not use these in a manner which persistently causes sedation or euphoria, level of function is increased rather than decreased, and medications are used as prescribed without loss of control over use.

From http://www.asam.org/asam50.htm, website of American Society of Addiction Medicine

II. Public Policy Statement on the Rights and Responsibilities of Physicians in the Use of Opioids for the Treatment of Pain

Adopted by the ASAM Board of Directors, April 1997.
Reprinted with permission American Society for Addiction Medicine, February 2, 1998.

Background

Physicians' concerns regarding possible legal, regulatory, licensing or other third party sanctions related to the prescription of opioids contribute significantly to the undertreatment of pain.

Physicians are obligated to relieve pain and suffering in their patients. Though many types of pain are best addressed by nonopioid interventions, opioids are often required as a component of effective pain treatment. In patients complaining of pain, which is a subjective phenomenon, it is often a difficult medical judgment as to whether opioid therapy is indicated.

This may be a particularly difficult judgment in patients with concurrent addictive disorders for whom exposure to potentially intoxicating substances may present special risks. It is, nonetheless, a medical judgment which must be made by a physician in the context of the doctor-patient relationship based on knowledge of the patient, awareness of the patient's medical and psychiatric conditions, and on observation of the patient's response to treatment. The selection of a particular opioid medication(s), and the determination of opioid dose and therapeutic schedule, similarly must be based on full clinical understanding of a particular situation and cannot be judged appropriate or inappropriate independent of such knowledge.

Despite appropriate medical practice, physicians who prescribe opioids for pain may occasionally be misled by skillful patients who wish to obtain medications for purposes other than pain treatment, such as diversion for profit, recreational abuse, or maintenance of an addicted state. The physician who is never duped by such patients may be denying appropriate relief to patients with significant pain all too often. It must be recognized that physicians who are willing to provide compassionate, ongoing medical care to challenging, psychosocially stressed patients may more often be faced with deception than physicians who decline to treat this difficult population.

Addiction to opioids may occur in the course of opioid therapy of pain in susceptible individuals under some conditions. Persistent failure to recognize and provide appropriate medical treatment for the disease of addiction is poor medical practice and may become grounds for practice concern. Similarly, persistent failure to use opioids effectively when they are indicated for the treatment of pain is poor medical practice and may also become grounds for practice concern. It is important to distinguish, however, between physicians who profit from diversion or other illegal prescribing activities and physicians who may inappropriately prescribe opioids due to misunderstandings regarding addiction or pain.

Physicians traditionally have received little or no education on addiction or clinical pain treatment in the course of medical training. This omission is likely a basis for inadequate detection and management of addiction and inadequate assessment and treatment of pain.

Recommendations

1. Physicians who prescribe opioids for the treatment of pain should use reasonable medical judgment to establish that a pain state exists and to determine whether opioids are an indicated component of treatment. Opioids should be prescribed in a legal and clinically sound manner, and patients should be followed at reasonable intervals for ongoing medical management and to confirm as nearly as is reasonable that the medications are used as prescribed. Such management should be appropriately documented.

2. Physicians who are practicing medicine in good faith and who use reasonable medical judgment regarding the prescription of opioids for the treatment of pain should not be held responsible for the willful and deceptive behavior of patients who successfully obtain opioids for nonmedical purposes. It is the appropriate role of the DEA, pharmacy boards and other regulatory agencies to inform physicians of the behavior of such patients when it is detected.

3. Physicians who consistently fail to recognize addictive disorders in their patients should be offered education, not sanction, as a first intervention.

4. Physicians who consistently fail to appropriately evaluate and treat pain in their patients should be offered education as a first-line intervention.

5. For the purpose of performing regulatory, legal, quality assurance and other clinical case reviews, it should be recognized that judgment regarding a) the medical appropriateness of the prescription of opioids for pain in a specific context, b) the selection of a particular opioid drug or drugs, and c) the determination of indicated opioid dosage and interval of medication administration can only be made properly with full and detailed understanding of a particular clinical case.

6. Regulatory, legal, quality assurance, and other reviews of clinical cases involving the use of opioids for the treatment of pain should be performed, when they are

indicated, by reviewers with a requisite level of understanding of pain medicine and addiction medicine.

7. Appropriate education in addiction medicine and pain medicine should be provided as part of the core curriculum at all medical schools.

8. Legal and/or licensing actions against physicians who are proven to profit from diversion of scheduled drugs or from other illegal prescribing activities are appropriate.

APPENDIX C

The FMS/MPS Petition

It is not sufficient to find enlightenment. You must then use what you have learned. One of the best ways to advocate is to work toward mandated training of medical school students in the diagnosis and treatment of FMS and MPS. This petition was designed for Joy Wu's website. To add your name to the FMS/MPS petition, mail to:

FibroWorld
P.O. Box 61924
Harrisburg, PA 17106-1924

Please include your

Name:

_____

Address:
City, State, and ZIP or Province/Territory, etc.

_____

_____

Country (if outside of the USA)

_____

Other Optional Information:

How many years have you have suffered with FMS, or been a significant other/caretaker/supporter:

_____

_____

If you are disabled or impaired from FMS:

_____

_____

Your occupation or former occupation:

_____

Any note or letter to Congress concerning your quality of life with FMS that you would like attached to the petition:

_____

_____

Sign by email at the FibroWorld website, or you can copy this petition and gather many signatures, sending a copy of the signed petition to your local medical school and your congressional representatives with a cover letter explaining how your life has been changed by your illness, and what you went through to get diagnosed and treated. You can make a difference!

Petition for Fibromyalgia Syndrome and Myofascial Pain Syndrome

This petition honors the memory of Janis "Jayelle" Murphy of Henderson, Nevada.

- Whereas Fibromyalgia Syndrome is associated with disability of a magnitude comparable to that of other chronic pain conditions and is a common and costly cause of work disability, and the quality of life of a person with Fibromyalgia Syndrome is less than those who suffer from Rheumatoid Arthritis, and Myofascial Pain Syndrome has been specified as incapacitating torture,

- Whereas Fibromyalgia Syndrome is prevalent in the population, the etiology of the Fibromyalgia Syndrome is yet unknown, and the perpetuating factors for myofascial trigger points have been ignored by the majority of the medical establishment,

- Whereas Juvenile Fibromyalgia and Myofascial Pain Syndrome present a unique challenge, cause our children to unduly suffer from their effects, and cause needless embarrassment at their schools due to the pathophysiology of these conditions being poorly understood,

- Whereas the majority of the medical and scientific community, the media, and our own government, even in the face of research, past and present findings, continue to trivialize Fibromyalgia Syndrome and Myofascial Pain Syndrome,

- Whereas people with the illnesses Fibromyalgia and Myofascial Pain Syndrome are inadequately treated for pain, which is the main focus of their fatigue and lack of quality sleep, or are treated with more invasive methods than are necessary,

- Whereas suicide is the leading cause of death from Fibromyalgia Syndrome and chronic Myofascial Pain Syndrome, and innumerable people with these nonterminal but devastating illnesses have chosen to end their interminable pain and suffering by taking their own lives, most notably two of whom, within ten months, have ended their suffering by using the services of Dr. Jack Kevorkian, and it is our sole intent to prevent any more tragic loss of life due to this disease entity, Fibromyalgia Syndrome and chronic Myofascial Pain Syndrome:

- We, the undersigned, do hereby demand that a significant increase in RESEARCH and EDUCATION Grants for Fibromyalgia Syndrome research be awarded by the United States Government; as repeatedly recommended by the Joint Congressional members of the Appropriations Committee 1993–94–95, and that special funds be allocated to address the unique and challenging problems of Juvenile Fibromyalgia and Myofascial Pain Syndrome.

- We do hereby demand that Fibromyalgia Syndrome and chronic Myofascial Pain Syndrome be listed as separate and distinct disabilities through the Social Security Administration, and that sufferers who attempt to continue to work be protected under the ADA (Americans with Disabilities Act) and the FMLA (Family Medical Leave Act.).

- We do hereby demand that the medical and scientific communities join in with the Fibromyalgia researchers to expand upon the research of biochemical abnormalities that have been discovered in the Fibromyalgia Syndrome, and to strive to ameliorate Fibromyalgia Syndrome and chronic Myofascial Pain Syndrome.

- We do hereby demand that the government and the scientific community cease and desist from awarding research grants to individuals attempting to label Fibromyalgia a psychogenic illness, as previous research has clearly shown otherwise, instead spending the resources available on addressing the biochemical abnormalities that are presently known and established.

- We do hereby demand that a government committee be set up to deal with the problems of Fibromyalgia Syndrome and chronic Myofascial Pain Syndrome, that Fibromyalgia Syndrome and chronic Myofascial Pain Syndrome be taken seriously as the devastating illnesses that they are, and not trivialized as "aches and pains" by the government, the medical and scientific communities, the media as a whole, and society itself.

- We do hereby demand that people with Fibromyalgia Syndrome and chronic Myofascial Pain Syndrome be treated properly for pain, to include narcotic pain medication when necessary, and that chronic/intractable pain patients, such as Fibromyalgia and chronic Myofascial Pain Syndrome patients, not be made to suffer when there is medication available that would alleviate such suffering, in place of being undertreated or treated with more invasive methods.

- We do hereby demand that, to provide a better quality of life for millions of Fibromyalgia Syndrome and chronic Myofascial Pain Syndrome sufferers, the new and updated findings and research on Fibromyalgia Syndrome be taught in the medical schools, and that the study of Travell and Simons' *Myofascial Pain and Dysfunction: The Trigger Point Manuals, Vol. I* and *Vol. II*, be made mandatory for medical schools, that these illnesses be recognized as the devastating conditions that they are, and that the wide range of symptoms associated with Fibromyalgia and chronic Myofascial Pain Syndrome, other than pain, also be recognized.

WE, THE UNDERSIGNED, SUPPORT THE FIBROMYALGIA SYNDROME/MYOFASCIAL PAIN SYNDROME PETITION TO THE U.S. CONGRESS:

Name   Street   City   State   Zip

_____

_____

_____

_____

_____

_____

_____

APPENDIX D

Fibromyalgia and Myofascial Pain Syndrome Functional Questionnaire

To: _____

Re: _____ (Name of Patient)

_____ (Social Security Number)

Please answer the following:

1. Nature, frequency, and length of contact with your patient:

_____

_____

2. Does your patient meet the American Rheumatological clinical testing criteria for Fibromyalgia? _____ Yes _____ No

3. List any other diagnosed impairments or coexisting conditions:

_____

_____

_____

4. Prognosis: _____

_____

5. Have your patient's impairments lasted or can they be expected to last at least 12 months?

_____ Yes   _____ No

6. Identify the clinical findings, the laboratory and test results that show your patient's medical impairments: _____

_____

_____

7. Identify all of your patient's symptoms:

_____ Multiple tender points   _____ Numbness and tingling

_____ Nonrestorative sleep   _____ Sicca symptoms

_____ Chronic fatigue   _____ Raynaud's phenomenon

_____ Morning stiffness   _____ Dysmenorrhea

_____ Subjective swelling   _____ Anxiety

_____ Irritable Bowel Syndrome   _____ Panic attacks

_____ Depression   _____ Frequent severe headaches

_____ Mitral valve prolapse   _____ Female Urethral Syndrome

_____ Hypothyroidism   _____ Premenstrual Syndrome

_____ Vestibular dysfunction   _____ Carpal Tunnel Syndrome

_____ Lack of coordination   _____ Chronic Fatigue Syndrome

_____ Cognitive Impairment   _____ TMJ Dysfunction

_____ Multiple trigger points   _____ Myofascial Pain Syndrome

_____ Difficulty communicating   _____ Dizziness

_____ Balance problems   _____ Headaches/migraines

_____ Shortness of breath   _____ Multiple chemical sensitivity

_____ Stress incontinence   _____ Free-floating anxiety

_____ Mood swings   _____ Unaccountable irritability

_____ Sensitivity to cold, heat,   _____ Problems climbing or going down stairs
humidity, noise, light

Explain nature of cognitive impairment(s) by circling those that apply: trouble concentrating, inability to get known words out, visual perception problems, short-term memory impairment, fugue states (staring into space before brain can function), inability to deal with multiple sensory stimuli, difficulty multitasking, other:

_____

_____

_____

8. If your patient has pain:

a) Identify the location of pain, including, where appropriate, an indication of affected areas:

_____ Lumbosacral spine   _____ Thoracic spine

_____ Cervical spine   _____ Chest

		Right	Left	Bilateral
_____	Shoulders	_____	_____	_____
_____	Arms	_____	_____	_____
_____	Hands/fingers	_____	_____	_____
_____	Hips	_____	_____	_____
_____	Legs	_____	_____	_____
_____	Knees/ankles/feet	_____	_____	_____

b) Describe the nature, frequency, and severity of your patient's pain:

_____

_____

_____

c) Identify any factors that precipitate pain:

_____ Changing weather   _____ Fatigue   _____ Movement/overuse

_____ Stress   _____ Hormonal changes   _____ Cold   _____ Heat

_____ Humidity   _____ Static position   _____ Allergy   _____ Other

_____

9. Is your patient a malingerer?   ____ Yes   ____ No

10. Do emotional factors contribute to the severity of your patient's symptoms and functional limitations?   _____ Yes   _____ No

11. Are your patient's physical impairments plus any emotional impairments reasonably consistent with symptoms and functional limitations described in this evaluation?

    _____ Yes   _____ No

12. How often is your patient's experience of pain sufficiently severe to interfere with attention and concentration?

    _____ Never   _____ Seldom   _____ Often   _____ Frequently   _____ Constantly

13. To what degree is your patient limited in the ability to deal with work stress?

    _____ No limitation   _____ Slight limitation   _____ Moderate limitation

    _____ Marked limitation   _____ Severe limitation

14. Identify the side effects of any medication which may have implications for working, e.g., dizziness, drowsiness, stomach upset, etc:

    _____

    _____

15. In view of your patient's impairments, estimate your patient's functional limitations if your patient were placed in a competitive work situation:

a) How many city blocks can your patient walk without rest or severe pain? _____

   Comment _____

b) Please circle the hours and/or minutes that your patient can continually sit and stand at one time without experiencing delayed onset symptoms:

Sit	Stand/walk		Sit	Stand/walk
_____	_____ Less than 2 hours		_____	_____ About 4 hours
_____	_____ About 2 hours		_____	_____ At least 6 hours

c) Does your patient need to include periods of walking during an 8 hour day?

   _____ Yes   _____ No   _____ Cannot work an 8 hr day

d) Does your patient need a job that permits shifting positions at-will from sitting, standing, or walking?   _____ Yes   _____ No

e) Will your patient sometimes need to lie down at unpredictable intervals during a work shift?   _____ Yes   _____ No

f) With prolonged sitting, should your patient's legs be elevated?

   _____ Yes   _____ No   _____ Cannot tolerate prolonged sitting

g) While engaged in occasional standing/walking, must your patient use a cane or other assistive device?   _____ Yes   _____ No

h) How many pounds can your patient carry in a competitive work situation without suffering delayed onset symptoms?

	Never	Occasionally	Frequently
_____ Less than 10 lbs	_____	_____	_____
_____ 10 lbs	_____	_____	_____
_____ 20 lbs	_____	_____	_____
_____ 50 lbs	_____	_____	_____

In an average workday, "occasionally" means less than one-third of a workday; "frequently" means between one-third to two-thirds of the workday.

i) Does your patient have any significant limitations in reaching, handling, or fingering?

_____ Yes   _____ No

If yes, please indicate the percentage of time during a workday on a competitive job that your patient can use hands/fingers/arms for the following repetitive activities:

Hands (grasp, turn, twist objects)   Right_____%   Left_____%

Fingers (fine manipulation)   Right_____%   Left_____%

Arms (reaching, including overhead)   Right_____%   Left_____%

j) Does your patient have difficulties with fine motor control?   _____ Yes   _____ No

16. On the average, how often do you anticipate that your patient's impairments and treatments would cause the patient to be absent from work?

_____ Never   _____ Less than once a month

_____ About twice a month   _____ About three times a month

_____ About once a month   _____ More than three times a month

17. Please describe any other limitations that would affect this patient's ability to work at a regular job on a sustained basis:

_____

_____

_____

_____

18. Does your patient have (Y or N):

____ nausea ____ cramps ____ buckling ankles ____ buckling knees

____ leg cramps ____ sciatica ____ muscle twitching ____ anxiety

____ lack of endurance ____ handwriting difficulties?

Date: _____ Signed: _____

Print/type name: _____

Address: _____

References

Abdel-Fattah, R. A. 1998. Craniomandibular Myofascial Pain: Diagnosis and Treatment Lecture: Travell Focus on Pain Seminar, San Antonio, March 12–15.

———. 1997. An introduction to occlusal biomechanics in temporomandibular disorder. *Cranio* 15(4): 349–350.

———. 1991. Considerations before and during occlusal equilibration. *J Gen Orthod* 2(2):18020.

Abraham, G. E., and J. D. Flechas. 1992. Management of fibromyalgia: rationale for the use of magnesium and malic acid. *J Nutritional Res* 3:39–59.

Acasuso-Diaz, M., and E. Collantes-Estevez. 1998. Joint hypermobility in patients with fibromyalgia syndrome. *Arth Care Res* 11(1):39–42.

Aikins Murphy, P. 1998. Alternative therapies for nausea and vomiting of pregnancy. *Obstet Gynecol* 91(1):149–155.

Airaksinen, O. and P. J. Pontinen. 1992. Effects of the electrical stimulation of myofascial trigger points with tension headache. *Acupunct Electrother Res* 17(4):285–290.

Alfven, G., B. de la Torre and K. Uvnas-Moberg. 1994. Depressed concentrations of oxytocin and cortisol in children with recurrent abdominal pain of non-organic origin. *Acta Paediatr* 83(10): 1076–1080.

Allegrante, J. P. 1996. The role of adjunctive therapy in the management of chronic nonmalignant pain. *Am J Med* 101(1A):33S–39S.

Alonzo-Ruiz, A., A. de la Hoz-Martinez and A. C. Zea-Mendoza. 1985. Fibromyalgia as a late complication of toxic oil syndrome. *J Rheumatol* 12(6):1207–1208.

Alvarez Lario B., J. L. Alonso Valdivieso, L. J. Alegre Lopez, S. C. Martel Soteres, J. L. Viejo Banuelos and A. Maranon Cabello. 1996. Fall in hemoglobin oxygenation in the arterial blood of fibromyalgia patients during sleep. *Am J Med* 101:54–60.

Andersen, S., and G. Leikersfeldt. 1996. Management of chronic non-malignant pain. *Br J Clin Pract* 50(6):324–330.

Anderson, R. A. 1992. Chromium, glucose tolerance, and diabetes. *Biol Trace Elem Res* 32:19–24.

Anderson, R. A., M. M. Polansky, N. A. Bryden, S. J. Bhathena and J. J. Canary. 1987. Effects of supplemental chromium on patients with symptoms of reactive hypoglycemia. *Metabolism* 36(4): 351–355.

Angarola, R. T. 1990. National and international regulation of opioid drugs: purpose, structures, benefits and risks. *J Pain Symptom Manage* 5(1 Suppl):S6–S11.

Angell, M. 1982. The quality of mercy. *N Engl J Med.* 306(2):98–99.

Aronson, M. D. 1997. Nonsteroidal anti-inflammatory drugs, traditional opioids, and tramadol: contrasting therapies for the treatment of chronic pain. *Clin Ther* 19(3):420–432.

Balfour, W. 1815. Observations on the pathology and cure of rheumatism. *Edin Med Surg* J 15:168–187.

Banahan, B. F., III and E. M. Kolassa. 1997. A physician survey on generic drugs and substitution of critical dose medications. *Arch Intern Med* 157(18):2080–2088.

Bani, D. 1997. Relaxin: a pleiotropic hormone. *Gen Pharmacol* 28(1):13–22).

Barlett, J. and J. Steele. 1994. *America: Who Really Pays the Taxes?* NY: Simon and Schuster.

Barnes, J. F. 1996. Myofascial release for craniomandibular pain and dysfunction. *Int J Orofacial Myology* 22:20–22.

Bassoe, C. F. 1995. The skinache syndrome. *J Royal Acad Med* 88:565–569.

Bates, T. and E. Grunwaldt. 1958. Myofascial pain in childhood. *J. Pediatrics* 53:198–209.

Becker, N., A. Bondegaard Thomsen, A. K. Olsen, P. Sjogren, P. Bech and J. Eriksen. 1997. Pain epidemiology and health-related quality of life in chronic non-malignant pain patients referred to a Danish multidisciplinary pain center. *Pain* 73(3):393–400.

Bendtsen, L., R. Jensen and J. Olesen. 1996. Qualitatively altered nociception in chronic myofascial pain. *Pain* 65(2–3):259–264.

Bendtsen, L., J. Norregaard, R. Jensen and J. Olesen. 1997. Evidence of qualitatively altered nociception in patients with fibromyalgia. *Arth Rheum* 40(1):98–102.

Bengtsson, A., G. Cederblad and J. Larsson. 1990. Carnitine levels in painful muscles of patients with fibromyalgia. *Clin Exper Rheum* 8(2):197–198.

Bennett, R. M. 1997. *Fibromyalgia Network Newsletter.* July, p. 5.

———. 1995a. Fibromyalgia the commonest cause of widespread pain. *Comp Ther* 21(6):269–275.

———. 1995b. IGF-assays and other GF tests in 500 fibromyalgia patients. *J Musculoskel Pain* 3(Suppl 1):109 (Abstract).

———. 1991. Symptoms of Raynaud's syndrome in patients with fibromyalgia. A study utilizing the Nielsen test, digital photopleysmography, and measurements of platelet alpha 2–adrenergic receptors. *Arth Rheum* 34(3):264–269.

———. 1987. Fibromyalgia. *JAMA* 257(20):2802–2803.

Bennett, R. M. and S. Jacobsen. 1994. Muscle function and origin of pain in fibromyalgia. *Baillieres Clin Rheumatol* 8(4):721–746.

Bennett, R. M., D. M. Cook, S. R. Clark, C. S. Burckhardt and S. M. Campbell. 1997. Hypothalamic-pituitary-insulin-like growth factor-I axis dysfunction in patients with fibromyalgia. *J Rheumatol* 24(7):1384–1389.

Bennett, R. M., S. C. Clark and J. Walczyk. 1998. A randomized, double-blind, placebo-controlled study of growth hormone in the treatment of fibromyalgia. *Am J Med* 104(3):227–231.

Birkmayer, W. and P. Riederer. 1989. *Understanding the Neurotransmitters: Key to the Workings of the Brain.* Translated from German by Karl Blau. NY: Springer-Verlag.

Blackman, J. D., V. L. Towle, G. F. Lewis, J. P. Spire and K. S. Polonsky. 1990. Hypoglycemic thresholds for cognitive dysfunction in humans. *Diabetes* 39:828–835.

Bluestone, R. 1998. Fibromyalgia in the workplace. *Workers' Compensation Quarterly* 11(1):7, 11–13 (published by the State Bar of California).

Bolles, R. N. 1992. *Job Hunting Tips for the So-Called Handicapped or People Who Have Disabilities.* Berkeley, CA: Ten Speed Press.

Bonaccorso, S., A. H. Lin, R. Verkerk, F. Van Hunsel, I. Libbrecht, S. Scharpe, L. DeClerck, M. Biondi, A. Janca and M. Maes. 1998. Immune markers in fibromyalgia: comparison with major depressed patients and normal volunteers. *J Affect Disord* 48(1):75–82.

Borg-Stein, J. and J. Stein. 1996. Trigger points and tender points: one and the same? Does injection treatment help? *Rheum Dis Clin N Am* 22(2):305–322.

Bou-Holaigah, I., H. Calkins, J. A. Flynn, C. Tunin, H. C. Chang, J. S. Kan and P. C. Rowe. 1997. Provocation of hypotension and pain during upright tilt table testing in adults with fibromyalgia. *Clin Exp Rheumatol* 15(3):239–246.

Branco, J., A. Atalaia and T. Paiva. 1994. Sleep cycles and alpha-delta sleep in fibromyalgia syndrome. *J Rheumatol* 21(6):1113–1117.

Brassell, W. R. 1994. *Belonging: A Guide to Overcoming Loneliness.* Oakland: New Harbinger Publications.

The Brattleboro Reformer, Brattleboro, VT. November 11, 1997, page 3.

Brenne, E., K. van der Hagen, E. Maehlum and S. Husebo. 1997. Treatment of chronic pain with amitriptyline. A double-blind dosage study with determination of serum level. *Tidsskr Nor Laegeforen* 117(24):3491–3494 (Norwegian).

Bueno, L., J. Fioramonti, M. Delvaux and J. Frexinos. 1997. Mediators and pharmacology of visceral sensitivity: from basic to clinical investigations. *Gastroenterology* 112(5):1714–1743.

Buhring, M. 1997. Special therapeutic practices from the viewpoint of naturopathy. *Z Arztl Forbild Qualitatssich* 91(7):674–681 (German).

Burckhardt, C. S., S. R. Clark and R. M. Bennett. 1993. Fibromyalgia and quality of life: a comparative analysis. *J Rheumatol* 20(3):475–479.

Burckhardt, C. S., S. R. Clark, S. M. Campbell, C. A. O'Reilly and R. M. Bennett. 1995. Events and co-morbidities associated with the onset of fibromyalgia. *J Musculoskel Pain* 3(Suppl 1):71 (Abstract).

Buskila, D., L. Neumann, E. Hershman, A. Gedalia, J. Press and S. Sukenik. 1995. Fibromyalgia syndrome in children—an outcome study. *J Rheumatol* 22(3):525–528.

Buskila, D., L. Neumann, D. Sibirski and P. Shvartzman. 1997. Awareness of diagnostic and clinical features of fibromyalgia among family physicians. *Fam Pract* 14(3):238–241.

Caidahl, K., M. Lurie, B. Bake, G. Johansson and H. Wetterqvist. 1989. Dyspnoea in chronic primary fibromyalgia. *J Intern Med* 226(4):265–270.

Candido, J., K. Lutfy, B. Billings, V. Sierra, A. Duttaroy, C. E. Inturrisi and B. C. Yoburn. 1992. Effect of adrenal and sex hormones on opioid analgesia and opioid receptor regulation. *Pharmacol Biochem Behav* 42(4):685–692.

Carrett, S., M. Dessureault and A. Belanger. 1992. Fibromyalgia and sex hormones. *J Rheumatol* 19(5):831.

Cassidy, C. M. 1998. Chinese medicine users in the United States. Part I: Utilization, satisfaction, medical plurality. *J Altern Complement Med* 4(1):17–27.

Chaitow, L. 1998. Positional release techniques in the treatment of muscle and joint dysfunction. *Clin Bul Myofas Ther* 3(1):25–35.

Charap, A. D. 1978. The knowledge, attitudes, and experience of medical personnel treating pain in the terminally ill. *Mt Sinai J Med* 45(4):561–580.

Check, J. H., H. G. Adelson and C. H. Wu. 1982. Improvement of cervical factor with guaifenesin. *Fertil Steril* 37(5):707–708.

Chen, S. M., J. T. Chen, T. S. Kuan and C-Z Hong. 1998. Myofascial trigger points in intercostal muscles secondary to herpes zoster infection of the intercostal nerve. *Arch Phys Med Rehabil* 79(3): 336–338.

Cho, Z. H., S. C. Chung, J. P. Jones, J. B. Park, H. J. Lee, E. K. Wong and B. I. Min. 1998. New findings of the correlation between acupoints and corresponding brain cortices using functional MRI. *Proc Natl Acad Sci USA* 95(5):2670–2673.

Christensen, L. 1997. The effect of carbohydrates on affect. *Nutrition* 13(6):503–514.

Clauw, D. J. 1995. Tilt table testing as a measure of dysautonomia in fibromyalgia. *J Musculoskel Pain* 3(Suppl 1):10 (Abstract).

Clayman, C. B., R. H. Curry and C. B. Mitchell. 1994. *American Medical Association Guide to Your Family's Symptoms*. New York, NY: Random House.

Cleveland, C. H. Jr., R. H. Fisher and E. E Brestel. 1992. The association between rhinitis and fibromyalgia. *J Allergy Clin Immunol* 89(1):358.

Coderre, T. J., J. Katz, A. L. Vaccarino and R. Melzack. 1993. Contribution of central neuroplasticity to pathological pain: review of clinical and experimental evidence. *Pain* 52(3):259–285.

Crofford, L. J., N. C. Engleberg and M. A. Demitrack. 1996. Neurohormonal perturbations in fibromyalgia. *Baillieres Clin Rheumatol* 10(2):365–378.

Cryer, P. E. 1996. Role of growth hormone in glucose counterregulation. *Horm Res* 46(4–5):192–194.

———. 1994. Hypoglycemia: the limiting factor in the management of IDDM. *Diabetes* 43(11):1426–1434 (Banting Lecture).

———. 1993. Glucose counterregulation: prevention and correction of hypoglycemia in humans. *Am J Physiol* 264 (2 pt 1):E149–E155.

Daost, J. and G. Daost. 1996. *Fat Burning Nutrition*. Del Mar, CA: Warton Publishing Co.

de Aloysio, D. and P. Penacchioni. 1992. Morning sickness control in early pregnancy by neuguan point acupressure. *Obstet Gyn* 80(5):852–854.

de Blecourt, A. C., A. A. Knipping, N. de Voogd and M. H. van Rijswijk. 1993. Weather conditions and complaints in fibromyalgia. *J Rheumatol* 20(11):1932–1034.

Deluze, C., L. Bosia, A. Zirbs, A. Chantraine and T. L. Vischer. 1992. Electroacupuncture in fibromyalgia: results of a controlled trial. *BMJ* 305(6864)1249–1252.

De Renzi, E., F. Lucchelli, S. Muggia and H. Spinnler. 1995. Persistent retrograde amnesia following a minor trauma. *Cortex* 31(3):531–542.

Dickenson, A. H. 1997. NMDA receptor antagonists: interactions with opioids. *Acta Anaesthesiol Scand* 41(1 Pt 2):112–115.

di Tomaso, E., M. Beltramo and D. Piomelli. 1996. Brain cannabinoids in chocolate. *Nature* 382(6593):667–678.

Drewes, A. M., K. Gade, K. D. Nielsen, K. Bjerregard, S. J. Taagholt and L. Svendsen. 1995. Clustering of sleep electroencephalographic patterns in patients with the fibromyalgia syndrome. *Brit J Rheumatol* 34(12):1151–1156.

Dubner, R. 1991a. Basic mechanisms of pain associated with deep tissues. *Can J Physiol Pharmacol* 69(5):607–609.

———. 1991b. Pain and hyperalgesia following tissue injury: New mechanisms and new treatments. *Pain* 44:213–214.

Dunteman, E., S. Turner and R. Swarm. 1996. Pseudo-spinal headache. *Reg Anesth* 21(4):358–360.

Eisinger, J. 1998. Metabolic abnormalities in fibromyalgia. *Clin Bul Myofas Ther* 3(1):3–21.

Eisinger, J., A. Plantamura and T. Ayavou. 1994. Glycolysis abnormalities in fibromyalgia. *J Am Col Nutri* 13(2)144–148.

Elam, M., G. Johansson and B. G. Wallin. 1992. Do patients with primary fibromyalgia have an altered sympathetic nerve activity? *Pain* 48(3):371–375.

Enestrom, S., A. Bengtsson and T. Frodin 1997. Dermal IgG deposits and increase of mast cells in patients with fibromyalgia—relevant findings for epiphenomena. *Scand J Rheumatol* 26(4):308–313.

Fannelli, G. M., Jr. and I. M. Weiner. 1975. Species variations among primates in responses to drugs which alter the renal excretion of uric acid *J Pharmacol Exp Ther* 193(2):363–375.

Faucett, J. A. 1994. Depression in painful chronic disorders: the role of pain and conflict about pain. *J Pain Symptom Manage* 9(8):520–526.

Ferguson, L. W. 1995. Treating shoulder dysfunction and "frozen shoulders." *Chiro Tech* 7(3):73–81.

Fernstrom, J. D. 1994. Dietary amino acids and brain function. *J Am Diet Assoc* 94(1):71–77.

———. 1991. Effects of the diet and other metabolic phenomena on brain tryptophan uptake and serotonin synthesis. *Adv Exp Med Biol* 294:369–376.

Fishbain, D. A., M. Goldberg, R. S. Rosomoff and H. Rosomoff. 1991. Completed suicide in chronic pain. *Clin J Pain* 7(1):29–36.

Fisher, A. A. 1998. Algometry in diagnosis of musculoskeletal pain and evaluation of treatment outcome: An update. *J Musculoskel Pain* 6(1):5–32.

Flax, H. J. 1995. Myofascial pain syndrome—the great mimicker. *Bol Assoc Med PR* 87(10–12):167–170.

Foley, K. M. 1985. The treatment of cancer pain. *N Engl J Med* 313(2):84–95.

Fricton, J. R. 1995. Management of masticatory myofascial pain. *Semin Orthod* 1(4):229–243.

———. 1994. Myofascial pain. *Ballieres Clin Rheumatol* 8(4):857–880.

Friedman, D. P. 1990. Perspectives on the medical use of drugs of abuse. *J Pain Symptom Manage* 5(1 Supp):S2–S5.

Frye, J. 1997. Homeopathy in office practice. *Prim Care* 24(4):845–865.

Gagliese, L. and R. Melzack. 1997. Chronic pain in elderly people. *Pain* 70(1):3–14.

Gamsa, A. 1990. Is emotional disturbance a precipitator or a consequence of chronic pain? *Pain* 42(2):183–195.

Garcia, J. and R. D. Altman. 1997a. Chronic pain states: pathophysiology and medical therapy. *Semin Arth Rheum* 27(1):1–16.

———. 1997b. Chronic pain states: invasive procedures. *Semin Arth Rheum* 27(3):156–160.

Gardner, G. C. and P. A. Simpkin. 1991. Adverse effects of NSAIDs. *Pharm Ther* 16:750–754.

Gardner, J. R. and G. Sandhu. 1997. The stigma and enigma of chronic non-malignant back pain (CNMBP) treated with long-term opioids (LTO). *Contemp Nurse* 6(2):61–66.

Gear, R. W., C. Miaskowski, N. C. Gordon, S. M. Paul and J. D. Levine. 1996. Kappa-opioids produce significantly greater analgesia in women than in men. *Nat Med* 2(11):1248–1250.

Gear, R. W., C. Miaskowski, S. M. Paul, P. H. Heller, N. C. Gordon and J. D. Levine. 1997. Benzodiazepine mediated antagonism of opioid analgesia. *Pain* 71(1):25–29.

Geddes, B. J. and A. J. Summerlee. 1995. The emerging concept of relaxin as a centrally acting peptide hormone with hemodynamic actions. *J Neuroendcrinol* 7(6):411–417.

Genter, P. M. 1994. Plasma glucose thresholds for counterregulation after an oral glucose load. *Metabolism* 43(1):98–103.

Genter, P. M. and E. Ipp. 1994. Accuracy of plasma glucose measurements in the hypoglycemic range. *Diabetes Care* 17(6):595–598.

Gerster, J. C. and A. Hadj-Djilani. 1984. Hearing and vestibular abnormalities in primary fibrositis syndrome. *J Rheumatol* 11(5):678–680.

Gloth, F. M., III. 1996. Concerns with chronic analgesic therapy in elderly patients. *Am J Med* 101(1A):19S-24S.

Godfrey, R. G. 1997. Fibromyalgia as a manifestation of petroleum fume toxicity in a family of four. *J Clin Rheum* 3:54–57

———. 1996. Fibromyalgia, chronic fatigue syndrome and myofascial pain syndrome. *Curr Opin Rheum* 8(2):113–123.

Graff-Radford, S. B., B. Jaeger and J. L. Reeves. 1986. Myofascial pain may present clinically as occipital neuralgia. *Neurosurgery* 19(4):610–613.

Greene, R. 1996. *Adenosine Control of Cholinergic Arousal Populations.* Sleep Research Society Bulletin 2(4).

Greenfield, S., M. A. Fitzcharles and J. M. Esdaile. 1992. Reactive fibromyalgia syndrome. *Arth Rheum* 35(6):678–681.

Griep, E. N., J. W. Boersma and E. R. de Kloet. 1994. Pituitary release of growth hormone and prolactin in the primary fibromyalgia syndrome. *J Rheumatol* 21(11):2125–2130.

Grigsby, J., N. L. Rosenberg and D. Busenbark. 1995. Chronic pain is associated with deficits in information processing. *Percept Mot Skills* 81(2):403–410.

Gritchnik, K. P. and F. M. Ferrante. 1991. The difference between acute and chronic pain. *Mt Sinai J Med* 58(3):217–220.

Gunn, C. C., F. G. Ditchburn, M. H. King and G. J. Renwick. 1976. Acupuncture loci: a proposal for their classification according to their relationship to known neural structures. *Am J Chin Med* 4(2):183–195.

Guttu, R. I., D. G. Page and D. M. Laskin. 1990. Delayed healing of muscle after injection of bupivacaine and steroid. *Ann Dent* 49:5–8.

Hagglund, K. J., W. E. Deuser, S. P. Buckelew, J. Hewett and D. R. Kay. 1994. Weather, beliefs about weather, and disease severity among patients with fibromyalgia. *Arth Care Res* 7(3):130–135.

Hainaut, K. and J. Duchateau. 1992. Neuromuscular electrical stimulation and voluntary exercise. *Sports Med* 14(2):100–113.

Hardie, D. G. 1991. *Biochemical Messengers: Hormones, Neurotransmitters and Growth Factors.* London: Chapman and Hall.

Harland, J. D. and R. P. Liburdy. 1997. Environmental magnetic fields inhibit the antiproliferative action of tamoxifen and melatonin in a human breast cancer cell line. *Bioelectromagnetics* 18(8):555–562.

Hawk, C., C. Long and A. Azad. 1997. Chiropractic care for women with chronic pelvic pain: a prospective single-group intervention study. *J Manip Physiol Ther* 20(2):73–79.

Hedenberg-Magnusson, B., M. Ernbrg and S. Kopp. 1997. Symptoms and signs of temporomandibular disorders in patients with fibromyalgia and local myalgia of the temporomandibular system. A comparative study. *Acta Odontol Scand* 55(6):344–349.

Heinrich, S. 1991. The role of physical therapy in craniofacial pain disorders: an adjunct to dental pain management. *Cranio* 9(1):71–75.

Helme, R. D., G. O. Littlejohn and C. Weinstein. 1987. Neurogenic flare responses in chronic rheumatic pain syndromes. *Clin Exp Neurol* 23:91–94.

Hendler, N. 1984. Depression caused by chronic pain. *J Clin Psychiatry* 45(3 Pt 2):30–38.

Henriksson, C., and C. Burckhardt. 1996. Impact of fibromyalgia on everyday life: a study of women in the USA and Sweden. *Disabil Rehabil* 18(5):241–248.

Heyes, M. P., C. L. Achim, C. A. Wiley, E. O. Major, K. Saito and S. P. Markey. 1996. Human microglia convert l-tryptophan into the neurotoxin quinolinic acid. *Biochem J* 320(2):595–597.

Heyes, M. P., C.Y. Chen, E. O. Major and K. Saito. 1997. Different kynurenine pathway enzymes limit quinolinic acid formation by various human cell types. *Biochem J* 326(2):351–356.

Hill, C. S., Jr. 1996. Government regulatory influences on opioid prescribing and their impact on the treatment of pain of nonmalignant origin. *J Pain Symptom Manage* 1(5):287–297.

———. 1993. The barriers to adequate pain management with opioid analgesics. *Semin Oncol* 20 (Suppl):1–5.

———. 1992. The Intractable Pain Treatment Act of Texas. *Tex Med* 88(2):70–72.

Hitchcock, L. S., B. R. Ferrell and M. McCaffrey 1994. The experience of chronic non-malignant pain. *J Pain Sympt Manage* 9(5):312–318.

Hong, C-Z. 1998. Algometry in evaluation of trigger points and referred pain. *J Musculoskel Pain* 6(1):47–59.

Hong, C-Z and T-C Hsueh. 1996. The difference in pain relief after trigger point injections in myofascial pain in patients with and without fibromyalgia. *Arch Phys Med Rehabil* 77(11):1161–1166.

Horne, J. A. and B. S. Shackell. 1991. Alpha-like EEG activity in non-REM sleep and the fibromyalgia (fibrositis) syndrome. *Electroenceph Clin Neurophysiol* 79(4):271–276.

Horning, M. R. 1997. Chronic opioids: a reassessment. *Alaska Med* 39(4):103–110.

Horven, A., T. C. Stiles, A. Holst and T. Moen. HLA antigens in primary fibromyalgia syndrome. *J Rheumatol* 19(8):1269–1270.

Hsueh, T. C., P. T. Cheng, T. S. Kuan and C-Z Hong. 1997. The immediate effectiveness of electrical nerve stimulation and electrical muscle stimulation on myofascial trigger points. 1997. *Am J Phys Med Rehabil* 76(6):471–476.

Hsueh, T. C., S. Yu, T. S. Kuan and C-Z Hong. 1998. Association of active myofascial trigger points and cervical disc lesions. *J Formos Med Assoc* 97(3):174–180.

Hvidberg, A., C. G. Fanelli, T. Hershey, C. Terkamp, S. Craft and P. E. Cryer. 1996. Impact of recent antecedent hypoglycemia on hypoglycemic cognitive dysfunction in nondiabetic humans. *Diabetes* 45(8):1030–1036.

Imamura, M., A. A. Fischer, S. T. Imamura, H. S. Kaziyama, A. E. Carvalho, Jr. and O. Salomao. 1998. Treatment of myofascial pain components in plantar fasciitis speeds up recovery: Documentation by algometry. *J Musculoskel Pain* 6(1):91–110.

Imamura, S. T., M. Riberto, A. A. Fischer, M. Imamura, H. H. Seguchi Kaziyama and M. J. Teixeira. 1998. Successful pain relief by treatment of myofascial components in patients with hip pathology scheduled for total hip replacement. *J Musculoskel Pain* 6(1):73–89.

Ingebrigtsen, T., B. Romner, K. Waterloo and J. H. Trumpy. 1996. Minor head injuries in sport. Occurrence, management, sequelae and prevention. *Tidsskr Nor Laegeforen* 116(30):3594–3597 (Norwegian).

Irwin, M., J. McClintick, C. Costlow, M. Fortner, J. White and C. Gillin. 1996. Partial night sleep deprivation reduces killer and cellular immune responses in humans. *FASEB J* 10(5):643–653.

Ishiura, S., I. Nonaka and H. Sugita. 1986. Biochemical aspects of bupivacaine-induced acute muscle degradation. *J Cell Sci* 83:197–212.

Jacobson, J. I. 1994 Pineal-hypothalamic tract mediation of picotesla magnetic fields in the treatment of neurological disorders. *Panminerva Med* 36(4):201–205.

Jensen, G. A., C. Roychoudhury and D. C. Cherkin. 1998. Employer-sponsored health insurance for chiropractic services. *Med Care* 36(4):544–553.

Jezova, D., E. Jurankova, A. Mosnarova, M. Kriska and I. Skultetyova. 1996. Neuroendocrine response during stress with relation to gender differences. *Acta Neurobiol Exp (Warsz)* 56(3):779–785.

Johansson, G., J. Risberg, U. Rosenhall, G. Orndahl, L. Svennerholm and S. Nystrom. 1995. Cerebral dysfunction in fibromyalgia: Evidence from regional cerebral blood flow measurements, otoneurological tests and cerebrospinal fluid analysis. *Acta Psychiatr Scand* 91(2):86–94.

Johannson, V. 1993. Does a fibromyalgia personality exist? *J Musculoskel Pain* 1(3/4):245–252.

Jones, R. C. 1996. Fibromyalgia: misdiagnosed, mistreated and misunderstood? *Am Fam Phys* 52(1):91–92.

Joos, E., R. Meeusen and K. de Meirleir. Measurement of physical capacity in fibromyalgia. *J Musculoskel Pain* 3(Suppl 1):87 (Abstract).

Joranson, D. E. 1994. Are health-care reimbursement policies a barrier to acute and cancer pain management? *J Pain Symptom Manage* 9(4):244–253.

———. 1990. Federal and state regulation of opioids. *J Pain Symptom Manage* 5(1 Suppl):S12–S23.

Jung, A. C., Staiger T. and Sullivan M. 1997. The efficacy of selective serotonin reuptake inhibitors for the management of chronic pain. *J Gen Intern Med* 12(6):384–389.

Kahn, M. 1995. *The Tao of Conversation.* Oakand, CA: New Harbinger Publications.

Kane, J. 1991. *Be Sick Well.* Oakland, CA: New Harbinger Publications.

Kaziyama, H. N. S., M. Miyazaki, M. Imamura, S. T. Imamura, L. R. Battistella, L. T. Yeng, M. J. Teixeira and M. Dourado. 1995. Fibromyalgia: continuous physical therapy program with or without long-term medical supervision. *J Musculoskel Pain* 3(Suppl 1):126 (Abstract).

Kelemen, J., E. Lang, G. Balint, M. Trocsanyi and W. Muller. 1998. Orthostatic sympathetic derangement of baroreflex in patients with fibromyalgia. *J Rheumatol* 25(4):823–825.

Kerr, S. J., P. J. Armati and B. J. Brew. 1995. Neurocytotoxicity of quinolinic acid in human brain cultures. *J Neurovirol* 1(5–6):375–380.

Koenig, Jr., W. C., J. J. Powers and E. W. Johnson. 1977. Does allergy play a role in fibrositis? *Arch Phys Med Rehab* 58(2):80–83.

Kosek, E. and P. Hansson 1997. Modulatory influence on somatosensory perception from vibration and heterotopic noxious conditioning stimulation (HNCS) in fibromyalgia patients and healthy subjects. *Pain* 70:41–51.

Kosek, E., J. Ekholm and P. Hannson. 1996. Sensory dysfunction in fibromyalgia patients with implications for pathogenic mechanisms. *Pain* 68(2–3):375–383.

———. 1995. Fibromyalgia patients have a generalized increase in pain sensibility which is not stimulus specific but related to the regional pain intensity. *J Musculoskel Pain* 3(Suppl 1):25 (Abstract).

Krabak, B. J., J. P. Borg-Stein, J. Oas and D. Dumais. 1996. Reduced dizziness and pain with treatment of cervical myofascial pain. *Arch Phys Med Rehabil* 77:940 (Abstract).

Kuch, K., B. J. Cox and R. J. Evans. 1996. Posttraumatic stress disorder and motor vehicle accidents: a multidisciplinary overview. *Can J Psychiatry* 41(7):429–434.

Lautenbacher, S. and G. B. Rollman. 1997. Possible deficiencies of pain modulation in fibromyalgia. *Clin J Pain* 13(3):189–196.

Leonetti, F., L. Morviducci, A. Giaccari, P. Sbraccia, S. Caiola, D. Zoretta, O. Lostia and G. Tamburrano. 1992. Idiopathic reactive hypoglycemia: a role for glucagon? *J Endocrinol Invest* 15(4): 273–278.

Leonetti, F., M. Foniciello, P. Iozzo, O. Riggio, M. Merli, P. Giovannetti, P. Sbraccia, A. Giaccari and G. Tamburrano. 1996. Increased nonoxidative glucose metabolism in ideopathic reactive hypoglycemia. *Metabolism* 45(5):606–610.

Levine, Stephen. 1982. *Who Dies?: An Investigation of Conscious Living and Conscious Dying.* NY: Anchor Press.

Liao, S. J. 1992. Acupuncture for low back pain in huang di nei jing su wen. (Yellow Emperor's Classic of Internal Medicine Book of Common Questions). *Acupunct Electrother Res* 17(4):249–258.

Liao, S. J. and M. K. Liao. 1985. Acupuncture and tele-electronic infra-red thermography. *Acupunct Electrother Res* 10(1–2):41–66.

Liebeskind, J. C. 1991. Pain can kill. *Pain* 44(1):3–4.

Littlejohn, G. O., C. Weinstein and R. D. Helme. 1987. Increased neurogenic inflammation in fibrositis syndrome. *J Rheumatol* 14(5):1022–1025.

London, Wayne. 1994. *Principles of Health.* 139 Main Street, Brattleboro, VT 05301: London Research.

Lurie, M., K. Caidahl and K. Johansson. 1990. Respiratory function in chronic fibromyalgia. *Scand J Rehabil Med* 22(3):151–155.

Mackner, L. M., R. H. Starr, Jr. and M. M. Black. 1997. The cumulative effect of neglect and failure to thrive on cognitive functioning. *Child Abuse Negl* 21(7):691–700.

Mann, J. J., K. M. Malone, D. A. Nielsen, D. Goldman, J. Erdos and J. Gelernter. 1997. Possible association of a polymorphism of the tryptophan hydroxylase gene with suicidal behavior in depressed patients. *Am J Psychiatry* 154(10):1451–1453.

Marks, R. M., and E. J. Sachar. 1973. Undertreatment of medical inpatients with narcotic analgesics. *Ann Intern Med* 78(2):173–181.

Martinez-Lavin, M., A. G. Hermosillo, C. Mendoza, R. Ortiz, J. C. Cajigas, C. Pineda, A. Nava and M. Vallejo. 1997. Orthostatic sympathetic derangement in subjects with fibromyalgia. *J Rheumatol* 24(4):714–718.

Masood, K., C. Wu, U. Brauneis and F. F. Weight. 1994. Differential ethanol sensitivity of recombinant N-methyl-D-aspartate receptor subunits. *Mol Pharmacol* 45(2):324–329.

Matthews, D. A., M. E. McCullough, D. B. Larson, H. G. Koenig, J. P. Swyers and M. G. Milano. 1998. "Religious committment and health status: a review of the research and implications for family medicine." *Arch Fam Med* 7(2):118–124.

May, K. P., S. G. West, M. R. Baker and D. W. Everett. 1993. Sleep apnea in male patients with the fibromyalgia syndrome. *Am J Med* 94(5):505–508.

Mazer, C., J. Muneyyirci, K. Taheny, N. Raio, A. Borella and P. Whitaker-Azmitia. 1997. Serotonin depletion during synaptogenesis leads to decreased synaptic density and learning deficits in the adult rat: a possible model of neurodevelopmental disorders with cognitive deficits. *Brain Res* 760(1–2):68–73.

McBride, J. L., G. Arthur, R. Brooks and L. Pilkington. 1998. The relationship between a patient's spirituality and health experiences. *Fam Med* 30(2):122–126.

McCaffery, M. and A. Beebe. 1989. *PAIN: A Clinical Manual for Nursing Practice*. St. Louis: C. V. Mosby Co.

McCaffery, M. and B. R. Ferrell. 1997. Nurses' knowledge of pain assessment and management: how much progress have we made? *J Pain Sympt Manage* 14(3):175–188.

McCarty, M. F. 1996. Chromium and other insulin sensitizers may enhance glucagon secretion: implications for hypoglycemia and weight control. *Med Hypo* 46(2):77–80.

McCrimmon, R. J., I. J. Deary, B. J. P. Huntly, K. J. MacLeod and B. M. Frier. 1996. Visual information processing during controlled hypoglycaemia in humans. *Brain* 119(4):1277–1287.

McDermid, A. J., G. B. Rollman and G. A. McCain. 1996. Generalized hypervigilance in fibromyalgia: evidence of perceptual amplification. *Pain* 66(2–3):133–144.

McKay, M., M. Davis and P. Fanning. 1997. *Thoughts and Feelings*, Second Edition. Oakland, CA: New Harbinger Publications.

McKay, M. and P. Fanning. 1997. *The Daily Relaxer*. Oakland, CA: New Harbinger Publications.

McQuay, H. J. and A. H. Dickenson. 1990. Implications of nervous system plasticity for pain management. *Anesth* 45(2):101–102.

Mercola, J. M., and D. L. Kirsch. 1995. The basis for microcurrent electrical therapy in conventional medical practice. *J Advan Med* 8(2):107–120.

Milano. 1998. Religious commitment and health status: A review of the research and implications for family medicine. *Arch Fam Med* 7(2):118–124.

Miranda, A. F., R. J. Boegman, R. J. Beninger and K. Jhamandas. 1997. Protection against quinolinic acid-mediated excitotoxicity in nigrostriatal dopaminergic neurons by endogenous kynurenic acid. *Neuroscience* 78(4):967–975.

Mock, L. E. 1998. Myofascial release treatment of specific muscles of the upper extremity (levels 3 and 4). Part IV. *Clin Bulletin of Myofas Ther* 3(1):71–93.

———. 1997. Myofascial release treatment of specific muscles of the upper extremity (levels 3 and 4). Parts I, II and III. *Clin Bulletin of Myofas Ther* 2(1):5–33; 2(2/3):5–22; 2(4):51–69.

Moldofsky, H. F. 1995. Sleep and the immune system. *Int J Immunopharmacol* 17(8):649–654.

———. 1994. Chronological influences on fibromyalgia syndrome. Theoretical and therapeutic influences. *Ballieres Clin Rheumatol* 8(4):801–810.

Moldofsky, H. F., A. Lue, C. Mously, W. J. Roth Schechterb and W. J. Reynolds. 1996. A study of Ambien (zolpidem) treatment of fibromyalgia: a medication in widespread use by fibromyalgia patients. *J Rheumatol* 23:529–533.

Montes Milina, R., A. Galen Tabernero and M. S. Martin Garcia. 1997. Spectral electromyographic changes during a muscular strengthening training based on electrical stimulation. *Electromyogr Clin Neurophysiol* 37(5):287–295.

Morley, J. S. 1993. Central neuroplasticity. *Pain* 54(3):363–365.

Mountz, J. M., L. A. Bradley, J. G. Modell, R. W. Alexander, M. Triana-Alexander, L. A. Aaron, K. E. Stewart, G. S. Alarcon and J. D. Mountz. 1995. Fibromyalgia in women. Abnormalities of regional cerebral blood flow in the thalamus and the caudate nucleus are associated with low pain threshold levels. *Arthritis Rheum* 38:926–938.

Neeck, G. and W. Reidel. Thyroid function in patients with fibromyalgia syndrome. *J Rhuematol* 19(7):1120–1122.

Nelson, D. V. and D. M. Novy. 1996. No unique psychological profile found for patients with reflex sympathetic dystrophy or myofascial pain syndrome. *Regional Anesth* 21(3):202–208.

Neoh, C-A 1997. Operation related myofascial pain syndrome—report and analysis of 57 cases. *Chin J Pain* 7:51–58.

———. 1995. Subjective shortness of breath and trigger points of levator scapular muscles. *J Musculoskel Pain* 3(Suppl 1):27 (Abstract).

Ng, E. H., C. Y. Ji, P. H. Tan, V. Lin, K. C. Soo and K. O. Lee. 1998. Altered serum levels of insulin-like growth factor binding proteins in breast cancer patients. *Ann Surg Oncol* 5(2):194–201.

Nicassio, P. M., C. Schuman, J. Kim, A. Cordova and M. H. Weisman. 1997. Psychosocial factors associated with complementary treatment use in fibromyalgia. *J Rheumatol* 24(10):2008–2013.

Nicolodi, M., A. R. Volpe and F. Sicuteri. 1998. Fibromyalgia and headache. Failure of serotonergic analgesia and N-methyl-D-aspartate-mediated neuronal plasticity: their common clues. *Cephalalgia* 18(Suppl 21):41–44.

Nikolaus, T. 1997. Assessment of chronic pain in elderly patients. *Ther Unsch* 54(6):340–344 (German).

Nilsson, N., H. W. Christensen and J. Hartvigsen. 1997. The effect of spinal manipulation in the treatment of cervicogenic headache. *J Manipulative Physiol Ther* 20(5):326–330.

Oberkalaid, F., D. Amos, C. Liu, F. Jarman, A. Sanson and M. Prior. 1997. "Growing pains": clinical and behavioral correlates in a community sample. *J Dev Behav Pediatr* 18(2):102–106.

O'Hara, V. 1995. *Wellness at Work*. Oakland, CA: New Harbinger Publications.

Olin, R. 1995. Fibromyalgia. A neuro-immuno-endocrinologic syndrome? *Lakartidningen* 92(8):755–758 (Swedish).

Ostensen, M., A. Rugelsjoen and S. H. Wigers. 1997. The effect of reproductive events and alterations of sex hormone levels or the symptoms of fibromyalgia. *Scand J Rheumatol* 26(5)355–360.

Paira, S. O. 1994. Fibromyalgia associated with female urethral syndrome. *Clin Rheumatol* 13(1):88–89.

Park, J. H., P. Phothimat, C. T. Oates, M. Hernanz-Schulman and N. J. Olsen. 1998. Use of P-31 magnetic resonance spectroscopy to detect metabolic abnormalities in muscles of patients with fibromyalgia. *Arth Rheum* 41(3):406–413.

Pellegrino, M., G. W. Waylonis and A. Sommer. 1989. Familial occurrence of primary fibromyalgia. *Arch Phys Med Rehab* 70(1):61–63.

Pellegrino, M. J., D. Van Fossen, C. Gordon, J. M. Ryan and G. W. Waylonis. 1989. Prevalence of mitral valve prolapse in primary fibromyalgia: a pilot investigation. *Arch Phys Med Rehabil* 70(7):541–543.

Pillemer, S. R., L. A. Bradley, L. J. Crofford, H. Moldofsky and G. P. Chrousos. 1997. The neuroscience and endocrinolgy of fibromyalgia. *Arth Rheum* 40(11):1928–1939.

Pioro-Boisset, M., J. M. Esdaile and M. A. Fitzcharles. 1996. Alternative medicine use in fibromyalgia syndrome. *Arth Care Res* 9(1):13–17.

Piotrowski, C. 1997. Hypoglycemia as a mitigating factor in vehicular accidents. *Perceptual Motor Skills* 84(3 Pt 2):1241–1242.

Polkington, B. S. 1998. Treatment of cervical disc protrusions via instrumental chiropractic adjustment. *J Manipulative Physiol Ther* 21(2):114–121.

Portenoy, R. K. 1996. Opioid therapy for chronic nonmalignant pain: a review of the critical issues. *J Pain Sympt Manage* 11(4):203–217.

Portenoy, R. K., V. Dole, H. Joseph, J. Lowinson, C. Rice, S. Segal and B. L. Richman. 1997. Pain management and chemical dependency. Evolving perspectives. *JAMA* 278(7):592–593.

Potter, J. W. 1994. Filing for Social Security Disability. *Fibromyalgia Network Newsletter* (July).

Potter-Effron, R. and P. Potter-Effron. 1995. *Letting Go of Anger*. Oakland, CA: New Harbinger Publications.

Powers, W. J., I. B. Hirsch and P. E. Cryer. 1996. Effect of stepped hypoglycemia on regional cerebral blood flow response to physiological brain activation. *Am J Physiol* 270(2 Pt. 2):H554–H559.

Prasanna, A. 1993. Myofascial pain as postoperative complication. *J Pain Sympt Manage* 8(7):450–451.

Press, J., M. Phillip, I. Neumann, R. Barak, Y. Segev, M. Abu-Shakra and D. Buskila. 1998. Normal melatonin levels in patients with fibromyalgia syndrome. *J Rheumatol* 25(3):551–555.

Radulovacki, M. 1995. Pharmacology of the adenosine system. The pharmacology of sleep. In *Handbook of Experimental Pharmacology*. Ed. A. Kales. 307–322. Berlin-Heidelberg: Springer-Verlag.

Radulovacki, M. 1991. Adenosine and Sleep. In *Adenosine and the Adenine Nucleotides as Regulators of Cellualar Function*. Ed. J. W. Phillips. 381–390. Boca Raton, FL: CRC Press Inc.

Raloff, J. 1997. Magnetic fields can diminish drug action. *Sci News* 152(22):342.

Ramsey, S. M. 1997. Holistic manual therapy techniques. *Prim Care* 24(4):759–786.

Rask, M. R. 1984. The omohyoideus myofascial pain syndrome: report of four patients. *J Craniomandib Pract* 2(3):256–262.

Reaven, G. M., R. J. Brand, Y. D. Chen, A. K. Mathur and I. Goldfine. 1993. Insulin resistance and insulin secretion are determinants of oral glucose tolerance in normal individuals. *Diabetes* 42(9): 1324–1332.

Regland, B., M. Andersson, L. Abrahamsson, J. Bagby, L. E. Dyrehag and C. G. Gottfries. 1997. Increased concentrations of homocysteine in the cerebrospinal fluid in patients with fibromyalgia and chronic fatigue syndrome. *Scand J Rheumatol* 26(4):301–307.

Reidenberg, M. M. and R. K. Portenoy. 1994. The need for an open mind about the treatment of chronic nonmalignant pain. *Clin Pharmacol* 55(4):367–369.

Riera, G., M. Vilardell, J. Vaque and C. Alonso. 1994. Fibromyalgia and abdominal pain. *Surgery* 116(1):117–118.

Rokas, S., M. Mavrikakis, A. Iliopoulou and S. Moulopoulos. 1992. Proarrhythmic effects of reactive hypoglycemia. *Pacing Clin Electrophysiol* 15(4):373–376.

Romano, T. J. 1991. Fibromyalgia in children: diagnosis and treatment. *W V Med J* 87 (3):112–114.

Rosenhall, U., G. Johannson and G. Orndahl. 1996. Otoneurologic and audiologic findings in fibromyalgia. *Scand J Rehabil Med* 28(4):225–232.

Russell, I. J. 1998a. Fibromyalgia syndrome: new insights from the clinic and the laboratory. Paper presented at the San Antionio, TX, Focus on Pain Seminar. Not published.

———. 1998b. The reliability of algometry in the assessment of patients with fibromyalgia syndrome. *J Musculoskel Pain* 6(1):139–152.

————. 1996. Neurochemical pathogenesis of fibromyalgia syndrome. 1996. *J Musculoskel Pain* 4(1/2): 61–92.

Sachs, C. and E. Svanborg. 1991. The exploding head syndrome: polysomnographic recordings and therapeutic suggestions. *Sleep* 14(3):263–266.

Saggini, R., M. A. Giamberardino, L. Gatteschi and L. Vecchiet. 1996. Myofascial pain syndrome of the peroneus longus: biomechanical approach. *Clin J Pain* 12(1):30–37.

Saito, K. 1995. Biochemical studies on AIDS dementia complex—possible contribution of quinolinic acid during brain damage. *Rinsho Byori* 43(9):891–901.

Saito, K., J. S. Crowley, S. P. Markey and M. P. Heyes. 1993. A mechanism for increased quinolinic acid formation following acute systemic immune stimulation. *J Biol Chem* 268(21):15496–15503.

Samborski, W., T. Stratz, T. Schochat, P. Mennet and W. Muller. 1996. Biochemical changes in fibromyalgia. *Z Rheumatol* 55(3):168–173 (German).

Sandyk, R. 1997a. Immediate recovery of cognitive functions and resolutions of fatigue by treatment with weak electromagnetic fields in a patient with multiple sclerosis. *Int J Neurosci* 90(1–2):59–74.

————. 1997b. Progressive cognitive improvement in multiple sclerosis from treatment with electromagnetic fields. *Int J Neurosci* 89(1–2):39–51.

————. 1996c. Suicidal behavior is attenuated in patients with multiple sclerosis by treatment with electromagnetic fields. *Int J Neurosci* 87(1–2):5–15.

Savage, S. R. 1996. Long-term opioid therapy: assessment of consequences and risks. *J Pain Symptom Manage* 11(5):274–286.

Schedle, A., P. Samorapoompichit, W. Fureder, X. H. Rausch-Fan, A. Franz, W. R. Sperr, et al. 1998. Metal ion-induced toxic histamine release from human basophils and mast cells. *J Biomed Mater Res* 39(4)560–567.

Schlenk, E. A., J. A. Erlen, J. Dunbar-Jacob, J. McDowell, S. Engberg, S. M. Sereika, J. M. Rohay and M. J. Bernier. 1998. Health-related quality of life in chronic disorders: a comparison across studies using the MOS SF-36. *Qual Life Res* 7(1):57–65.

Schneider, M. J. 1995. Tender Points/fibromyalgia vs. trigger points/myofascial pain syndrome: a need for clarity in terminology and differential diagnosis. *J Manip Physiol Ther* 18(6):398–406.

————. 1992. Soft tissue effects of sacroiliac and lumbosacral joint manipulation. *Chiro Tech* 4(4): 136–142.

Schneider, M. J. and J. H. Cohen. 1992. Nimmo Receptor Tonus Technique: A Chiropractic Approach to Trigger Point Therapy. In *Chiropractic Family Practice Manual*. Ed J. J. Sweere. Section 3, chapter 3, 1–18. Gaithersburg, MD: Aspen Publication.

Schwarcz, R., C. Speciale and E. D. French. 1987. Hippocampal kynurenines as etiological factors in seizure disorders. *Pol J Pharmacol Pharm* 39(5):485–494.

Scudds, R. A. 1998. Lecture: Fibromyalgia and Myofascial Pain: Differential Diagnosis and Differences. Travell Seminar: Focus on Pain, San Antonio, TX, March 13–15.

Sears, B. 1997a. *Zone Perfect Meals in Minutes*. NY: ReganBooks, HarperCollins.

————. 1997b. *Mastering the Zone*. NY: HarperCollins.

Sears, B. and B. Lawren. 1995. *Enter the Zone*. NY: HarperCollins.

Sees, K. L. and H. W. Clark. 1993. Opioid use in the treatment of chronic pain: assessment of addiction. J *Pain Symptom Manage* 8(5):257–264.

Seibold, J. R., P. J. Clements, D. E. Furst, M. D. Mayes, D. A. McCloskey, L. W. Moreland, B. White, F. M. Wigley, S. Rocco, M. Erikson, et al. 1998. Safety and pharmacokinetics of recombinant human relaxin in systemic sclerosis. *J Rheumatol* 25(2):302–307.

Sendrowski, D. P., E. A. Buker and S. S. Gee. 1997. An investigation of sympathetic hypersensitivity in chronic fatigue syndrome. *Optom Vis Sci* 74(8):660–663.

Shankland, II, W. E. 1996. *TMJ: Its Many Faces*. Columbus: Anadem Publishers.

———. 1995. Craniofacial pain syndromes that mimic temporomandibular joint disorders. *Ann Acad Med Singapore* 24(1):83–112.

———. 1983. Craniomandibular pain: current treatment options. *Ohio Dent* 57(7):53–57.

Shapiro, R. S. 1994. Legal bases for the control of analgesic drugs. *J Pain Symptom Manage* 9(3): 153–159.

Shear, D.A., J. Dong, K. L. Haik-Creguer, T. J. Bazzett, R. L. Albin and G. L. Dunbar. 1998. Chronic administration of quinolinic acid in the rat stratum causes spatial learning deficits in a radial arm water maze task. *Exp Neurol* 150(2):305–311.

Sheehan, J., J. McKay, M. Ryan, N. Walsh and D. O'Keefe. 1996. What cost chronic pain? *Ir Med J* 89(6):218–219.

Siegan, J. B., A. T. Hama and J. Sagen. 1997. Suppression of neuropathic pain by a naturally derived peptide with NMDA antagonist activity. *Brain Res* 755(2):331–334.

Siegel, D. M., D. Janeway and J. Baum. 1998. Fibromyalgia syndrome in children and adolescents: clinical features at presentation and status at follow-up. *Pediatrics* 101(3 Pt 1):377–382.

Simms, R. W. 1996. Is there muscle pathology in fibromyalgia syndrome? *Rheum Dis Clin North Am* 22(2):245–266.

Simms, R. W. and D. I. Goldenberg. 1988. Symptoms mimicking neurologic disorders in fibromyalgia syndrome. *J Rheumatol* 15(8):1271–1273.

Simms, R. W., C. A. Zerbini, N. Ferrante, J. Anthony, D. T. Felson and D. E. Craven. 1992. Fibromyalgia syndrome in patients infected with human immunodeficiency virus. Boston City Hospital Clinical AIDS Team. *Am J Med* 92(4):368–374.

Simons, D. G. 1997. Myofascial trigger points: the critical experiment. *J Musculoskel Pain* 5(4):113–118.

———. 1987. Myofascial pain syndrome due to trigger points. *Internat Rehab Med Assn Monograph Series 1.* Available from Gebauer (800) 321–9348.

Simons, D. G. and S. Mense. 1998. Understanding and measurement of muscle tone as related to clinical muscle pain. *Pain* 75(1):1–17.

Simons, D. G. and L. S. Simons. 1989. Chronic myofascial pain syndrome. In *Handbook of Chronic Pain Management.* Eds. C. D. Tollison, J. R. Satterswaite, J. W. Tollison and C. G. Trent. Baltimore: Williams and Wilkins.

Simons, D. G., J. G., Travell, and L. S. Simons. Publication Pending. *Travell & Simons' Myofascial Pain And Dysfunction: The Trigger Point Manual, Volume 1, Edition 2.* Baltimore: Williams & Wilkins.

Simpson, L. O. 1997. Myalgic encephalomyelitis (ME): a haemorheological disorder manifested as impaired capillary blood flow. *J Orthomolecular Med* 12:69–76.

Simunovic, Z. 1996. Low level laser therapy with trigger points technique: a clinical study on 243 patients. *J Clin Laser Med Surg* 14(4):163–167.

Singh, G., D. R. Ramey, D. Morfeld, H. Shi, H. T. Hatoum and J. F. Fries. 1996. Gastrointestinal tract complications of nonsteroidal anti-inflammatory drug treatment in rheumatoid arthritis. A prospective observational cohort study. *Arch Intern Med* 156(14):1530–1536

Sivri, A., A. Cindas, F. Dincer and B. Sivri. 1996. Bowel dysfunction and irritable bowel syndrome in fibromyalgia patients. *Clin Rheumatol* 15(3):283–286.

Sjolund, K. F., A. Sollevi, M. Segerdahl and T. Lundeberg. 1997. Intrathecal adenosine analog administration reduces substance P in cerebrospinal fluid along with behavioral effects that suggest antinociception in rats. *Anesth Analg* 85(3):627–632.

Skargren, E. I., B. E. Oberg, P. G. Carlsson and M. Gade. 1997. Cost and effectiveness analysis of chiropractic and physiotherapy treatment for low back and neck pain. Six-month follow-up. *Spine* 22(18):2167–2177.

Slotkoff, A. T., D. A. Radulovic and D. J. Clauw. 1997. The relationship between fibromyalgia and the multiple chemical sensitivity syndrome. *Scand J Rheumatol* 26(5):364–367.

Smart, P. A., G. W. Waylonis and K. V. Hackshaw. 1997. Immunologic profile of patients with fibromyalgia. *Am J Phys Med Rehabil* 76(3):231–234.

Smythe, H. 1998. Examination for tenderness: learning to use 4 kg force. *J Rheumatol* 25(1):149–151.

Sorensen, J., A. Bengtsson, E. Backman, K. G. Henriksson and M. Bengtsson. 1995. Pain analysis in patients with fibromyalgia. Effects of intravenous morphine, lidocaine, and ketamine. *Scand J Rheumatol* 24(6):360–365.

Sorensen, J., A. Bengtsson, J. Ahlner, K. G. Henriksson, L. Ekselius and M. Bengtsson. 1997. Fibromyalgia—are there different mechanisms in the processing of pain? A double blind crossover comparison of analgesic drugs. *J Rheumatol* 24(8):1615–1621.

Sorensen, J., T. Graven-Nielsen, K. G. Henriksson, M. Bengtsson and L. Arendt-Nielsen. 1998. Hyperexcitability in fibromyalgia. *J Rheumatol* 25(1):152–155.

Sprott, H. 1998. Efficiency of acupuncture in patients with fibromyalgia. *Clin Bul Myofas Ther* 3(1):37–43.

Sprott, H., A. Muller and H. Heine. 1997. Collagen crosslinks in fibromyalgia. *Arth Rheum* 40(8):1450–1454.

Srinivasan, R., S. Smolinske and D. Greenbaum. 1997. Probable gastrointesinal toxicity of Kombucha tea: is this beverage healthy or harmful? *J Gen Intern Med* 12(10):643–644.

St. Amand, R. P. and C. Potter. 1997. The use of uricosuric agents in fibromyalgia: theory, practice and a rebuttal to the Oregon study of guaifenesin treatment. *Clin Bul Myofas Ther* 2(4):5–17.

Starlanyl, D. J. and M. E. Copeland. 1996. *Fibromyalgia & Chronic Myofascial Pain Syndrome: A Survival Manual*. Oakland: New Harbinger Publications.

Starlanyl, D. J. 1997. *Chronic Myofascial Pain Syndrome: A Guide to the Trigger Points*. Two-hour video. Oakland, CA: New Harbinger.

Stewart, D. P., J. Kaylor and E. Koutanis. 1996. Cognitive deficits in presumed minor head injured patients. *Acad Emerg Med* 3(1):21–26.

Sztark, F., O. Tueux, P. Erny, P. Dabadie and J. P. Mazat. 1994. Effects of bupivacaine on cellular oxygen consumption and adenine nucleotide metabolism. *Anesth Analg* 78(2):335–339.

Tavoni, A., G. Jeracitano and G. Cirigliano. 1998. Evaluation of S-adenosylmethionine in secondary fibromyalgia: a double-blind study. *Clin Exp Rheumatol* 16(1):106–107.

Thomas, S. A. and R. D. Palmiter. 1997a. Disruption of the dopamine beta-hydroxylase gene in mice suggests roles for norepinephrine in motor function, learning, and memory. *Behav Neurosci* 111(3):579–589.

———. 1997b. Impaired maternal behavior in mice lacking norepinephrine and epinephrine. *Cell* 91(5):583–592.

Teitelbaum, J. 1996. *From Fatigue to Fantastic*. Garden City Park, NY: Avery Publishing Group.

Torpy, D. J. and G. P. Chrousos. 1996. The three-way interactions between the hypothalamic-pituitary-adrenal and gonadal axes and the immune system. *Baillieres Clin Rheumatol* 10(2):181–198.

Travell, J. G. 1968. *Office Hours Day and Night*. NY: World Publishing Co.

Travell, J. G., S. Rinzler and M. Herman. 1942. Pain and disability of the shoulder and arm, treatment by intermuscular infiltration with procaine hydrochloride. *JAMA* 120(6):417–22.

Travell, W. and J. G. Travell. 1946. Therapy of low back pain by manipulation and of referred pain in the lower extremity by procaine infiltration. *Arch Phys Med* XXVII:537–47.

Travell, J. G. and D. G. Simons. 1992. *Myofascial Pain and Dysfunction: The Trigger Point Manual, Volume II: The Lower Body*. Baltimore: Williams and Wilkins.

———. 1983. *Myofascial Pain and Dysfunction: The Trigger Point Manual, Volume I: The Upper Body*. Baltimore: Williams and Wilkins (revision in process).

Triadafilopoulus, G., R. W. Simms and D. I. Goldenberg. 1991. Bowel dysfunction in fibromyalgia syndrome. *Digest Dis Sci* 36(1):1237–1248.

Tsai, G. and J. T. Coyle. 1998. The role of glutamatergic neurotransmission in the pathophysiology of alcoholism. *Ann Rev Med* 49:173–184.

Tsen, L. C. and W. R. Camann. 1997. Trigger point injections for myofascial pain during epidural analgesia for labor. *Reg Anesth* 22(5):466–468.

Tuncer, T., B. Buntun, M. Arman, A. Akyokus and A. Doseyen. 1997. Primary fibromyalgia and allergy. *Clin Rheumatol* 16(1):9–12.

Uvnas-Moberg, K., G. Bruzelius, P. Alster and T. Lundeberg. 1993. The antinociceptive effect of nonnoxious sensory stimulation is mediated partly through oxytocinergic mechanisms. *Acta Physiol Scand* 149(2):199–204.

Vaeroy, H., A. Abrahamsen, O. Forre and E. Kass. 1989. Treatment of fibromyalgia (fibrositis syndrome): a parallel double blind trial with carisoprodol, paracetamol and caffeine (Somadril comp) versus placebo. *Clin Rheumatol* 8(2):245–250.

Vallance, A. K. 1998. Can biological activity be maintained at ultra-high dilution? An overview of homeopathy, evidence and Bayesian philosophy. *J Altern Complement Med* 4(1):49–76.

Van Loon, E. 1995. Fibromyalgic (FMS) depression (DEPR): Surely it's all in her head? *J Musculoskel Pain* 3(Suppl 1):141 (Abstract).

Vecchiet, L., M. A. Giamberdino and R. Saggini. 1991. Myofascial pain syndrome, clinical and pathological aspects. *Clin J Pain* 7(Suppl1):S16–S22.

Vecchiet, L., E. Pizzigallo, S. Iezzi, A. Giannapia, J. Vecchiet and M. A. Giamberardino. 1998. Differentiation of sensitivity in different tissues and its clinical significance. *J Musculoskel Pain* 6(1):33–45.

Wallace, D. J. 1990. Genitourinary manifestations of fibrositis and increased association with female urethral syndrome. *J Rheumatol* 17(2):238–239.

Ward, A. A. 1996. Spontaneous electrical activity at combined acupuncture and myofascial trigger point sites. *Acupunct Med* 14(2):75–79.

Waylonis, G. W. and W. Heck. 1992. Fibromyalgia syndrome. New associations. *Am J Phys Med Rehabil* 71(6):343–348.

Weiner, S. R. 1983. Growing pains. *Am Fam Physician* 27(1):189–191.

Weiss, D. J., T. Kreck and R. K. Albert. 1998. Dyspnea resulting from fibromyalgia. *Chest* 113(1):246–249.

Weissman, D. E. 1993. Doctors, opioids, and the law; the effect of controlled substances regulations on cancer pain management. *Semin Oncol* 20(1 Supp 1):53–58.

Wellington, N. and M. J. Rieder. 1993. Attitudes and practices regarding analgesia for newborn circumcision. *Pediatrics* 92(4):541–543.

Westley, B. R., S. J. Slayton, M. R. Daws, C. A. Molloy and F. E. May. 1998. Interactions between the oestrogen and insulin-like growth factor signalling pathways in the control of breast epithelial cell proliferation. *Biochem Soc Symp* 63:5–44.

White, A. 1995. The fibromyalgia syndrome: electroacupuncture is a potentially valuable treatment. *Brit Med J* 310(6991):1406.

White, A. R., K. L. Resch and E. Ernst. 1997. Complementary medicine: use and attitudes among GPs. *Fam Pract* 14(4):302–306.

Wilke, W. S. 1995. Treatment of "resistant" fibromyalgia. *Rheum Dis Clin N Am* 21(1):247–260.

Wolfe, F., H. A. Smythe, M. B. Yunus, R. M. Bennett, C. Bombardier, D. L. Goldenberg, P. Tugwell, S. M. Campbell, M. Ables, P. Clark, et al. 1990. The American College of Rheumatology 1990 Criteria for the Classification of Fibromyalgia. Report of the Multicenter Criteria Committee. *Arth Rheum* 33(2):160–172.

Wolfe, F., K. Ross, J. Anderson, I. J. Russell and L. Herbert. 1995. Prevalence and characteristics of fibromyalgia in the general population. *Arth Rheum* 38(1):19–28.

Wu, H.Q., F. G. Salituro and R. Schwarcz. 1997. Enzyme-catalyzed production of the neuroprotective NMDA receptor antagonist 7–chlorokynurenic acid in the rat brain in vivo. *Eur J Pharmacol* 319(1):13–20.

Yang, J. 1994. Intrathecal administration of oxytocin induces analgesia in low back pain involving the endogenous opiate peptide system. *Spine* 19(8):867–871.

Yunus, M. B. 1992. Towards a model of pathophysiology of fibromyalgia: Aberrant central pain mechanisms with peripheral modulation. *J Rheumatol* 19:6:846–850.

———. 1988. Diagnosis, etiology and management of fibromyalgia syndrome: An update. *Compr Ther* 14(4):8–20.

Zborovskii, A. B. and A. R. Babaeva. 1996. New trends in the study of the primary fibromyalgia syndrome. *Vestn Ross Akad Med Nauk* 11:52–56 (Russian).

Zenz, M., M. Strumpf and M. Tryba. 1992. Long-term oral opioid therapy in patients with chronic non-malignant pain. *J Pain Sympt Manag* 7(2):69–77.

Bibliography

Aarflot, T. and D. Bruusgaard. 1996. Association between chronic widespread musculoskeletal complaints and thyroid autoimmunity. Results from a community survey. *Scand J Prim Health Care* 14(2):111–115.

Affleck, G., S. Urrows, H. Tennen, P. Higgins and M. Abeles. 1996. Sequential daily relations of sleep, pain intensity, and attention to pain among women with fibromyalgia. *Pain* 68(2–3):363–368.

Aftimos, S. 1989. Myofascial pain in children. *N Z Med J* 102(874):440–441.

Ahmadpour, S. and U. M. Kabadi. 1997. Pancreatic alpha-cell function in idiopathic reactive hypoglycemia. *Metabolism* 46(6):639–643.

Alagiri, M., S. Chottiner, V. Ratner, D. Slade, and P. M. Hanno. 1997. Interstitial cystitis: unexplained associations with other chronic disease and pain syndromes. *Urol* 49(5A Suppl):52–57.

Allen, B. J., S. D. Rogers, J. R. Ghilardi, P. M. Menning, M. A. Kuskowski, A. I. Basbaum, D. A. Simone and P. W. Mantyh. 1997. Noxious cutaneous thermal stimuli induce a graded release of endogenous substance P in the spinal cord; imaging peptide action in vivo. *J Neurosci* 17(15):5921–5927.

Ambrogetti, A., L. G. Olson and N. A. Saunders. 1991. Disorders of movement and behavior during sleep. *Med J Aust* 155(5):336–340.

American Academy of Pain Medicine and American Pain Society. 1997. The use of opioids for the treatment of chronic pain. *Clin J Pain* 13(3):6–8.

American Journal of Health System Pharm. 1996. Oral morphine eases chronic non-cancer pain, with little risk of addiction. 53(8):836.

American Society of Anesthesiologists Task Force on Pain Management, Chronic Pain Section. 1997. Practice guidelines for chronic pain management. *Anesthesiology* 86(4):995–1004.

Amir, M., Z. Kaplan, L. Neuman, R. Sharabani, N. Shani and D. Buskila. 1997. Posttraumatic stress disorder, tenderness and fibromyalgia. *J Psychosom Res* 42(6):607–613.

Andersson, H. I., G. Ejlertsson, I. Leden and C. Rosenberg. 1996. Compared to patients with regional MPS pain, patients with widespread pain have lower work capacity and a worse prognosis. *Scand J Rheumatol* 25(3):146–154.

Antelman, S. M. 1994. Time-dependent sensitization in animals: a possible model of multiple chemical sensitivity in humans. *Toxicol Indus Health.* 10(4/5):335–342.

Appelboom, T. and A. Schoutens. 1990. High bone turnover in fibromyalgia. *Calcif Tis Internat* 46(5): 314–317.

Ashburn, M. A. and P. G. Fine. Persistent pain following trauma. *Mil Med* 154(2):86–89.

Atkinson, L. 1996. Pain management for children and infants. *Contemp Nurse* 5(2):64–70.

Auleciems, L. M. 1995. Myofascial pain syndrome: a multidisciplinary approach. *Nurse Pract* 20(4):18.

Avery, D. H., K. Dahl, M. V. Savage, G. L. Brengelmann, L. H. Larsen, M. A. Kenny, D. N. Eder, M. V. Vitiello and P. N. Prinz. 1997. Circadian temperature and cortisol rhythms during a constant routine are phase-delayed in hypersomnic winter depression. *Biol Psychiatry* 41(11):1109–1123.

Awerbuch, M. 1994. Fibromyalgia in the workplace. *Ann Rheum Dis* 3(4):285.

Bagge, E., B. A. Bengtsson, L. Carlsson and J. Carlsson. 1998. Low growth secretion in patients with fibromyalgia—a preliminary report on 10 patients and 10 controls. *J Rheumatol* 25(1):145–148.

Baker, B. A. 1986. The muscle trigger: evidence of overload injury. *J Neuro Ortho Med Surg* 7(1):35–44.

Barrett, K., N. Buxton, A. D. Redmond, J. Hones, A. Boughey and A. B. Ward. 1995. A comparison of symptoms experienced following minor head injury and acute neck strain (whiplash injury). *J Accid Emerg Med* 12(3):173–176.

Baumstark, K. E., S. P. Bucklew and K. J. Sher. 1993. Pain behavior predictors among fibromyalgia patients. *Pain* 339–346.

Belilos, E. and S. Carsons. Rheumatologic disorders in women. 82(1):77–101.

Bell, D. S., K. M. Bell and P. R. Chesney. 1994. Primary juvenile fibromyalgia syndrome and chronic fatigue syndrome in adolescents. *Clin Infect Disease* 18(Suppl 1):S21–S28.

Bengtsson, A., E. Backman, B. Lindblom and T. Skogh. 1994. Long-term follow-up of fibromyalgia patients: clinical symptoms, muscular function, laboratory tests an eight-year comparison study. *J Musculoskel Pain* 2(2):67–80

Bengtsson, A., J. Ernerudh, M. Vrethem and T. Skogh. 1990. Absence of autoantibodies in primary fibromyalgia. *J Rheumatol* 17(12):1682–1683.

Bengtsson, A., K. G. Henriksson and J. Larsson. 1986. Reduced high-energy phosphate levels in the painful muscles of patients with primary fibromyalgia. *Arth Rheum* 29(7)817–821.

Bennett, R. M. 1996. Fibromyalgia and the disability dilemma. A new era in understanding a complex, multidimensional pain syndrome. *Arth Rheum* 39(10):1627–1634.

——. 1994. Exercise and exercise testing in fibromyalgia patients: lessons learned and suggestions for further studies. *J Musculoskel Pain* 2(3):143–152.

——. 1993. Disabling fibromyalgia: appearance versus reality. *J Rheumatol.* 20(11):1821–1824.

Bennett, R. M., S. R. Clark, S. M. Campbell and C. S. Burckhardt. 1992. Low levels of somatomedin-C in patients with the fibromyalgia syndrome. A possible link between sleep and muscle pain. *Arth Rheum* 35(10):1113–1116.

Bennett, R. M., H. A. Smith and F. Wolf. 1992. Recognizing fibromyalgia. *Patient Care* 211–218.

Bernstein, J. E. 1991. Capsaicin and substance P. *Clin Dermatol* 9(4):497–503.

Bertoluci, L. E. and B. di Dario. 1995. Efficacy of a portable acustimulation device in controlling sea-sickness. *Aviat Space Environ* 66(12):1155–1158.

Billington, L. and B. M. Carlson. 1996. The recovery of long-term denerved rat muscles after Marcaine treatment and grafting. *J Neurol Sci* 144(1–2):147–155.

Blunz, K. L., M. R. Rajwani and R. C. Guerriero. 1997. The effectiveness of chiropractic management of fibromyalgia patients: a pilot study. *J Manip Physiol Ther* 20(6):389–399.

Boisset-Poiro, M. H., J. M. Esdaile and M. A. Fitzcharles. 1995. Sexual and physical abuse with fibromyalgia syndrome. *Arth Rheum* 38(2):235–241.

Bolwijn, P. H., M. H. van Santen-Hoeufft, H. M. Barrs, C. D. Kaplan and S. van der Linden. 1996. The social network characteristics of fibromyalgia patients compared with healthy controls. *Arth Care Res* 9(1):18–26.

Bombardier, C. H. and D. Buchwald. 1996. Chronic fatigue, chronic fatigue syndrome and fibromyalgia. Disability and health care use. *Med Care* 34(9):924–930.

Bonica, John J., J. D. Loeser, C. R. Chapman and W. E. Fordyce. 1990. *The Management of Pain*. Baltimore: Williams and Wilkins. (Originally published by Lea and Febiger.)

Borenstein, D. 1995. Prevalence and treatment outcome in primary and secondary fibromyalgia in patients with spinal pain. *Spine* 20(7):1821–1824.

Borg-Stein, J., P. Bell Adar and D. L. Goldenberg. 1995. The role of the occupational therapist in fibromyalgia rehabilitation. *J Musculoskel Pain* 3(Suppl 1):158 (Abstract).

Born, J., T. Lange, K. Hansen, M. Molle and H. L. Fehm. 1997. Effects of sleep and circadian rhythm on human circulating immune cells. *J Immunol* 158(9):4454–4464.

Boyr, T. 1995. A long-term follow-up on post-traumatic fibromyalgia patients. *Am J Phys Med and Rehab* 74(6):476–477.

Brault, J. R., J. B. Wheeler, G. P. Siegmund and E. J. Brault. 1998. Clinical response of human subjects to rear-end automobile collisions. *Arch Phys Med Rehabil* 79(1):72–80.

Bridges, A. J. 1993. Fibromyalgia, antinuclear antibodies and clinical features of connective tissue disease. *Clin Exper Rheumatol* 11(6):696–697.

Bronstein, A. C. 1995. Multiple chemical sensitivities—new paradigm needed. *J Toxicol Clin Toxicol* 33(2):93–94.

Bruce, E. 1995. Myofascial pain syndrome: early recognition and comprehensive management. *AAOHN* 43(9):469–474.

Bruusgaard, D., A. R. Evensen and T. Bjerkedal. 1993. Fibromyalgia—a new cause for disability pension. *Scand J Soc Med* 21(2):116–119.

Buchwald, D. 1996. Fibromyalgia and chronic fatigue syndrome: similarities and differences. *Rheum Dis Clin North Am* 22(2):219–243.

Buchwald, D., J. Umali and M. Stene. 1996. Insulin-like growth factor-1 (somatomedin C) levels in chronic fatigue syndrome and fibromyalgia. *J Rheum* 23(4):730–742.

Buchwald, D. and D. Garrity. 1994. Comparison of patients with chronic fatigue syndrome, fibromyalgia and multiple chemical sensitivities. *Arch Int Med* 154(18):2049–203.

Burk, O. 1989. Effect of homeopathic treatment of fibromyalgia. *Brit Med J* 299:685.

Burckhardt, C. S., K. D. Jones and S. R. Clark. 1998. Soft tissue problems associated with rheumatic disease. *Prim Care Pract* 2(1):20–29.

Burckhardt, C. S., S. R. Clark S. M. Campbell, C. A. O'Reilly and R. M. Bennett. 1995. The pain coping strategies of women with fibromyalgia. *J Musculoskel Pain* 3(Suppl 1):72 (Abstract).

Burckhardt, C. S., S. R. Clark and R. M. Bennett. 1991. The fibromyalgia impact questionnaire: development and validation. *J Rheumatol* 18(5):728–733.

Buskila, D., A. Shnaider, L. Neumann, D. Zilberman, N. Hilzenrat and E. Sikuler. 1997. Fibromyalgia in hepatitis C virus infection. Another infectious disease relationship. *Arch Intern Med* 157(21):2497–2500.

Buskila, D. and L. Neumann. 1997. Fibromyalgia syndrome (FM) and nonarticular tenderness in relatives of patients with FM. *J Rheumatol* 24(5):941–944.

Buskila, D., L. Neumann, G. Vaisberg, D. Alkalay and F. Wolfe. 1997. Increased rates of fibromyalgia following cervical spine injury. A controlled study of 161 cases of traumatic injury. *Arth Rheum* 40(3):446–452.

Buskila, D., L. Neumann, I. Hazanov and R. Carmi. 1996. Familial aggregation in the fibromyalgia syndrome. *Semin Arthritis Rheum* 26(3):605–611.

Buskila, D., D. D. Gladman, K. V. Straaton, P. Langevitz, S. Urowicz and H. A. Smythe. 1990. Fibromyalgia in human immunodeficiency syndrome virus infection. *J Rheumatol* 17(9): 1202–1206.

Cagnacci, A., S. Arangino, M. Angiolucci, E. Maschio, G. Longu and G. B. Melis. 1997. Potentially beneficial cardiovascular effects of melatonin administration in women. *J Pineal Res* 22(1):16–19.

Calabro, J. J. 1986. Fibromyalgia in children. *Am J Med* 81: 3A:57–59.

Cameron, R. S. 1995. The cost of long-term disability due to fibromyalgia, chronic fatigue syndrome and repetitive strain injury. The private insurance perspective. *J Musculoskel Pain* 3(2):169–172.

Capen, K. 1995. The courts, expert witnesses and fibromyalgia. *Can Med Assn J* 153(2):206–228.

Carette, S., G. Oakson, C. Guimont and M. Steriade. 1995. Sleep electroencephalography and the clinical response to amitriptyline in patients with fibromyalgia. *Arth Rheum* 38(9):1211–1217.

Carette, S. and L. Lefrancois. 1988. Fibrositis and primary hypothyroidism. *J Rheumatol* 15(9): 1418–1421.

Carlson, C. R., J. P. Okeson, D. A. Falace, A. J. Nitz and J. E. Lindroth. 1993. Reduction of pain and EMG activity in the masseter region by trapezius trigger point injection. *Pain* 55(3):397–400.

Cassisi, J. E., G. W. Sypert, L. Lagana, E. M. Friedman and M. E. Robinson. 1993. Pain, disability, and psychological functioning chronic low-back pain subgroups: Myofascial versus herniated disc syndrome. *Neurosurgery* 33:379–385.

Caterina, M. J., M. A. Schumacher, M. Tominaga, T. A. Rosen, J. D. Levine and D. Julius. 1997. The capsaicin receptor: a heat-activated ion channel in the pain pathway. *Nature* 389(6653):816–824.

Champion, G. D., M. L. Cohen and J. L. Quinter. 1993. Fibromyalgia in the workplace. *Ann Rheum Dis* 52(11):836–837.

Chandra, S. and R. K. Chandra. 1986. Nutrition, immune response, and outcome. *Prog Food Nutr Sci* 10(1–2):1–65.

Chaplan, S. R., F. W. Bach, S. L. Shafer and T. L. Yaksh. 1995. Prolonged alleviation of tactile allodynia by intravenous lidocaine in neuropathic rats. *Anesthesiology* 83(4):775–785.

Cheshire, W. P., S. W. Abashian and J. D. Mann. 1994. Botulinum toxin in the treatment of myofascial pain syndrome. *Pain* 59(1):65–69.

Christiansen, E., B. Dannerskiold-Samsoe, B. Lund and R. B. Andersen. 1982. Regional muscle tension and pain (fibrositis) effect of massage on myoglobin in plasma. *Scand J Rehab Med* 15:17–20.

Clark, G. T., D. A. Seligman, W. K. Solberg and A. G. Pullinger. 1990. Guidelines for the treatment of temporomandibular disorders. *J Craniomandib Disord* 4(2):80–88.

Clauw, D. J. 1995a. Fibromyalgia: more than just a musculoskeletal disease. *Am Fam Phy* 52(2): 843–851.

———. 1995b. The pathogenisis of chronic pain and fatigue syndromes, with special reference to fibromyalgia. *Med Hyp* 44(5):369–378.

Cleare, A. J., J. Bearn, T. Allain, A. McGregor, S. Wessely, R. M. Murray and V. O'Keane. 1995. Contrasting neuroendocrine responses in depression and chronic fatigue syndrome. *J Affect Disord* 34(4):283–289.

Cohen, M. I., R. B. Sheather-Reid, A. F. Arroyo and G. D. Champion. 1995. Evidence for abnormal nociception in fibromyalgia and repetative strain injury. *J Musculoskel Pain* 3(2):49–58.

Collee, G., B. A. Dijkmans, J. P. Vandenbroucke and A. Cats. 1991. Iliac crest pain syndrome in low back pain. A double blind, randomized study of local injection therapy. *J Rheumatol* 18(7): 1060–1063.

Colquhoun, D. 1990. Re-analysis of clinical trial of homeopathic treatment in fibrositis. *Lancet* 336: 441–442.

Conigliaro, D. A. 1996. Opioids for chronic non-malignant pain. *J Fla Med Assoc* 83(10):708–711.

Cooperstein, R. and M. S. Schneider. 1996. Assessments of chiropractic techniques and procedures. *Top Clin Chiro* 3(1):44–51.

Corran, T. M., M. J. Farrell, R. D. Helme and S. J. Gibson. 1997. The classification of patients with chronic pain: age as a contributing factor. *Clin J Pain* 13(3):207–214.

Corrigan, F. M., S. MacDonald, A. Brown, K. Armstrong and E. M. Armstrong. 1994. Neurasthenic fatigue, chemical sensitivity and GABAa receptor toxins. *Med Hyp* 43(4):195–200.

Cote, K.A. and M. Moldofsky. 1997. Sleep, daytime symptoms, and cognitive performance in patients with fibromyalgia. *J Rheumatol* 24(10):2014–2023.

Craig, K. D., C. M. Lilley and C. A. Gilbert. 1996. Social barriers to optimal pain management in infants and children. *Clin J Pain* 12(3):232–242.

Crofford, L. J. and M. A. Demitrack. 1996. Evidence that abnormalities of central neurohormonal systems are key to understanding fibromyalgia and chronic fatigue syndrome. *Rheum Dis Clin North Am* 22(2):267–284.

Crofford, L. J. 1994. Neuroendocrine aspects of fibromyalgia. *J Musculoskel Pain* 2(3):125–133.

Croft, P., J. Burk, J. Schollum, E. Thomas, G. Macfarland and A. Stilman. 1996. More pain, more tender points: Is fibromyalgia just one end of a continuous spectrum. *Ann Rheum Dis* 55(7):482–485.

Culclasure, T. E., R. J. Enzenauer and S. G. West. 1993. Post-traumatic stress disorder presenting as fibromyalgia. *Am J Med* 94(5):548–549.

Cunningham, M. E. 1996. Becoming familiar with fibromyalgia. *Orthop Nurs* 15(2):33–36.

Dafinova, Y. 1995. Low intensity laser treatment of myofascial pain. *J Musculoskel Pain* 3(Suppl 1):101 (Abstract).

Danneskiold-Samsoe, B., E. Christiansen and R. B. Anderson. 1986. Myofascial pain and the role of myoglobin. *Scand J Rheumatol* 5:174–178.

Danneskiold-Samsoe, B., E. Christiansen, B. Lund and R. B. Andersen. 1982. Regional muscle tension and pain (fibrositis). Effect of massage on myoplasma. *Scand J Rehab Med* 15:17–20.

Davies, H. T., I. K. Crombie, J. H. Brown and C. Martin. 1997. Diminishing returns or appropriate treatment strategy?—an analysis of short-term outcomes after pain clinic treatment. *Pain* 70(2–3): 203–208.

Davis, A. E.1996. Primary care management of chronic musculoskeletal pain. *Nurse Pract* 21(8):72.

Davis, J. R. 1990. Fibrositis: a legal and medical enigma. *Trauma* 32(1):7–15.

Dawson, D. and N. Encel. 1993. Melatonin and sleep in humans. *J Pineal Res* 15(1):1–12.

Dean, B. Z., F. H. Williams, J. C. King and M. J. Goddard. 1994. Pain rehabilitation Part 4. Therapeutic options in pain management. *Arch Phys Med Rehabil* 75(5 Spec No):S21–S30.

de Giorlamo, G. 1991. Epidemiology and social costs of low back pain and fibromyalgia. *Clin J Pain* 7(Suppl 1):S1–S7.

Dellasega, C. and C. L. Keiser. 1997. Pharmacologic approaches to chronic pain in the older adult. *Nurse Pract* 22(5):20–24.

Demitrack, M. A. and L. J. Crofford. 1995. Hypothalamic-pituitary-adrenal dysregulation in fibromyalgia and chronic fatigue syndrome. An overview and hypothesis. *J Musculoskel Pain* 3(2):67–74.

Deodhar, A. A., R. A. Fisher, C. V. Blacker and A. D. Woolfe. 1994. Fluid retention syndrome and fibromyalgia. *Br J Rheumatol* 33(6):576–582.

Dertwinkel, R., A. Weibalck, M. Zenz and M. Strumpf. 1996. Oral opioids for long-term treatment of chronic non-cancer pain. *Anaesthesist* 45(6):495–505 (German).

Diakow, P. 1992. Differentiation of active and latent trigger points by thermography. *J Manip Physiol Ther* 15(7):439–441.

Dinerman, H. and A. C. Stere. 1992. Lyme disease associated with fibromyalgia. *Ann Int Med* 117(4): 281–285.

Disla, E., H. R. Rhim, A. Reddy, I. Karten and A. Taranta. 1994. Costochondritis. A prospective analysis in an emergency department setting. *Arch Intern Med* 154(21):2466–2469.

Di Stefano, G. and B. P. Radanov. 1995. Course of attention and memory after common whiplash: a two-years' prospective study with age, education and gender pair-matched patients. *Acta Neurol Scand* 91(5):346–352.

Djurica, S. 1995. Glomerular filtration in patients suffering from reactive hypoglycemia. *Clin Nephrol* 43(3):201–202.

Dobrenbusch, R., R. Gruterich and M. Genth. 1996. Fibromyalgia and Sjogren's syndrome: clinical and methodological aspects. *Z Rheumatol* 55:19–27.

Dole, V. P. 1992. Hazards of process regulations. The example of methadone maintenance. *JAMA* 267(16):2234–2235.

Dommerholt, J. 1998. Biomechanics of Low Speed Rear-end Collisions. Paper presented at the Focus on Pain Seminar in San Antonio, TX, March 12–15.

Drewes, A. M., K. D. Neilsen, S. J. Taagholt, K. Bierregaard, L. Svendsen and J. Gade. 1995. Slow wave sleep in fibromyalgia. *J Musculoskel Pain* 3(Suppl 1):29 (Abstract).

Drewes, A. M., K. D. Nielsen, S. J. Taagholt, K. Bjerregard, L. Svendsen and J. Gade. 1995. Sleep intensity in fibromyalgia: focus on the microstructure of the sleep process. *Brit J Rheum* 34(7):692–635.

Drewes, A. M., A. Andreseasen, H. D. Schroder, B. Hogsaa and P. Jennum. 1993. Pathology of skeletal muscle in fibromyalgia: a histo-immunochemical and ultrastructural study. *Brit J Rheumatol* 32(6):479–483.

Dubner, R. 1992. Hyperalgesia and expanded receptive fields. *Pain* 48:3–4.

Dubner, R. and K. M. Hargreaves. 1989. The neurobiology of pain and its modulation. *Clin J Pain* 5(Suppl 2):S1–S4.

Dubray, C., A. Alloui, L. Bardin, E. Rock, A. Mazur, Y. Rayssiguier, A. Eschalier and J. Lavarenne. 1997. Magnesium deficiency induces an hyperalgesia reversed by the NMDA receptor antagonist MK801. *Neuroreport* 8(6):1383–1386.

Durette, M. R., A. A. Rodriquez, J. C. Agre and J. L. Silverman. 1991. Needle electromylgraphic evaluation of patients with myofascial or fibromyalgic pain. *Am J Phys Med Rehabil* 70(3):154–156.

Eisinger, J., C. Gandalfo, H. Zakarian and T. Ayavou. 1997. Reactive oxygen species, antioxidant status and fibromyalgia. *J Musculoskel Pain* 5(4):5–15.

Eisinger, J., H. Zakarian, A. Plantamura, D. Bendahan and T. Ayayou. 1995. Mitochondrial respiratory chain in fibromyalgia. *J Musculoskel Pain* 3(Suppl 1):11 (Abstract).

Elert, J. E., S. B. Rantapaa-Dahlquist, L. Henriksson-Larsen, R. Lorentsan and B. U. Gerdle. 1992. Muscle performance, electromyography and fibre type composition in fibromyalgia and work-related myalgia. *Scand J Rheumatol* 21(1):28–34.

English, T. 1991. Skeptical of skeptics. *JAMA* 265(8):964.

Escobar, P. L. and J. Ballesteros. 1987. Myofascial pain syndrome. *Orthop Rev* 16(10):708–713.

Evans, R. W., R. I. Evans and M. J. Sharp. 1994. The physician survey on the post-concussion and whiplash syndromes. *Headache* 34(5):268–274.

Evans, R. W. 1992. Some observations on whiplash injuries. *Neurol Clin* 10(4):975–997.

Fernstrom, J. D. 1987. Food-induced changes in brain-serotonin synthesis: Is there a relationship to appetite for specific macro-nutrients? *Appetite* 8(3):163–182.

Ferraccioli, G., E. S. Fontanna and E. Scita. 1989. EMG-biofeedback training in fibromyalgia syndrome. *J Rheumatol* 16(7):1013–1014.

Fine, P. G. 1987. Myofascial trigger point pain in children. 111(4):547–548.

Finestone, D. H., B. A. Sawyer and S. K. Ober. 1991. Periodic leg movements during sleep in patients with fibromyalgia. *Ann Clin Psych* 3(3).

Fishbain, D. A. 1996. Myofascial pain syndrome and post-traumatic fibromyalgia: comment on the article by Wolfe. *Arth Care Res* 9(2):157–158.

Fishbain, D. A., H. L. Rosomoff and R. S. Rosomoff. 1992. Drug abuse, dependence, and addiction in chronic pain patients. *Clin J Pain* 8(2):77–85.

Fitzcharles, M. A. and J. M. Esdaile. 1997. The overdiagnosis of fibromyalgia syndrome. *Am J Med* 103(1):44–50.

Fitzcharles, M. A., S. Greenfield and J. M. Esdaile. 1992. Reactive fibromyalgia syndrome. *Arth Rheum* 35(6):678–681.

FitzGerald, R. T. D. 1991. Observations on trigger points, fibromyalgia, recurrent headaches and the cervical syndrome. *J Man Med* 6(4):124–129.

Flato, B., A. Aasland, I. H. Vandvik and O. Forre. 1997. Outcome and predictive factors in children with chronic idiopathic musculoskeletal pain. *Clin Exp Rheumatol* 15(5):567–577.

Freese, A. and K. J. Swartz. 1990. Kynurenine metabolites of tryptophan: implications for neurologic diseases. *Neurol* 40(4):691–695.

Fricton, J. R. 1994. Myofascial pain. *Balliere's Clin Rheumatol* 8(4):857–880.

Friedman, M. J. 1994. Neurobiological sensitization models of post-traumatic stress disorder: their possible relevance to multiple chemical sensitivity syndrome. *Toxicol Indus Health* 10(4/5): 449–462.

Friedman, P. J. 1997. Predictors of work disability in work-related upper-extremity disorders. *J Occip Environ Med* 39(4):339–343.

Gaby, A. R. 1996. Dehydroepiandrosterone: biological effects and clinical significance. *Alternative Med Rev* 1(2):60–69.

Galloway, J. 1990. Maintaining serenity in chronic illness. *NY State J Med* 90(7):366–367.

Garopian, M. B. 1995. The ultrastructure of myogenic trigger points in patients with contracture of mimetic muscles. *J Musculoskel Pain* 3(Suppl 1):23 (Abstract).

Garvey, T. A., M. R. Marks and S. W. Wiesel. 1989. A prospective, randomized, double-blind evaluation of trigger point injection therapy for low-back pain. *Spine* 14(9):962–964.

Gedalia, A., J. Press, M. Klein and D. Buskila. 1993. Joint hypermobility and fibromyalgia in school-children. *Ann Rheum Dis* 52(7):494–496.

Geel, S. E. 1994. The fibromyalgia syndrome: Musculoskeletal pathophysiology. *Sem Arth Rheum* 23(5):353.

Gerwin, R. and L. Feinberg. Ultrasound and EMG Identification of the Myofascial Trigger Point. 1998. Paper presented at the Focus on Pain Seminar Series lectures, San Antonio, TX. March 12–15.

Gerwin, R. 1997. Myofascial pain syndromes in the upper extremity. *J Hand Ther* 10:130–136.

Gerwin, R. and D. Duranleau. 1997. Ultrasound identification of the myofascial trigger point. *Muscle Nerve* 20(6):767–768.

Gerwin, R. 1995a. Chronic myofascial pain: iron insufficiency and coldness as risk factors. *J Musculoskel Pain* 3(Suppl 1):120 (Abstract).

———. 1995b. Myofascial back and neck pain. *Phys Med Rehab: State Art Rev* 9(3):657–671.

———. 1995c. A study of 96 subjects examined both for fibromyalgia and myofascial pain. *J Musculoskel Pain* 3(Suppl 1):121 (Abstract).

Giovengo, S. L., I. J. Russell and A. A. Larson. 1995. Amino acids in cerebrospinal fluid (CSF) of patients with fibromyalgia. *J Musculoskel Pain* 3(Suppl 1):9.

Gladman, D. D., M. B. Urowitz, J. Gough and A. MacKinnon. 1997. Fibromyalgia is a major contributor to quality of life in lupus. 24(11):2145–2148.

Godfrey, R. G. 1996. A guide to the understanding and use of tricyclic antidepressants in the overall management of fibromyalgia and other chronic pain disorders. *Arch Int Med* 156(10):1047–1052.

Goldberg, G. M., R. D. Kerns and R. Rosenberg. 1993. Pain-relevant support as a buffer from depression among chronic pain patients low in instrumental activity. *Clin J Pain* 9(1):34–40.

Goldberg, R.T. and W. N. Pachas. 1995. Childhood psychological traumas of patients with myofascial pain, fibromyalgia, fascial pain and other soft tissue disorders. *J Musculoskel Pain* 3(Suppl 1):80 (Abstract).

Goldenberg, D. L. 1997. Fibromyalgia, chronic fatigue syndrome, and myofascial pain syndrome. *Curr Opin Rheumatol* 9(2):135–143.

Goldenberg, D., M. Mayskiy, C. Mossey, R. Ruthazer and C. Schmid. 1996. Treatment: a randomized, double-blind crossover trial of fluoxetine and amitriptyline in the treatment of fibromyalgia. *Arth Rheum* 39:1852–1859.

Goldenberg, D. L. 1994a. Fibromyalgia and chronic fatigue syndrome. *J Musculoskel Pain* 2(3):51–55.

———. 1994b. Medications/clinical trials in fibromyalgia. *J Musculoskel Pain* 2(3):135–142.

———. 1993. Do infections trigger fibromyalgia? *Arth Rheum* 36(11):1489–1492.

Goldman, J. A. 1991. Hypermobility and deconditioning: important links to fibromyalgia/fibrositis. *South Med J* 84(10):1192–1196.

Goldman, L. B. and N. L. Rosenberg. 1991. Myofascial pain and fibromyalgia. *Sem Neuro* 11(3): 274–280.

Golsch, S., E. Vocks, J. Rakoski, K. Brockow and J. Ring. 1997. Reversible increase in photosensitivity to UV-B caused by St. John's wort extract. *Hautarzt* 48(4):249–253 (German).

Gorman, A. L., K. J. Elliot and C. E. Inturrisi. 1997. The d- and l-isomers of methadone bind to the non-competitive site on the N-methyl-Daspartate (NMDA) receptor in rat forebrain and spinal cord. *Neurosci Lett* 223(1):5–8.

Gowers, W. R. 1904. Lumbago: its lessons and analogues. *Brit Med J* 1:117–121.

Graff-Radford, S. B., J. L. Reeves, R. L. Baker and D. Chiu. 1989. Effects of transcutaneous electrical nerve stimulation on myofascial pain and trigger point sensitivity. *Pain* 37(1):1–5.

Grassi, W., P. Core, G. Corlino, F. Salaffi and C. Cervini. 1994. Capillary permeability in fibromyalgia. *J Rheumatol* 21(7):1328–1331.

Graven-Nielsen, T., L. Arendt-Neilsen, P. Svensson and T. S. Jensen. 1997. Experimental muscle pain: a quantitative study of local and referred pain in humans following the injection of hypertonic saline. *J Musculoskel Pain* 5(1):49–69.

Graziotti, P. J. and C. R. Goucke. The use of oral opioids in patients with chronic non-cancer pain. Management stragegies. *Med J Aust* 167(1):30–34.

Griep, E. N. 1993. Altered reactivity of hypothalmic-pituitary-adrenal axis in the primary fibromyalgia syndrome. *J Rheumatol* 20 (3):469–474.

Grontved, A., T. Brask, J. Kambskard and E. Hentzer. 1988. Ginger root against seasickness. A controlled trial on the open sea. *Acta Otolaryngol* 105(1/2):45–49.

Habirov, F., V. Veselovsky, R. Abashev and Z. Isanova. 1995. Role of axoplasmatic transport disturbance in formation of myofascial pain syndrome. *J Musculoskel Pain* 3(Suppl 1):157 (Abstract).

Hader, N., D. Rimon, A. Kinarty and N. Lahat. 1991. Altered interleukin-2 secretion in patients with primary fibromyalgia syndrome. *Arth Rheum* 34(7):866–872.

Hallmark, M. A., T. H. Reynolds, C. A. DeSouza, C. O. Dotson, R. A. Anderson and M. A. Rogers. 1996. Effects of chromium and resistive training on muscle strength and body composition. *Med Sci Sports Exerc* 28(1):139–144.

Han, S. C. and P. Harrison. 1997. Myofascial pain syndrome and trigger-point management. *Reg Anesth* 22(1):89–101.

Hannen, H. C., H. T. Hoenderdos, L. K. van Romunde, W. C. Hop, C. Mallee, J. P. Terwiel and G. B. Hekster. Controlled trial of hypnotherapy in the treatment of refractory fibromyalgia. *J Rheumatol* 18(1):72–75.

Harvey, C. K. 1993. Fibromyalgia Part II. Prevalence in the podiatric patient population. *J Am Podiat Med Assn* 83(7):416–417.

Hawley, D. J. and F. Wolfe. 1994. Effects of light and season on pain and depression in subjects with rheumatic disorders. *Pain* 59(2):227–234.

Hawley, D. J., F. Wolfe and M. A. Cathey. 1988. Pain, functional disability, and psychological status: a 12–month study of severity in fibromyalgia. *J Rheumatol* 15(10):1551–1556.

Helme, R. D., S. Gibson and Z. Khalil. 1990. Neural pathways in chronic pain. *Med J Aust* 153(7):400–406.

Henriksson, C. M. 1995a. Living with continuous muscular pain—patient perspectives. Part II: Strategies for daily life. *Scand J Caring Sci* 9(2):77–86.

———. 1995b. Living with continuous muscular pain—patient perspectives. Part I: Encounters and consequences. *Scand J Caring Sci* 9(2):67–76.

———. C. M. 1994. Long-term effects of fibromyalgia on everyday life. A study of 56 patients. *Scand J Rheumatol* 23(1):36–41.

Henriksson, C. M., I. Gundmark, A. Bengtsson and A. C. Ek. 1992. Living with fibromyalgia, consequences for everyday life. *Clin J Pain* 8(2):138–144.

Heppelmann, B., K. Messlinger, H. G. Schaible and R. F. Schmidt. 1991. Nociception and pain. *Curr Opin Neurobiol* 1(2):192–197.

Hesse, J., B. Mogelvang and H. Simonsen. 1994. Acupuncture versus metoptolol in migraine prophylaxis: a randomized trial of trigger point inactivation. *J Intern Med* 235(5):451–456.

Heuser, G. and A. Vojdani. 1997. Enhancement of natural killer cell activity and T and B cell function by buffered vitamin C in patients exposed to toxic chemicals: the role of protein kinase-C. *Immunopharmacol Immunotoxicol* 19(3):291–312.

Heyes, M. P. 1993. Quinolinic acid and kynurenine pathway metabolism in inflammatory and non-inflammatory neurologic disease. *Brain* 115(5):1249–1273.

Heyes, M. P., K. Saito and S. P. Markey. 1992. Human macrophages convert L-tryptophan into the neurotoxin quinolinic acid. *Biochem J* 283(Pt 3):633–635.

Hitchcock, L. S., B. R. Ferrell and M. McCaffery. 1994 The experience of chronic non-malignant pain. *J Pain Sympt Manage* 9(5):312–318

Holsten, F. and B. Bjorvaten. 1997. Phototherapy. An alternative for seasonal affective disorders of sleep disorders. *Tidsskr Nor Laegeforen* 117(17):2484–2488. (Norwegian).

Honeyman, G. S. 1997. Metabolic therapy for hypothyroid and euthyroid fibromyalgia: two case reports. *Clin B Myofasc Ther* 2(4):19–49.

Hong, C-Z, T. S. Kuan, J. T. Chen and S. M. Chen. 1997. Referred pain elicited by palpation and by needling of myofascial trigger points: a comparison. *Arch Phys Med Rehabil* 78(9):957–960.

Hong, C-Z. 1996. Pathophysiology of myofascial trigger points. *J Formos Med Assoc* 95:93–104.

Hong, C-Z, J. T. Chen, S. M. Chen, J. J. Yan and Y. J. Su. 1996. Histological findings of responsive loci in a myofascial trigger spot of rabbit skeletal muscle from where localized twitch responses could be elicited. *Arch Phys Med Rehabil* 77:962 (Abstract).

Hong, C-Z, Y. Torigoe and J. Yu. 1995. The localized twitch responses in responsive taut bands of rabbit skeletal muscle fibers are related to the reflexes at spinal cord level. *J Musculoskel Pain* 3(1):15–34.

Hong, C-Z, T-C Hsueh, S. Yu and V. Lin. 1997. Recurrent myofascial trigger points related to traumatic cervical disc bulging. *J Musculoskel Pain* 3(Suppl 1):21 (Abstract).

Hong, C-Z. 1994a. Considerations and recommendations regarding myofascial trigger point injection. *J Musculoskel Pain* 2(1):29–59.

———. 1994b. Lidocaine injection versus dry needling to myofascial trigger point: the importance of the local twitch response. *Am J Phys Med Rehabil* 73:256–263.

———. 1994c. Reply to Dr. Starlanyl. *J Musculoskel Pain* 2(2):143.

———. 1993. Myofascial trigger point injection. *Critical Reviews in Phys Med Rehabil* 5:203–217.

Hong, C-Z, Y-C Chen, C. H. Pon and J. Yu. 1993. Immediate effects of various physical medicine modalities on pain threshold of an active myofascial trigger point. *J Musculoskel Pain* 1(2):37–53.

Hong, C-Z and Simons D. G. 1992. Response to treatment for pectoralis minor myofascial pain syndrome after whiplash. *J Musculoskel Pain* 1(1):89–131.

Hopwood, M. B. and S. E. Abram. 1994. Factors associated with failure of trigger point injections. *Clin J Pain* 10(3):227–234.

Hsu, V. M., S. J. Patella and L. H. Sigal. 1993. "Chronic Lyme disease" as the incorrect diagnosis in patients with fibromyalgia. *Arth Rheum* 36(11):1493–1500.

Hubbard, D. R. and G. Berkoff. 1993. Myofascial trigger points show spontaneous needle EMG activity. *Spine* 18(13):1803–1807.

Hudson, J. I. and H. G. Pope, Jr. 1995. Does childhood sexual abuse cause fibromyalgia? *Arth Rheum* 38(2):161–163.

Hudson, N., M. R. Starr, J. M. Esdaile and M. A. Fitzcharles. Diagnostic associations with hypermobility in rheumatology patients. *Br J Rheumatol* 34(12):1157–1161.

Huether, G. 1994. Melatonin synthesis in the gastrointestinal tract and the impact of nutritional factors on circulating melatonin. *Ann NY Acad Sci* 19:146–158.

Hyppa, M. T. and E. Kronholm. 1995. Nocturnal motor activity in fibromyalgia patients with poor sleep quality. *J Phychosom Res* 39(1):85–91.

Inturrisi, C. E., W. A. Colburn, R. F. Kaiko, R. W. Honde and K. M. Foley. 1987. Pharmacokinetics and pharmacodynamics of methadone in patients with chronic pain. *Clin Pharmacol Ther* 41(4): 392–401.

Irwin, M., A. Mascovich, J. C. Gillin, R. Willoughby, J. Pike and T. L. Smith. 1994. Partial sleep deprivation reduces natural killer cell activity in humans. *Psychosom Med* 56(6):493–498.

Journal Occupational Medicine. Does fibromyalgia qualify as a work-related injury? 1992. *J Occupa Med* 34(10):968.

Jacobsen, S., K. Main, B. Danneskiold-Samsoe and N. E. Skakkebaek. 1995. A controlled study on serum insulin-like growth factor-1 and urinary excretion of growth hormone in fibromyalgia. *J Rheumatol* 22(6):1138–1140.

Jacobsen, S. 1994. Chronic widespread musculoskeletal pain—the fibromyalgia syndrome. *Dan Med Bul* 41(5):541–564.

Jacobsen, S., A. Gam, C. Egsmose, M. Olsen, B. Danneskiold-Samsoe and G. F. Jensen. 1993. Bone mass and turnover in fibromyalgia. *J Rheumatol* 20(5):856–859.

Jacobsen, S. and B. Danneskiold-Samsoe. 1992. Dynamic muscular endurance in primary fibromyalgia compared with chronic myofascial pain syndrome. *Arch Phys Med Rehab* 73(2):170–173.

Jaeger, B. 1989. Are "cervicogenic" headaches due to myofascial pain and cervical spine dysfunction? *Cephalalgia* 9(3):157–164.

Jaeger, B. and J. L. Reeves. 1986. Quantification of changes in myofascial trigger point sensitivity with the pressure algometer following passive stretch. *Pain* 27(2):203–210.

Jager, C., H. Sprott, C. H. Anders, H. C. H. Scholle and G. Hein. 1995. EMG-mapping in fibromyalgia. *J Musculoskel Pain* 3(Suppl 1):67 (Abstract).

Jamison, R. N. 1996. Comprehensive pretreatment and outcome assessment for chronic opioid therapy in nonmalignant pain. *J Pain Symptom Manage* 11(4):231–241.

Jamison, R. N., K. O. Anderson, C. Peeters-Asdourian and F. M. Ferrante. 1994. Survey of opioid use in chronic nonmalignant pain patients. *Reg Anesth* 19(4):225–230.

Jayson, M. I. 1996. Fibromyalgia and trigger point injections. *Bul Hosp Joint Dis* 55(4):176–177.

Jeal, W. and P. Benfield. 1997. Transdermal fentanyl. A review of its pharmacological properties and therapeutic efficacy in pain control. 53(1):109–138.

Jean, T. 1992. Stemming the office epidemic. *Risk Manag* 39(1):34–38.

Jennum, P., A. M. Drewes and A. Andreasen. 1993. Sleep and other problems in primary fibromyalgia and in healthy controls. *J Rheumatol* 20(10):1756–1759.

Jensen, K. 1995. Human cerebral blood flow changes during ischemic muscular pain. *J Musculoskel Pain* 3(Suppl 1):43 (Abstract).

Jensen, M. D., M. L. Martin, P. E. Cryer and I. R. Roust. 1994. Effects of estrogen on free fatty acid metabolism in humans. *Am J Physiol* 266(6 Pt 1):E914–E920.

Jeschonneck, M., H. Sprott, G. Grohmann and G. Hein. 1995. Temperature and laser-flow-measuring above tender points in fibromyalgia. *J Musculoskel Pain* 3(Suppl 1):17 (Abstract).

Johnson, M., M. L. Pannanen, P. Rahinantti, and P. Hannonen. 1995. Self-esteem and fibromyalgia. *J Musculoskel Pain* 3(Suppl 1):35 (Abstract).

Joos, E., R. Meeusen and L. de Meirleir. Measurement of physical capacity in fibromyalgia. *J Musculoskel Pain* 3(Suppl 1):87 (Abstract).

Joyce, E., S. Blumenthal and S. Wessely. 1996. Memory, attention and executive function in chronic fatigue syndrome. *J Neurol Neurosurg Psychiatry* 60(5):459–503.

Jubrias, S. A., R. M. Bennett and G. A. Klug. 1994. Increased incidence of resonance in the phosphodiester region of 31P nuclear magnetic resonance spectra in the skeletal muscle of fibromyalgia patients. *Arth Rheum* 37(6):801–807.

Kanakamedalia, R. V. and C-Z Hong. 1989. Peroneal nerve entrapment at the knee localized by short segment stimulation. *Am J Phys Med Rehabil* 68(3):116–122.

Karlsten, R. and T. Gordh, Jr. 1995. An A1–selective adenosine agonist abolishes allodynia elicited by vibration and touch after intrathecal injection. *Anesth Analg* 80(4):844–847.

Karoliussen, O. H. and L. Kvalheim. 1995. Effects of mexiletine on pain and other symptoms in primary fibromyalgia. *J Musculoskel Pain* 3(Suppl 1):26 (Abstract).

Kaufmann, H. 1997. Neurally mediated syncope and syncope due to autonomic failure: differences and similarities. *J Clin Neurophysiol* 14(3):183–196.

Kaunaite, D. 1995. Pathogenesis of chest muscular pain syndrome in patients with coronary heart disease. *J Musculoskel Pain* 3(Suppl 1):153 (Abstract).

Kelley, P. and P. Clifford. 1997. Coping with chronic pain: assessing narrative approaches. *Sco Work* 42(3)266–277.

Kemple, K. 1989. Fingernail pits: Clinical markers for fibromyalgia? *Mod Med* 57(5):58–59.

Kennedy, M. and D. T. Felson 1996. A prospective long-term study of fibromyalgia syndrome. *Arthritis Rheum* 39(4):682–685.

Kerb, R., J. Brockmoller, B. Staffeldt, M. Ploch and I. Roots. 1996. Single-dose and steady-state pharmacokinetics of hypericin and pseudohypericin. *Antimicrob Agents Chemother* 40(9):2087–2093.

Kermode-Scott, B. 1997. Chronic non-malignant pain. Consider using opioids. *Can Fam Physician* 43:1011–1013.

Kerns, R. D., R. Rosenberg, R. N. Jamison, M. S. Caudill and J. Haythornthwaite. 1997. Readiness to adopt a self-management approach to chronic pain: the Pain Stages of Change Questionnaire. *Pain* 72(1–2):227–234.

Khalil, T. M., S. S. Asfour, L. M. Martinez, S. M. Waly, R. S. Rosomoff and H. L. Rosomoff. 1992. Stretching in the rehabilitation of low-back pain patients. *Spine* 17(3):311–317.

King, J. C. and M. J. Goddard. 1994. Pain rehabilitation. 2. Chronic pain syndrome and myofascial pain. *Arch Phys Med Rehabil* 75(5 Spec No):S9–S14.

Kischka, U., T. Ettlin, S. Heim and G. Schmid. 1991. Cerebral symptoms following whiplash injury. *Eur Neural* 31(3):136–140.

Kiselev, M. O. and M. B. Gariphianova. 1995. The satellite trigger points in muscles of pelvis bottom in patients with contracture of mimetic muscles. *J Musculoskel Pain* 3(Suppl 1):24 (Abstract).

Klein, R. and P. A. Berg. 1994. A comparative study on antibodies to nucleoli and 5–hydroxytryptamine in patients with fibromyalgia syndrome and tryptophan-induced eosinophilia-myalgia syndrome. *Clin Investig* 72(7):541–549.

Klepstad, P. and P. C. Borchgrevink. 1997. Four years' treatment with ketamine and a trial of dextromethorphan in a patient with severe post-herpetic neuralgia. *Acta Anasthesiol Scand* 41(3): 422–426.

Kosek, E., J. Ekholm and P. Hansson. 1995. Increased pressure pain sensibility in fibromyalgia patients is located deep to the skin but not restricted to muscle tissue. *Pain* 63(3):335–339.

Kovacs, F. M., V. Abraira, F. Pozo, D. G. Kleinbaum, J. Beltran, I. Mateo, C. Perez de Ayala, A. Pena, A. Zea, M. Gonzalez-Lanza and L. Morillas. 1997. Local and remote sustained trigger point therapy for exacerbations of chronic low back pain. A randomized, double-blind, controlled, multicenter trial. *Spine* 22(7):786–797.

Kramis, R. C., W. J. Roberts and R. G. Gillette. 1996. Non-nociceptive aspects of persistent musculoskeletal pain. *J Orthop Sports Phys Ther* 24(4):255–267.

Krapac, L., M. Stadoljev, D. Sacer and D. Sakie. 1997. Rheumatic complaints and musculoskeletal disorders in workers of a meat processing industry. *Arch Hig Rada Toksikol* 48(2):211–217.

Kronn, E. 1993. The incidence of TMJ dysfunction in patients who have suffered a cervical whiplash injury following a traffic accident. *J Orofac Pain* 7(2):209–213.

Kruse, R. A., Jr. and J. A. Christiansen. 1992. Thermographic imaging of myofascial trigger points: a follow-up study. *Arch Phys Med Rehabil* 73(9):819–823.

Kuch, K., B. Cox, R. J. Evans, P. C. Watson and C. Bubela. 1993. To what extent do anxiety and depression interact with chronic pain? *Can J Psychiatry* 38(1):36–38.

Langley, P. 1997. Scapular instability associated with brachial plexus irritation: a proposed causative relationship with treatment implications. *J Hand Therapy* 10(1):35–40.

Lapossy, E., R. Maleizke, P. Hyrcaj, W. Mennet and W. Muller. The frequency of transition of chronic low back pain to fibromyalgia. *Scand J Rheumatol* 24(1):29–33.

Lebovits, A. H., I. Florence, R. Bathina, V. Hunko, M. T. Fox and C. Y. Bramble. 1997. Pain knowledge and attitudes of healthcare providers: practice characteristic differences. *Clin J Pain* 13(3): 237–243.

Lee, J. C., D. T. Lin and C-Z Hong. 1997. The effectiveness of simultaneous thermotherapy with ultrasound and electrotherapy with combined AC and DC current on the immediate pain relief of myofascial trigger points. *J Musculoskel Pain* 5(1):81–90.

Lehman, R. Assessment of hypoglycemia. 1994. *Schweitz Med Wochenschr* 124(26):1155–1161.

Lentjes, E. G., E. N. Griep, J. W. Boersma, F. P. Romijn and E. R. de Kloet. 1997. Glucocorticoid receptors, fibromyalgia and low back pain. *Psychoneuroendocrinology* 22(8):603–614.

Leonetti, F. 1996. Increased nonoxidative glucose metabolism in idiopathic reactive hypoglycemia. *Metabolism* 45(5):606–610.

Lewis, P. J. 1996. A review of prayer within the role of the holistic nurse. *J Holist Nurs* 14(4):308–315.

———. 1993. Electroacupuncture in fibromyalgia. *Brit Med J* 306(6874):393.

Liebenson, C. 1996. Rehabilitation and chiropractic practice. *J Manip Physiol Ther* 19(2):134–140.

Lightfoot, R.W., Jr., B. J. Luft, D. W. Rahn, A. C. Steere, L. H. Sigal, D. C. Zoschke, P. Gardner, M. C. Britton and R. L. Kaufman. 1993. Empiric parenteral antibiotic treatment of patients with fibromyalgia and fatigue and a positive serologic result for Lyme disease. *Ann Intern Med* 119(6):503–509.

Lin, T.Y., M. J. Teixeira, P. Stump, H. J. Pai, G. C. B. Castro, A. T. Ungaretti, J. A. Figueiro, H. H. S. Kaziyama, C. V. Hort, C. A. Simoes and E. Queiroz. 1995. Chronic abdominal pain of unknown origin. The role of myofascial pain syndrome. *J Musculoskel Pain* 3(Suppl 1):32 (Abstract).

Lin, T.Y., M. J. Texiera, P. Stump, H. J. Pai, A. Ungaretti, Jr., G. C. B. Castro, H. H. S. Kaziyama, J. A. Figueiro, L. A. K. Yoshihara, C. V. Horta and R. M. Marcon. 1995. Pelvic pain of uncertain aetiology—clinical and therapeutic aspects. *J Musculoskel Pain* 3(Suppl 1):33 (Abstract).

Lin, T.Y., M. J. Teixeira, H. J. Pai, H. A. S. Kaziyama, E. Guedes, P. Stump, R. Bergel, J. A. Figueiro, R. J. Azze, R. Mattar, Jr., S. T. Imamura, E.T. Saito and S. Abramicus. Cumulative trauma disorders (CTD). The role of myofascial pain syndromes in the aetiology of pain. *J Musculoskel Pain* 3(Suppl 1):149 (Abstract).

Lin, T.Y., M. J. Teixeira, H. H. S. Kaziyama, H. J. Pai, P. Stump, C. Horta, R. J. Azze, R. Mattar, Jr., and S. Imamura. 1995. Myofascial Pain Syndrome (MPS) associated with reflex sympathetic dystrophy. *J Musculoskel Pain* 3(Suppl 1):150 (Abstract).

Lind-Olesen, L. H. and K. Lund-Olesen. 1994. The etiology and possible treatment of chronic fatigue syndrome/fibromyalgia. *Med Hypoth* 43:55–58.

Linde, K., G. Ramirez, C. D. Mulrow, A. Pauls, W. Weidenhammer and D. Melchart. 1996. St. John's wort for depression—an overview and meta-analysis of randomized clinical trials. *BMJ* 313(7052):253–258.

Lindgren, M., B. Eckert, G. Stenberg and C. D. Agardh. 1996. Restitution of neurophysiological functions, performance, and subjective symptoms after moderate insulin-induced hypoglycemia in non-diabetic men. *Diabetic Medicine* 13:218–225.

Lister, B. J. 1996. Dilemmas in the treatment of chronic pain. *Am J Ned* 101(1A):2S-5S.

Littlejohn, G. O. 1989. Medicolegal aspects of fibrositis syndrome. *J Rheumatol* 16(Suppl 19):169–173.

Liu, H., P. W. Mantyh and A. I. Basbaum. 1997. NMDA-receptor regulation of substance P release from primary afferent nociceptors. *Nature* 386(6626):721–724.

Lorenzen, I. 1994. Fibromyalgia: a clinical challenge. *J Int Med* 235(3):199–203.

Lotter, N. 1995. Natural killer cells and early diagnosis of fibromyalgia. *J Musculoskel Pain* 3(Suppl 1):89 (Abstract).

Lovy, M. R., G. Starkebaum and S. Uberoi. 1996. Hepatitis C infection presenting with rheumatic manifestations: a mimic of rheumatoid arthritis. *J Rheumatol* 23(6):979–983.

Lowe, J. C., A. J. Reichman, G. S. Honeyman, and J. Yellin. 1997. Thyroid status of fibromyalgia patients. *Clin Bulletin Myofas Ther* 3(1):69–70 (Abstract).

Lowe, J. C., R. Garrison, A. Reichman, J. Yellin, M. Thompson and D. Kaufman. 1997. Effectiveness and safety of T3 (triiodthyronine) therapy for euthyroid fibromyalgia: a double-blind placebo-controlled response-driven crossover study. *Clin Bulletin Myofas Ther* 2(2/3):31–57.

Lowe, J. C., A. J. Reichman and J. Yellin. 1998. A case-control study of metabolic therapy for fibromyalgia: long-term follow-up comparison of treated and untreated patients. *Clin Bulletin Myofas Ther* 3(1):23–24 (Abstract).

Lowe, J. C., A. Reichman and J. Yellin. 1997. The process of change during T3 treatment for euthyroid fibromyalgia: a double-blind placebo-controlled crossover study. *Clin Bull Myofas Ther* 2(2/3): 91–124.

Lowe, J. C., M. E. Cullum, L. H. Graf, Jr.and J. Yellin. 1997. Mutations in the c-erbA beta gene: do they underlie euthyroid fibromyalgia? *Med Hypo* 48(2):125–135.

Lue, E. A. 1994. Sleep and fibromyalgia. *J Rheumatol* 2(3):89–100.

Lupien, S. J. and B. S. McEwen. 1997. The acute effects of corticosteroids on cognition: integration of animal and human model studies. *Brain Res Brain Res Rev* 24(1):1–27.

Lykkegaard, J. J., A. H. Hansen and B. Danneskiold-Samsoe. 1997. Prevalence of joint hypermobility in patients with fibromyalgia. *J Musculoskel Pain* 3(Suppl 1):117 (Abstract).

Macarthur, C., J. G. Wright, R. Srivastava, W. Rosser and W. Feldman. 1996. Variability in physicians' reported ordering and perceived reassurance value of diagnostic tests in children with "growing pains." *Arch Pediatr Adolesc Med* 150(10):1072–1076.

MacFarlane, J. G., B. Shahal, C. Mously and H. Moldofsky. 1996. Periodic K/alpha sleep EC activity and periodic limb movements during sleep: comparisons of clinical features of sleep parameters. *Sleep* 19:200–204.

Mackley, R. J. 1990. Role of trigger points in the management of head, neck and face pain. *Funct Orthod* 7(5):4–14.

Majewski, M. D. 1995. Neuronal actions of dehydroepiandrosterone. Possible roles in brain development, angina, memory, and affect. *Ann NY Acad Sci* 774:111–120.

Makela, M. and M. Heliovaara. 1991. Prevalence of primary fibromyalgia in the Finnish population. *Brit Med J* 303:216–219.

Malleson, P. N., M. al-Matar and R. E. Petty. 1992. Idiopathic musculoskeletal pain syndromes in children. *J Rheumatol* 19(11):1786–1789.

Mandel, L. M. and S. J. Berlin. 1982. Myofascial pain syndrome and its effect on the lower extremities. *J Foot Surg* 21(1):74–79.

Mantyh, P. W., S. D. Rogers, P. Honore, B. J. Allen, J. R. Ghilardi, J. Li, R. D. Daughters, D. A. Lappi, R. G. Wiley and D. A. Simone. 1997. Inhibition of hyperalgesia by ablation of lamina I spinal neurons expressing the substance P receptor. *Science* 278(5336):275–279.

Mantyh, P. W. 1991. Substance P and the inflammatory and immune response. *Ann NY Acad Sci* 632:263–271.

Manu, P., T. J. Lane, D. A. Matthews, R. J. Castriotta, R. K. Watson and M. Ables. Alpha-delta sleep in patients with a chief complaint of chronic fatigue. *South Med J* 87(4):465–470.

Margolis, F. R., K. A. Hudson and Y. Michel. 1995. Beliefs and perceptions about children in pain: a survey. *Pediatric Nurs* 21(2):111–115.

Marwick, C. 1996. Medical records privacy a patient rights issue. *JAMA* 276(23):1861–1862.

———. 1995. Should physicians prescribe prayer for health? Spiritual aspects of well-being considered. *JAMA* 273(20):1561–1562.

Maryon, F. 1991. Fibrositis (fibromyalgia syndrome) and the dental clinician. *J Craniomandib Dis* 9(1):63–70.

Masi, A. T. 1994. An intuitive person-centered perspective on fibromyalgia syndrome and its management. *Ballieres Clin Rheumatol* 8(4):957–993.

Mason, J., S. L. Silverman and A. L. Weaver. 1991. Fibromyalgia Impact Assessment Form. *Arth Care Res* 4:523.

Maurizio, S. J. and R. L. Rogers. 1997. Recognizing and treating fibromyalgia. *Nurse Pract* 22(12):18–26.

Mayou, R. and B. P. Radanov. 1996. Whiplash neck injury. *J Psychosom Res* 40(5):461–474.

McArdle, A., C. I. A. Jack, R. H. T. Edwards and M. J. Jackson. 1995. Microdialysis measurements of pain-producing substances in muscle during ischemia and reperfusion. *J Musculoskel Pain* 3(Suppl 1):6 (Abstract).

McCaffrey, M. and C. L. Pasero. 1997. Pain ratings: the fifth vital sign. 1997. *Am J Nurs* 97(2):15–16.

McCain, G. A. 1994. Treatment of the fibromyalgia syndrome. *J Musculoskel Pain* 2(1):93–104.

McCain, G. A., R. Cameron and J. C. Kennedy. 1989. The problem of long-term disability payments and litigation in primary fibromyalgia syndrome: the Canadian perspective. *J Rheumatol* 16(Suppl 19):174–176.

McClaflin, R. R. 1994. Myofascial pain syndrome. Primary care strategies for early intervention. *Postgrad Med* 96(2):56–59.

McCormack, K. 1994. Non-steroidal anti-inflammatory drugs and spinal nociceptive processing. *Pain* 59(1):9–43.

McCracken, L. M. and R. T. Gross. 1993. Does anxiety affect coping with chronic pain? *Clin J Pain* 9(4):253–259.

McMillan, A. S. and B. Blasberg. 1994. Pain-pressure threshold in painful jaw muscles following trigger point injection. *J Orofac Pain* 8(4):384–390.

McSherry, J. A. 1989. Cognitive impairment after head injury. *Am Fam Phys* 40(4):186–190.

Meggs, W. J. 1995. Neurogenic switching: a hypothesis for a mechanism for shifting the site of inflammation in allergy and chemical sensitivity. *Environ Health Perspect* 103(1):54–56.

Mengshoel, A. M., E. Saugan, O. Forre and N. K. Vollestad. 1995. Muscle fatigue in early fibromyalgia. *J Rheumatol* 22(1):43–50.

Mengshoel, A. M., O. Forre and H. B. Konmaesh. 1990. Muscle strength and aerobic capacity in primary fibromyalgia. *Clin Exper Rheumatol* 8(5):475–479.

The Merck Manual. 1992. Rahway NJ: Merck & Co.

Mense, S. 1996. Biochemical pathogenesis of myofascial pain. *J Musculoskel Pain* 4(1/2):145–162.

———. 1993. Nociception from skeletal muscle in relation to clinical muscle pain. *Pain* 54(3):241–289.

Middleton, G. D., J. E. McFarlin and P. E. Lipsky. 1994. The prevalence and clinical impact of fibromyalgia in systemic lupus erythematosus. *Arth and Rheum* 37(8):181–188.

Mikkelsson, M., J. J. Salminen and H. Kautiainen. 1997. Non-specific musculoskeletal pain in preadolescents. Prevalence and 1–year persistence. *Pain* 73(1):29–35.

Moldofsky, H. 1995. Sleep, neuroimmune and neuroendocrine functions in fibromyalgia and chronic fatigue syndrome. *Advan Neuroimmun* 5(1):39–56.

———. 1993. Fibromyalgia, sleep disorder and chronic fatigue syndrome. *Ciba Found Symp* 173: 262–271.

———. 1989a. Sleep and fibrositis syndrome. *Rheum Dis Clin N Am* 15(1):1701–1704.

———. 1989b. Sleep-wake mechanisms in fibrositis. *J Rheumatol* 16(Supp 19):47–48.

Moldofsky, H., R. Gilbert, F. A. Lue and A. W. MacLean. 1995. Sleep-related violence. *Sleep* 18(9):731–739.

Moldofsky, H., M. Wong and F. Lue. 1994. Litigation, sleep, symptoms and disabilities in post-accident pain (fibromyalgia). *J Rheumatol* 20:1935–1940.

Morand, E. F., M. H. Miller, S. Whittingham and G. O. Littlejohn. 1994. Fibromyalgia syndrome and disease activity in systemic lupus erythematosus. *Lupus* 3(3):187–191.

Mufson, M. and Q. R. Regestein. 1993. The spectrum of fibromyalgia disorders. *Arth Rheum* 36(5): 647–650.

Mukerji, B., V. Mukerji, M. A. Alpert and R. Sekular. 1995. The prevalence of rheumatologic disorders in patients with chest pain and angiographically normal coronary arteries. *Angiol* 46(5):425–430.

Murphy, B. A. and N. J. Dawson. 1995. The assessment of intramuscular discrimination using signal detection theory: its potential contribution to chiropractic. *J Manip Physiol Ther* 18(9):572–576.

Nasr, F. W. 1995. The fibromyalgia syndrome. *J Med Liban* 43(1):23–25.

Neoh, C. A. 1995. The importance of trigger points in cancer pain management. In *Management of Pain: A World Perspective*. Eds. P. R.-J. Erdine and D. NivMonduzzi. 85–88. Monduzzi Editore: Bologna, Italy.

New, P. W., T. C. Lim, S. T. Hill and D. J. Brown. 1997. A survey of pain during rehabilitation after acute spinal cord injury. *Spinal Cord* 35(10):658–663.

Ng, S. C. 1992. The fibromyalgia syndrome. *Sing Med J* 33(3):294–295.

Nielson, W. R., C. Walker and G. A. McCain. 1992. Cognitive behavioral treatment of fibromyalgia syndrome: preliminary findings. *J Rheumatol* 19(1):98–103.

Nielson, W. R., G. M. Grace, M. Hopkins and M. Berg. 1995. Concentration and memory deficits in patients with fibromyalgia syndrome. *J Musculoskel Pain* 3(Suppl 1):123 (Abstract).

Nishikai, M. 1992. Fibromyalgia in Japanese. *J Rheumatol* 19(1):110–114.

Njoo, K. H. and E. Van der Does. The occurrence and inter-rater reliability of myofascial trigger points in the quadratus lumborum and gluteus medius: a prospective study in non-specific low back pain patients and controls in general practice. *Pain* 59(3):317–323.

Nordstrom, D. 1994. Disabling fibromyalgia. Appearance vs. reality. *J Rheumatol* 21(8):1776.

Okifuji, A., D. C. Turk, J. D. Sinclair, T. W. Starz and D. A. Marcus. 1997. A standard manual tender point survey. I. Development and determination of a threshold point for the identification of positive tender points in fibromyalgia syndrome. *J Rheumatol* 24(2):377–383.

Older, S. A., D. F. Battafarano, C. L. Danning, J. A. Ward, E. P. Grady, S. Derman and I. J. Russell. 1995. Delta wave sleep interruption and fibromyalgia symptoms in healthy subjects. *J Musculoskel Pain* 3(Suppl 1):159 (Abstract).

Ostensen, M., A. Rugelsjoen and S. H. Wigers. 1997. The effect of reproductive events and alterations of sex hormone levels on the symptoms of fibromyalgia. *Scand J Rheumatol* 26(5):355–360.

Ostuni, P. A. Acupuncture vs. low-dose myanserine in primary fibromyalgia syndrome. 1995. *J Musculoskel Pain* 3(Suppl 1):88 (Abstract).

Owada, K., T. Wasada, Y. Miyazono, H. Yoshino, S. Hasumi, H. Kuroki, K. Yano, A. Maruyama, K. Kawai and Y. Omori. 1995. Highly increased insulin secretion in a patient with postprandial hypoglycemia: role of glucagon-like peptide-1 (7–36) amide. *Endocr J* 42(2):147–151.

Pappagallo, M. and L. J. Heinberg. 1997. Ethical issues in the management of chronic nonmalignant pain. *Semin Neurol* 17(3):203–211.

Parziale, J. R. and J. J. Chen. 1996. Fibromyalgia. *Med Health RI* 79(5):188–192.

Pascarelli, E. F. and J. J. Kella. 1993. Soft-tissue injuries related to use of the computer keyboard. A clinical study of 53 severely injured persons. *J Occup Med* 35(5):522–532.

Pasero, C. L. and M. McCaffery. 1997. Pain control. *Am J Nurs* 97(6):20–21.

Perlis, M. L., D. E. Giles, R. R. Bootzin, Z. V. Dikman, G. M. Fleming, S. P. Drummond and M. W. Rose. 1997. Alpha sleep and information processing, perception of sleep, pain, and arousability in fibromyalgia. *Int J Neurosci* 89(3–4):265–280.

Piometti, D. 1994. Eicosanoids in synaptic transmission. *Crit Rev Neurobiol* 8(1–2):65–83.

Pollman, L. 1994. Fibromyalgia. Chronobiological aspects. *Chronobio Internat* 1(6):393–396.

Portenoy, R. K. and S.R. Savage. 1997. Clinical realities and economic considerations: special therapeutic issues in intrathecal therapy—tolerances and addiction. *J Pain Sympt Manage* 14(3 Suppl): S27–S35.

Portenoy, R. K. 1990. Chronic opioid therapy in nonmalignant pain. *J Pain Sympt Manage* 5(1 Suppl): S46–S62.

Porter, F. L., C. M. Wolf, J. Gold, D. Lotsoff and J. P. Miller. 1997. Pain and pain management in newborn infants: A survey of physicians and nurses. *Pediatrics* 100(4):626–632.

Porter, J. and H. Jick. 1980. Addiction rare in patients treated with narcotics. *New Eng J Med* 302:123.

Potter, J. W. 1992. Helping fibromyalgia patients obtain Social Security benefits. *J Musculoskel Med* 9(9):65–74. (Available ttp://wavecom.net/~lrandall/index.html Lois Randall website.)

Potts, M. K. and S. L. Silverman. 1990. The importance of aspects of treatment for fibromyalgia (fibrositis). Differences between patient and physician views. *Arth Care Res* 3(1):11–18.

Powers, R. 1993. Fibromyalgia: an age-old malady begging for respect. *J Gen Int Med* 8(2):93–105.

Prescott, E., S. Jacobsen, M. Kjoller, P. M. Bulow, B. Danneskiold-Samsoe and F. Kamper-Jorgensen. 1993. Fibromyalgia in the adult Danish population II. A study of clinical features. *Scand J Rheum* 22(5):238–242.

Rachlin, E. C. 1997. Importance of trigger point management in orthopedic practice. *Phys Med & Rehab Clin N Am* 8(1):171–177.

Radanov, B. P., S. Begre, M. Sturzeneggar and K. F. Augustiny. 1996. Course of psychological variables in whiplash injury–a two-year follow-up with age, gender and education pair-matched patients. *Pain* 64(3):429–434.

Reid, G. D. 1994. Disabling fibromyalgia. Appearance vs. reality. *J Rheumatol* 21(8):1578–1579.

Reid, G. J., B. A. Lang and P. J. McGrath. 1997. Primary juvenile fibromyalgia: psychological adjustment, family functioning, coping and functional disability. *Arth Rheum* 40(4):752–760.

Reiffenberger, D. H. and L. H. Amundson. 1996. Fibromyalgia syndrome: a review. *Am Fam Phys* 53(5):1698–1712.

Reilly, P. A. 1993. Fibromyalgia in the workplace: a "management" problem. *Ann Rheum Dis* 52(4):249–251.

Reitinger, A., H. Radner, H. Tilscher, M. Hanna, A. Windsch and W. Feigl. 1996. Morphologische Untersuchung an Triggerpunkten (Morphological Study of Trigger Points). *Manuelle Medizin* 34:256–262 (German).

Reville, J. D. 1997. Soft-tissue rheumatism: diagnosis and treatment. *Am J Med* 102(1A):23S-29S.

Reynolds, M. D. 1984. Myofascial trigger points in persistent posttraumatic shoulder pain. *South Med J* 77(10):1277–1280.

Rivera J., A. De Diego, M. Trinchet and A. Garcia Monforte. 1997. Fibromyalgia-associated hepatitis C virus infection. *Br J Rheumatol* 36(9):981–985.

Robel, P. and E. E. Baulieu. 1995. Dehydroepiandrosterone (DHEA) is a neuroactive neurosteriod. *Ann NY Acad Sci* 774:82–110.

Rogers, N., C. van den Heuvel and D. Dawson. 1997. Effect of melatonin and corticosteroid on in vitro cellular immune function in humans. *J Pineal Res* 22(2):75–80.

Roistacher, S. L. and D. Tannenbaum. 1986. Myofascial pain associated with oropharyngeal cancer. *Oral Surg Oral Med Oral Pathol* 61(5):459–462.

Roizenblatt, S., S. Tufik, J. Goldenberg, L. R. Pinto, M. P. Hilario and D. Feldman. 1997. Juvenile fibromyalgia: clinical and polysomnographic aspects. *J Rheumatol* 24(3):579–585.

Romano, T. J. 1997. Myofascial pain and fibromyalgia syndrome. *Neurology* 48(6):1739–1740.

———. 1995. Abnormal central nervous system neurodiagnostic testing in post-traumatic fibromyalgia. *J Musculoskel Pain* 3(Suppl 1):106 (Abstract).

———. 1993. The usefulness of cranial electrotherapy in the treatment of headache in fibromyalgia patients. *Am J Pain Manag* 3(1):15–19.

———. 1988a. The fibromyalgia syndrome. It's the real thing. *Postgrad Med* 83(5):231–232.

———. 1988b. Fibrositis in men. *WV Med J* 84:235–237

Rosen, N. B. 1994. Physical medicine and rehabilitation approaches to the management of myofascial pain and fibromyalgia syndrome. *Ballieres Clin Rheumatol* 8(4):881–916.

Rosenhall, U., G. Johannson and G. Orndahl. 1987. Eye motility dysfunction in chronic primary fibromyalgia with dysthesia. *Scand J Rehabil Med* 19(4):139–145.

Ruben, I. L. and J. R. Sanes. 1996. Neuronal and glial cell biology *Curr Opin Neurobiol* 6(5):573–575.

Ruiz-Moral, R., M. Munoz Alamo, L. Perula de Torres and M. Aguayo Galcote. 1997. Biopsychosocial features of patients with widespread chronic musculoskeletal pain in family medicine clinics. *Fam Pract* 14(3):242–248.

Russell, A. S. and J. S. Percy. 1994. Disabling fibromyalgia. Appearance vs. reality. *J Rheumatol* 21(8):1580.

Russell I. J. 1996a. Fibromyalgia syndrome: approaches to management. *Bul Rheum Dis* 45(3):1–4.

———. Ed. 1996b. *Clinical Overview and Pathogenesis of the Fibromyalgia Syndrome, Myofascial Pain Syndrome, and other Pain Syndromes.* Binghamton, NY: Haworth Press.

———. 1995. Neurohormonal: abnormal laboratory findings related to pain and fatigue in fibromyalgia. *J Musculoskel Pain* 3(2):59–66.

———. 1994. Biochemical abnormalities in fibromyalgia syndrome. *J Musculoskel Pain* 2(3):101–115.

———. 1990. Treatment of patients with fibromyalgia syndrome: considerations of the whys and wherefores. *Advance Pain Res Ther* 17:303–314.

———. 1989. Neurohormonal aspects of fibromyalgia syndrome. *Rheum Dis Clin N Am* 15(1):149–168.

Russell, I. J., J. E. Michalek, J. D. Flechas and G. E. Abraham. 1995. Treatment of fibromyalgia syndrome with Super Malic; a randomized, double-blind, placebo-controlled, crossover pilot study. *J Rheumatol* 22(5):953–958.

Russell, I. J., M. D. Orr, B. Littman, G. A. Vipraio, D. Alboukrek, J. E. Michalek, Y. Lopez and F. MacKillip. 1994. Elevated cerebrospinal levels of substance P in patients with the fibromyalgia syndrome. *Arth Rheum* 37(11):1593–1601.

Russell, I. J., J. E. Michalek, G. A. Vipraio, E. M. Fletcher and K. Wall. 1989. Serum amino acids in fibrositis/fibromyalgia. *J Rheumatol* Suppl 19:158–163.

Ryan, K. S. and J. Milles. Use of a posture training device as an adjunctive treatment of myofascial pain. *J Musculoskel Pain* 3(Suppl 1):53 (Abstract).

Ryan, S. 1995. Fibromyalgia: what help can nurses give? *Nursing Stand* 9(37):25–28.

Santandrea, S., F. Montrone, P. Sarzi-Puttini, L. Boccassini and I. Caruso. 1993. A double-blind crossover study of two cyclobenzaprine regimens in primary fibromyalgia syndrome. *J Int Med Res* 21(2):74–80.

Sarnoch, H., F. Adler and O. B. Scholz. 1997. Relevance of muscular sensitivity, muscular activity, and cognitive variables for pain reduction associated with EMG biofeedback in fibromyalgia. *Percept Motor Skills* 84(3 Pt 1):1043–1050.

Schafer, K. M. 1997. Health patterns of women with fibromyalgia. *J Adv Nurs* 26(3):565–571.

———. 1995. Struggling to maintain balance: a study of women living with fibromyalgia. *J Advance Nurs* 21:95–102.

Schmelz, M., R. Schmidt, A. Bickel, H. O. Handwerker and H. E. Torebjork. 1997. Specific C-receptors for itch in human skin. *J Neurosci* 17(20):8003–8008.

Schneider, M. J. 1990. Snapping hip syndrome in a marathon runner: treatment by manual trigger point therapy—a case study. *Chir Sports Med* 4(2):54–58.

Schochat, T., P. Croft and H. Raspe. 1994. The epidemiology of fibromyalgia. Workshop of the Standing Committee on European League Against Rheumatism. (EULAR). Held at Bad Sackingen, Germany. *Brit J Rheum* 33(8):783–786.

Schwarcz, R. 1993. Metabolism and function of brain kynurenines. *Biochem Soc Trans* 21(1):77–82.

Schwarcz, R. and F. Du 1991. Quinolinic acid and kynurenic acid in the mammalian brain. *Adv Exp Med Biol* 284:185–199.

Scicchitano, J., B. Rounsefell and I. Pilowsky. 1996. Baseline correlates of the response to the treatment of chronic localized myofascial pain syndrome by injection of local anesthetic. *J Psychosom Res* 40(1):75–85.

Scudds, R. A., M. Landry, T. Burmingham, J. Buchan and K. Griffin. 1995. The frequency of referred signs from muscle pressure in normal healthy subjects. *J Musculoskel Pain* 3(Suppl 1):99 (Abstract).

Scudds, R. A., L. C. Traschel, B. J. Luckhurst and J. S. Percy. 1989. A comparative study of pain, sleep quality and pain responsiveness in fibrositis and myofascial pain syndrome. *J Rheumatol* 16(Suppl 19):120–126.

Second World Congress on Myofascial Pain and Fibromyalgia August 17–20, 1992. Consensus Document on Fibromyalgia: The Copenhagen Declaration. 1992. *Lancet*, vol. 340, Sept. 12, 1992, and incorporated into the World Health Organization's 10th revision of the International Statistical

Classification of Diseases and Related Problems, ICD 10, Jan. 1, 1993. *J Musculoskel Pain* 1(3–4), 1993:295–312.

Seers, K. 1996. The patients' experiences of their chronic non-malignant pain. *J Adv Nurs* 24(6):1160–1168.

Shaver, J. L., M. Lentz, C. A. Landis, M. M. Heitkamper, D. S. Buchwald and N. F. Woods. 1997. Sleep, psychological distress, and stress arousal in women with fibromyalgia. *Res Nurs Health* 20(3): 247–257.

Shealy, N. 1995. A review of dehydroepiandrosterone (DHEA). *Integrat Physiol Behav Sci* 30(4):308–313.

Sherry, D. D. 1997. Musculoskeletal pain in children. *Curr Opin Rheumatol* 9(5):465–470.

Shi, D., O. Nikodijevic, K. A. Jacobson and J. W. Daly. 1994. Effects of chronic caffeine on adenosine, dopamine and acetylcholine systems in mice. *Arch Int Pharmacodyn Ther* 328(3):261–287.

———. 1993. Chronic caffeine alters the density of adenosine, adrenergic, cholinergic, GABA and serotonin receptors and calcium channels in the mouse brain. *Cell Mol Neurobiol* 13(3):247–261.

Sietsema, K. E., D. M. Cooper and X. Caro. 1993. Oxygen uptake during exercise in patients with primary fibromyalgia syndrome. *J Rheumatol* (5):860–865.

Silverman, S. L. and J. H. Mason. 1992. Measuring the functional impact of fibromyalgia. *J Musculoskel Med* 9(7):15–24.

Simms, R. W., L. Cahill and M. Prashker. 1995. The direct costs of fibromyalgia treatment: comparison with rheumatoid arthritis and osteoarthritis. *J Musculoskel Pain* 3(2):127–132.

Simms, R. W. 1994. Controlled trials of therapy in fibromyalgia syndrome. *Ballieres Clin Rheumatol* 8(4):917–934.

Simons, D. G. 1996. Clinical and etiological update of myofascial pain from trigger points. *J Musculoskel Pain* 4(1/2):97–125.

———. 1995. Myofascial pain syndrome: One term but two concepts; a new understanding. *J Musculoskel Pain* 3(1):7–14.

———. 1993. Referred phenomena of myofascial trigger points. Chap 28 in *New Trends in Referred Pain and Hyperalgesia*. Eds. L. Vecchiet, D. Albe-Fessard, U. Lindblom and M. A. Giamberardino. 341–357. No. 27 in the series Pain Research and Clinical Management. Amsterdam: Elsevier Science Publishers.

———. 1990. Familial fibromyalgia and/or myofascial pain syndrome? *Arch Phys Med Rehab* 71(3):258–259.

Simons, D. G., C-Z Hong and L. S. Simons. 1995a. Nature of myofascial trigger points active loci. *J Musculoskel Pain* 3(Suppl 1):62 (Abstract).

———. 1995b. Prevalence of spontaneous electrical activity at trigger spots and control sites in rabbit muscle. *J Musculoskel Pain* 3(1):35–49.

———. 1995c. Spike activity in trigger points. *J Musculoskel Pain* 3(Suppl 1):125 (Abstract).

———. 1994. Understanding myofascial pain syndromes. *J Musculoskel Pain* 2(l):143–146.

Simons, D. G. and Hong C. Z. 1994. Reply to Dr. Quintner. *J Musculoskel Pain* 2(2):137–140.

Skootsky, S. A., B. Jaeger and R. K. Oye. 1989. Prevalence of myofascial pain in general internal medicine practice. *West J Med* 151(2):157–160.

Sletvold H., T. C. Stiles and N. I. Landro. 1995. Information processing in primary fibromyalgia, major depression, and healthy controls. *J Rheumatol* 22:137–142.

Smiley, W. M., Jr., J. R. Cram, M. S. Margoles, T. J. Romano and J. Stiller. 1992. Innovations in soft-tissue jurispridence. *Trial Diplomacy J* 15:199–208.

Smythe, H. 1992. Links between fibromyalgia and myofascial pain syndromes. *J Rheumatol* 19(6): 842–843.

Soderberg, S., B. Lundman and A. Norberg. 1997. Living with fibromyalgia: sense of coherence, perception of well-being, and stress in daily life. *Res Nurs Health* 20(6):495–503.

Spath, M., B. Obermair-Kusser, P. Fischer and D. Pongratz. 1995. Are point mutations or deletions of mitochondrial DNA of any significance for fibromyalgia? *J Musculoskel Pain* 3(Suppl 1):116 (Abstract).

Spiegelman, I. and E. Puil. 1991. Substance P actions on sensory neurons. *Ann NY Acad Sci* 632: 220–228.

Sprott, H., H. Kluge, S. Franke and G. Hein. 1995. Altered serotonin-levels in patients with fibromyalgia. *J Musculoskel Pain* 3(Suppl 1):64 (Abstract).

Stacy, B. R. 1996. Effective management of chronic pain. The analgesic dilemma. *Postgrad Med* 100(3): 281–284.

Starlanyl, D. J. 1997. Fibromyalgia and myofascial pain syndrome: A special challenge. *Clin Bull Myofas Ther* 2(2/3):75–89.

———. 1995. Comment on Granges and Littlejohn's prevalence of myofascial pain syndrome in fibromyalgia and regional pain syndrome: A comparative study. *J Musculoskel Pain* 3(1):129–132.

———. 1994. Comment on article by Hong, Chen, Pon and Yu. Intermediate effects of various physical medicine modalities on pain threshold of an active myofascial trigger point. *J Musculoskel Pain* 2(2):141–142.

Stedman's Medical Dictionary, 25th Edition. 1990. Baltimore, MD: Williams & Wilkins.

Stone, T. W. 1993. Neuropharmacology of quinolinic and kynurenic acids. *Pharm Rev* 45(3):309–379.

Stone, T. W. and J. H. Connick. 1991. Effects of quinolinic acid and kynurenic acid on central neurons. *Adv Exp Med Bio* 294:329–336.

Stoner, B. P. and R. Corey. 1992. Chronic fatigue syndrome: a practical approach. *N Carol Med J* 53(6):267–270.

Stormorken, H. and E. Brosstad. 1992. Fibromyalgia: family clustering and sensory urgency with early onset indicate genetic predisposition and thus a true disease. *Scand J Rheumatol* 21(4):207.

Stratz, T., T. Schochat, L. Farber, C. Schweiger and W. Muller. 1995. Are there subgroups in fibromyalgia? *J Musculoskel Pain* 3(Suppl 1):15 (Abstract).

Stratz, T., T. Schochat, P. Hrycaj, C. Schweiger, P. Mennet, L. Fabber, P. Mennet and W. Muller. 1995. The blockade of 5–HT3 receptors in fibromyalga. A new therapy concept? *J Musculoskel Pain* 3(Suppl 1):64 (Abstract).

Striffler, J. S., J. S. Law, M. M. Polansky, S. J. Bhathena and R. A. Anderson. 1995. Chromium improves insulin response to glucose in rats. *Metabolism* 44(10):1314–1320.

Strobel, E. S., M. Krapf, M. Suckfull, W. Bruckle, W. Fleckenstein and W. Muller. Tissue oxygen measurement and 31P magnetic resonance spectroscopy in patients with muscle tension and fibromyalgia. *Rheumatol Int* 16(5):175–180.

Sturzenegger, M., B. P. Radanov and G. Di Stefano. 1995. The effect of accidental mechanisms and initial findings on the long-term course of whiplash injury. *J Neurol* 242(7):443–449.

Sturzenegger, M., G. Di Stefano, B. P. Radanov and A. Schnidrig. 1994. Presenting symptoms and signs after whiplash injury: the influence of accident mechanisms. *Neurology* 44(4):688–693.

Sucher, B. M. 1993. Myofascial release of carpal tunnel syndrome. *J Am Osteopath Assoc* 93(1):92–94.

Swedo, S. E., A. J. Allen, C. A. Glod, C. H. Clark, M. H. Teicher, D. Richter, C. Hoffman, S. D. Hamburger, S. Dow, C. Brown and N. E. Rosenthal. 1997. A controlled trial of light therapy for the treatment of pediatric seasonal affective disorder. *J Am Acad Child Adolesc Psychiatry* 36(6): 816–821.

Tanis, B. C., G. J. Westendorp and H. M. Smelt. 1996. Effect of thyroid substitution on hypercholesterolaemia in patients with subclinical hypothyroidism: a reanalysis of intervention studies. *Clin Endocrinol (Oxf)* 44(6):643–649.

Tavares, V. and J. Branco. 1995. Relation of sleep-related complaints with tender points and pain intensity in fibromyalgia syndrome (FMS). *J Musculoskel Pain* 3(Suppl 1):138 (Abstract).

Taylor, M. I., D. R. Trotter and M. E. Csuka. 1995. The prevalence of sexual abuse in women with fibromyalgia. *Arth Rheum* 38(2):229–234.

Thompson, J. M. 1990. Tension myalgia as a diagnosis at the Mayo Clinic and its relationship to fibrositis, fibromyalgia and myofascial pain syndrome. *Mayo Clin Proc* 65(9):1237–1248.

Tishler, M., Y. Barak, D. Paran and M. Yaron. 1997. Sleep disturbances, fibromyalgia and primary Sjogren's syndrome. *Clin Exp Rheumatol* 15(1):71–74.

Triano, J. J., M. McGregor and D. R. Skogsbergh. 1997. Use of chiropractic manipulation in lumbar rehabilitation. *J Rehabil Res Dev* 34(4):394–404.

Trojan, D. A and N. R. Cashman. 1995. Fibromyalgia is common in a postpolio clinic. *Arch Neuro* 52(6):620–624.

Tschopp, K. P. and C. Gysin. 1996. Local injection therapy in 107 patients with myofascial pain syndrome of the head and neck. *ORL J Otorhinolaryngol Relat Spec* 58(6):306–310.

Turk, D. C., A. Okifuji, T. W. Starz and J. D. Sinclair. 1996. Effects of type of symptom onset on psychological distress and disability in fibromyalgia syndrome patients. *Pain* 68(2–3):423–430.

Vaeroy, H., T. Sakuruda, O. Forre, E. Kass and L. Terenius. 1989. Modulation of pain in fibromyalgia (fibrositis syndrome): cerebrospinal fluid (CSF) investigation of pain-related neuropeptides with special references to calcitonin gene related peptide (CGRP). *J Rheumatol* Supp 19:94–97.

Vallbona, C., C. F. Hazelwood and G. Jurida. 1997. Response of pain to static magnetic fields in postpolio patients: a double-blind pilot study. *Arch Phys Med Rehabil* 78(11):1200–1203.

van Denderen, J. C., J. W. Boersma, P. Zeinstra, A. P. Hollander and B. R. van Neerbos. 1992. Physiological effects of exhaustive physical exercise in primary fibromyalgia syndrome (PFS): Is PFS a disorder of neuroendocrine reactivity? *Scand J Rheumatol* 21(1):35–37.

Van Fossen, D. and C. Gordon. 1989. Prevalence of mitral valve prolapse in primary fibromyalgia. *Arch Phys Med Rehab* 70(1):541–543.

van Why, R. 1997. *Fibromyalgia Syndrome and Manual Therapy: Issues and Opportunities*. Richard van Why. 123 East Eighth Street #212, Frederick, MD 21701.

Veale, D., G. Kavanaugh, J. F. Fielding and O. Fitzgerald. 1991. Primary fibromyalgia and the irritible bowel syndrome: different expressions of a common pathogenic process. *Brit J Rheumatol* 30(3): 220–222.

Verstappen, F. T. J., H. M. S. van Santen-Hoeuftt, P. H. Bolwijn, S. Van der Linden and H. Kuiper. 1997. Effects of a group activity program for fibromyalgia patients on physical fitness and well-being. *J Musculoskel Pain* 5(4):17–28.

Vitali, C., A. Ravoni, B. Rossi, E. Bibolotti, C. Giannini, L. Puzzuoli, R. Cacialli and G. Pasero. 1989. Evidence of neuromuscular hyperexcitability features in patients with primary fibromyalgia. *Clin Exp Rheumatol* 7(4):385–390.

Vitanen, J.V., H. Kautiainen and H. Isomaki. 1993. Pain intensity in patients with fibromyalgia and rheumatoid arthritis. *Scand J Rheumatol* 22(3):131–135.

Wadsworth, R., S. Kennedy, A. Bradlow, D. Barlow and J. David 1995. Gynaecological symptoms in fibromyalgia. *Brit J Rheumatol* 34(9):888–889.

Wagner, M. L., A. S. Walters, R. G. Coleman, W. A. Hening, K. Grasing and S. Choroverty. 1996. Randomized, double-blind, placebo-controlled study of clonidine in restless legs syndrome. *Sleep* 19(1):52–58.

Waksman, B. H. 1990. Psychoimmunology. *R I Med* 73(11):555–559.

Walker, E. A., W. J. Keegan, G. Gardner and M. Sullivan. 1997. Predictors of physician frustration in the care of patients with rheumatological complaints. *Gen Hosp Psychiatry* 19(5):315–323.

Wallace, D. J. 1997. The fibromyalgia syndrome. *Ann Med* 29(1):9–12.

Walters, A. S. 1995. Toward a better definition of the restless legs syndrome. The International Restless Legs Syndrome Study Group. *Mov Disord* 10(5):634–642.

Warner, E., al-N. Keshavjee, N. R. Shupak and A. Bellini. 1997. Rheumatic symptoms following adjuvant therapy for breast cancer. *Am J Clin Oncol* 20(3):322–326.

Wasada, T. 1996. Lack of C-peptide suppression by hyperinsulinemia in subjects with symptoms suggesting reactive hypoglycemia. *Endocr J* 43(6)639–644.

Watson, C. P. 1994. Topical capsaicin as an adjuvant analgesic. *J Pain Symptom Manage* 9(7):425–533.

Waxman, J. and S. M. Zatckis. 1986. Fibromyalgia and menopause. Examination of the relationship. *Postgrad Med* 80(4):165–167, 170–171.

Waylonis, G. W., P. G. Roman and C. Gordon. 1994. A profile of fibromyalgia in occupational environments. *Am J Phys Med Rehab* 73(2):112–115.

Waylonis, G. W. and R. H. Perkins. 1994. Post-Traumatic fibromyalgia. A long-term follow-up. *Am J Phys Med Rehab* 73(6):403–412.

Weight, F. F. , L. G. Aguayo, G. White, D. M. Lovinger and R. W. Peoples. GABA- and glutamate-gated ion channel as molecular sites of alcohol and anesthetic action. *Adv Biochem Psychopharmacol* 47:335–347.

Welin, M., B. Bragee, F. Nyberg and M. Kristiansson. 1995. Elevated substance P levels are contrasted by a decrease in met-enkephalin-arg-phe levels in CSF from fibromyalgia patients. *J Musculoskel Pain* 3(Suppl 1):4 (Abstract).

Welin, M., M. L. Lowenertz and B. Bragee. 1995. Is the pain in fibromyalgia NMDA-receptor mediated? *J Musculoskel Pain* 3(Suppl 1):8 (Abstract).

Westgaard, R. H., C. Jensen, D. Bansevicius and O. Vasselein. 1995. Differential surface EMG responses of the trapezius in fibromyalgia or myofascial pain. *J Musculoskel Pain* 3(Suppl 1):49 (Abstract).

Weverman, I. 1997. A functional approach to the treatment of fibromyalgia in a physical therapy and stress management setting. *J Musculoskel Pain* 3(Suppl 1):31 (Abstract).

White, K. P., M. Harth and R. W. Teasell. 1995. Work disability evaluation and the fibromyalgia syndrome. *Sem Arth Rheum* 24(6):371–381.

Wigers, S. H., T. C. Stiles and P. A. Bogel. 1996. Effects of aerobic exercise versus stress management treatment in fibromyalgia: A 4.5 year prospective study. *Scand J Rheum* 25:77–86.

Wilke, W. S. 1996. Fibromyalgia: Recognizing and addressing the multiple interrelated factors. *Postgrad Med* 110(1):153–156, 159, 163–166.

Wilson, P. R. 1994. Myofascial pain, fibromyalgia and chronic fatigue. *Clin J Pain* 10(3):169–170.

Wiseman, S. A., J. T. Powell, S. E. Humphries and M. Press. 1993. The magnitude of the hypercholesterolemia of hypothyroidism is associated with variation in the low density lipoprotein receptor gene. *J Clin Endocrinol Metab* 77(1):108–112.

Wolfe, F. 1996. Vancouver Fibromyalgia Consensus Group: the fibromyalgia syndrome: a consensus report on fibromyalgia and disability. *J Rheumatol* 23:534–539

———. 1993. Disability and the dimensions of distress fibromyalgia. *J Musculoskel Pain* 1(2):65–67.

Wolfe, F., J. Anderson, D. Harkness, R. M. Bennett, X. J. Caro, D. L. Goldenberg, I. J. Russell and M. B. Yunus. 1997. Health status and disease severity in fibromyalgia: results of a six-center longitudinal study. *Arthritis Rheum* 40(9):1571–1579.

Wolfe, F., I. J. Russell, G. Vipraio, K. Ross and J. Anderson. 1997. Serotonin levels, pain threshold, and fibromyalgia symptoms in the general population. *J Rheumatol* 24(3):555–559.

Wolfe, F., R. Aarflot, D. Bruusgaard, K. G. Henriksson, G. Littlejohn, H. Moldofsky, H. Raspe and H. Vaeroy. 1995. Fibromyalgia and disability. Report of the Moss International Working Group on medico-legal aspects of chronic widespread musculoskeletal pain complaints and fibromyalgia. *Scand J Rheumatol* 24(2):112–118.

Wolfe, F., J. Anderson, D. Harkness, D. J. Hawley, R. M. Bennett, X. Caro, D. Goldenberg, I. J. Russell and M. B. Yunus. 1995. The work and disability status of persons with fibromyalgia. *J Musculoskel Pain* 3(Suppl 1):155 (Abstract).

Wolfe, F., D. G. Simons, J. Fricton, R. M. Bennett, D. I. Goldenberg, R. Gerwin, D. Hathaway, G. A. McCain, I. J. Russell, H. O. Sanders, et al. 1992. The fibromyalgia and myofascial pain syndromes: a preliminary study of tender points and trigger points in persons with fibromyalgia, myofascial pain syndrome and no disease. *J Rheumatol* 19(6):944–951.

Wolfe, F. and M. A. Cathey. 1990. Assessment of functional ability in patients with fibromyalgia. *Arch Intern Med* 150(2):460.

Wortman, R. I. 1994. Searching for the cause of fibromyalgia syndrome. Is there a defect in energy metabolism? *Arth Rheum* 37(6):790–793.

Wreje, U. and B. Brorsson. 1995. A multicenter randomized controlled trial of injections of sterile water and saline for chronic myofascial pain syndromes. *Pain* 61(3):441–444.

Yaron, I., D. Buskila, I. Sharazi, L. Neumann, O. Elkayam, D. Paran and M. Yaron. 1997. Elevated levels of hyaluronic acid in the sera of women with fibromyalgia. *J Rheumatol* 24(11):2221–2224.

Yellin, J. 1997. Why is substance P high in fibromyalgia? *Clin Bull Myofas Ther* 2(2/3):23–27.

Yue, S. K. 1995. Initial experience in the use of botulinum toxin A for the treatment of myofascial related muscle dysfunctions. *J Musculoskel Pain* 3(Suppl 1):22 (Abstract).

Yunus, M. B. and J. C. Aldag. 1996. Restless legs syndrome and leg cramps in fibromyalgia syndrome: a controlled study. *Br Med J* 312:1339.

Yunus, M. B. 1994. Fibromyalgia syndrome: clinical features and spectrum. *J Musculoskel Pain* 2(3):5–21.

Yunus, M. B., F. X. Hussey and J. C. Aldag. 1993. Antinuclear antibodies and connective disease features in fibromyalgia syndrome: A controlled study. *J Rheumatol* 20(9):1557–1560.

Ziegler, D. K. 1997. Opioids in headache treatment. Is there a role? *Neurol Clin* 15(1):199–207.

Ziem, G. and J. McTamney. 1997. Profile of patients with chemical injury and sensitivity. *Environ Health Perspect* 105(Suppl 2):417–436.

Zimmermann, M. 1991. Pathophysiological mechanisms of fibromyalgia. *Clin J Pain* 7(Suppl 1):S8–Sl5.

Zweben, J. E. and J. L Sorensen. 1988. Misunderstandings about methadone. *J Psychoactive Drugs* 20(3):275–281.

Advocate's Reading List

Alberti, Robert E. and Michael L. Emmons. 1995. *Your Perfect Right: A Guide to Assertive Living.* 7th ed. San Luis Obispo, CA: Impact Publishers.

American Self-Help Clearinghouse. 1998. *The Self-Help Sourcebook: Your Guide to Community and Online Support Groups.* Denville, NJ 07834-2995: Northwest Covenant Medical Center.

Backstrom, Gayle. 1995 *When Muscle Pain Won't Go Away.* 2212 Ft. Worth Drive, Denton, TX 76205.

Beisser, Arnold R. 1989. *Flying Without Wings: Personal Reflections on Being Disabled.* NY: Doubleday.

Bolles, Richard N. 1991. *Job-Hunting Tips for the So-Called Handicapped or People Who Have Disabilities.* Berkeley, CA: Ten Speed Press.

Brassell, W. R. 1994. *Belonging: A Guide to Overcoming Loneliness.* Oakland, CA: New Harbinger Publications.

Butler, Sharon J. 1996. *Conquering Carpal Tunnel Syndrome and Other Repetitive Strain Injuries.* Oakland, CA: New Harbinger Publications.

Catalano, Ellen M. and Kimeron N. Hardin. 1996. *The Chronic Pain Control Workbook.* Oakland, CA: New Harbinger Publications.

Catalano, Ellen M. 1990. *Getting to Sleep.* Oakland, CA: New Harbinger Publications.

Cohen, Don. 1995. *An Introduction to Craniosacral Therapy: Anatomy, Function and Treatment.* Berkeley, CA: North Atlantic Press.

Cohen, Ken 1997. *The Way of Qigong: The Art and Science of Chinese Energy Healing.* NY: Ballentine Books.

Copeland, Mary Ellen. 1994. *Living Without Depression and Manic Depression.* Oakland, CA: New Harbinger Publications.

———. 1992. *The Depression Workbook: A Guide to Living with Depression and Manic Depression.* Oakland, CA: New Harbinger Publications.

———. 1997. *Wellness Recovery Action Plan.* Peach Press. P.O. Box 6237, Battleboro, VT 05302.

Davis, Martha, Elizabeth Robins Eshelman and Matthew McKay. 1995. *The Relaxation & Stress Reduction Workbook.* 4th ed. Oakland, CA: New Harbinger Publications.

Donoghue, Paul J. and Mary E. Siegel. 1992. *Sick and Tired of Feeling Sick and Tired: Living with Chronic Invisible Illness.* NY: Norton.

Freedman, Jacqueline and Susan Gersten. 1987. *Travelling . . . Like Everybody Else: A Practical Guide for Disabled Travelers.* 306 W. 38 Street, New York, NY 10018: Adama Books.

Fibromyalgia Network Newsletter. P. O. B. 31750, Tucson, AZ 85751-1750. (800) 853-2929. Editor Kristin Thorson.

Fibromyalgia Syndrome and Chronic Fatigue Syndrome in Young People, and *Getting the Most Out of Your Medicines* from the Fibromyalgia Network. P. O. Box 31750, Tucson, AZ 85751.

Fransen, Jenny and I. Jon Russell. 1996. *The Fibromyalgia Helpbook: Practical Guide to Living with Fibromyalgia.* Saint Paul, MN: Smith House.

Kahn, Michael. 1995. *The Tao of Conversation.* Oakland, CA: New Harbinger Publications.

Kane, Jeff. 1991. *Be Sick Well.* Oakland, CA: New Harbinger Publications.

LeMaistre, JoAnn. 1993. *Beyond Rage: Mastering Unavoidable Health Changes.* Oak Park, IL: Alpine Guild.

Marcus, Norman J. and Jean S. Arbeiter 1995. *Freedom from Pain.* NY: Simon and Schuster.

McKay, Matthew and Patrick Fanning. 1997. *The Daily Relaxer.* Oakland, CA: New Harbinger Publications.

McKay Matthew, Peter D. Rogers and Judith McKay. 1989. *When Anger Hurts.* Oakland, CA: New Harbinger Publications.

McKay Matthew, Martha Davis and Patrick Fanning. 1997. *Thoughts and Feelings.* Oakland, CA: New Harbinger Publications.

O'Hara, Valerie. *Wellness at Work.* 1995. Oakland, CA: New Harbinger Publications.

Pelligrino, Mark J. 1993. *Fibromyalgia: Managing the Pain.* 3620 N. High St., Columbus, OH 43214: Anadem Publishing.

Pitzele, Sefra K. 1985. *We Are Not Alone: Learning to Live with Chronic Illness.* NY: Workman Publishing.

Potter, J. W. 1995. "Swimming upstream." *Fibromyalgia Network Newsletter* (April).

———. 1994. "Filing for Social Security Disability." *Fibromyalgia Network Newsletter* (July).

Potter-Efron, Ron and Pat Potter-Efron. *Letting Go of Anger.* 1995. Oakland, CA: New Harbinger Publications.

Saathoff, Mary Anne. *The Fibromyalgia Syndrome.* Central Ohio FMS Assn, P.O. Box 21988, Columbus, OH 43221.

Scott, Gini Graham. *Resolving Conflict.* 1990. Oakland, CA: New Harbinger Publications.

Sears, Barry. 1997. *Mastering the Zone.* NY: Regan Books HarperCollins.

———. 1997. *Zone Perfect Meals: 150 Fast and Simple Healthy Recipes.* NY: HarperCollins.

Solomon, Muriel. 1990. *Working with Difficult People.* Engelwood Cliffs, NJ: Prentice Hall.

Stack, Michelle. 1994. *Handling Insurance Claims.* Fibromyalgia Network Newsletter (April).

Starlanyl, D. J. 1997. *Chronic Myofascial Pain Syndrome: A Guide to the Trigger Points.* Two-hour video. Oakland, CA: New Harbinger Publications.

Starlanyl, D. J. and M. E. Copeland. 1996. *Fibromyalgia & Chronic Myofascial Pain Syndrome: A Survival Manual.* Oakland, CA: New Harbinger Publications.

Stolman, Marc D. 1994. *A Guide to Legal Rights for People with Disabilities.* NY: Demos Publications.

Strong, Maggie. 1988. *Mainstay: For the Well Spouse of the Chronically Ill.* Boston: Little, Brown and Co.

Teitelbaum, Jacob. 1996. *From Fatigued to Fantastic.* Garden City Park, NJ: Avery Press.

Whalen, Freda. 1996. *Hypoglycemia and Diabetes Wellness Guide.* Lake Charles, LA: Body Care Publications.

Williams, Mary. 1996. *Cool Cats, Calm Kids: Relaxation and Stress Management for Young People*. San Luis Obispo, CA: Impact Publishers Inc. (ages 7-12).

Williamson, Miryam E. 1996. *Fibromyalgia: A Comprehensive Approach*. NY: Walker and Co.

Zuercher-White, Elke. 1995. *An End to Panic*. Oakland, CA: New Harbinger Publications.

Further Reading

The following recommendations are for the adventurous who would like further insight. These publications may be easier to find through interlibrary loan requests.

Birkmayer, W. and P. Riederer. 1989. *Understanding the Neurotransmitters: Key to the Workings of the Brain*. Translated from the German by Karl Blau. New York: Springer-Verlag.

Braun, Stephen. 1996. *Buzz : The Science and Lore of Alcohol and Caffeine*. Oxford: Oxford University Press.

Hardie, D.G. 1991. *Biochemical Messengers: Hormones, Neurotransmitters and Growth Factors*. London: Chapman and Hall.

Juhan, Deane. 1987. *Job's Body*. Barrytown, NY: Station Hill Press.

Orlock, Carol. 1995. *Know Your Body Clock*. NY: Citadel Press.

Shea, Michael J. and Dale Schmidt. 1996. *The Myofascial Release Textbook*. Shea Educational Group, Inc. 13878 Oleander Avenue, Juno Beach, FL 33408-1626. Phone: (800) 717-7432; fax: (561) 625-3775.

Thayer, R. E. 1996. *Mood: The Origin of Everyday Moods*. Oxford: Oxford University Press.

Travell, Janet G. 1968. *Office Hours Day and Night*. NY: World Publishing Co.

van Why, Richard 1994. *Fibromyalgia Syndrome and Massage Therapy: Issues and Opportunities*. Richard R. van Why, 123 East 8th Street, Frederick, NM 21701.

Titles from the Society of Automotive Engineers

The studies done by the Society of Automotive Engineers are among the best-kept secrets in the world. Patients, doctors, and lawyers should know that they exist and know how to access them. Insurance lawyers frequently try to tie human accident injury claims to the amount of auto damage incurred, and these studies prove that method is false.

If your health has been worsened by an auto accident you, or your advocates, should check out the following website. I have listed some of the more interesting SAE papers that may be valuable resources for you, but there are many more available.

Important titles available from the Society of Automotive Engineers 400 E. Commonwealth Drive, Warrendale PA 15096-0001. Phone: (724) 766-4970; fax: (724) 776-0790; custsvc@sec org website

<http://www.sae.org/PRODSERV/TECHPAPE/individu.htm>

Papers are listed by SEC document number:

970277 *The Effect of Driver Age on Traffic Accidents*

970394 *Human Subject Responses to Repeated Low-Speed Impacts Using Utility Vehicles.*

970494 *Lack of Relationship Between Vehicle Damage and Occupant Injury*

973322 *Pelvic Injuries in Side Impact Collisions: A Field Accident Analysis and Dynamic Tests on Isolated Pelvic Bones*

973318 *Injury Risk Curves for Children and Adults in Frontal and Rear Collisions*

973329 *The Position and Movement of the Foot in Emergency Maneuvers and the Influence of Tension in the Achilles Tendon*

970123 *The Relationship Between Car Size and Occupant Injury in Traffic Accidents in Japan*

970120 *Vehicle and Occupant Response in Heavy-Truck-to-Car Low-Speed Rear Impacts*

973320 *Chestband Analysis of Human Tolerance to Side Impact*

973340 *Cervical Injury Mechanism Based on the Analysis of Human Cervical Vertebral Motion and Head-Neck-Torso Kinematics During Low-Speed Rear Impacts*

940532 *Human Occupant Response to Low-Speed Rear-End Impacts*

Videos

"Power Up" Your Body and Relax Your Mind with Qi gong and Taoist Meditation. 60 min. video. Deer Mountain T'ai Chi Health Academy P.O. Box 19835, Asheville, NC 28815. (Related videos available.)

Coming For Doctors

Simons, D. G. and L. S. Simons. Travell and Simons' *Myofascial Pain and Dysfunction: The Trigger Point Manual.* 1999. Vol. I, 2nd Ed. Baltimore MD: Williams & Wilkins.

Resources

This section lists a number of agencies and organizations that both you and your health care team will find helpful.

Agencies and Organizations

Acupressure Institute. 1533 Shattuck Avenue, Berkeley, CA 94709. Phone: (510) 854-1059.

Academy for Myofascial Trigger Point Therapy. 1512 East Carson Street, Pittsburgh, PA. Phone: (412) 281-2555 or (412)-481-2555.

American Academy of Environmental Medicine. P. O. Box 16106, Denver, CO 80216. Phone: (800) LET-HEAL.

American Association of Naturopathic Physicians. P. O. Box 20386, Seattle, WA 98102. Phone: (206) 328-8510.

American Chiropractic Association. 1701 Clarendon Blvd., Arlington, VA 22209. Phone: (703) 276-8800.

American Chronic Pain Association. P. O. Box 850, Rocklin, CA 95677-0850. Phone: (916) 632-0922: email ACPA@pacbell.net Penney Cowan.

American Massage Therapy Association. 802 Davis Street, Suite 100, Evanston, IL 60201-4444. Phone: (847) 864-0123.

American Occupational Therapy Association. 4720 Montgomery Lane or P.O. Box 31220 Bethesda, MD 20824-1220. Phone: (301) 652-2682.

American Osteopathic Association. 142 E. Ontario Street, Chicago, IL 60611. Phone: (800) 621-1773 or (312)4 280-5854.

American Physical Therapy Association. 1111 North Fairfax Street, Alexandria, VA 22314. Phone: (703) 684-2782.

Fibromyalgia Network. P. O. Box 31750, Tucson, AZ 85752-1750. Phone: (602) 290-5508. Owner/Publisher/Editor: Kristin Thorson. (They publish the *Fibromyalgia Network Newsletter*. Phone: (800) 853-2929.)

Hypoglycemia Association, Inc. Box 165, Ashton, MD 20861-0165. Phone: (202) 544-4044.

Internet listserv guaifenesin support group: listserv@MAELSTROM.STJOHNS.EDU Contact this email address with the command sub guai-support Jenni Cat (substituting your name).

Internet listserv FMS/MPS support group: listserv@MITVMA@MIT.EDU
Contact this email address with the command
subscribe Elliot Cat (substituting your name) FIBROM-L alone in the body of the letter.

National Association of Trigger Point Myotherapists. P.O. Box 68, Yarmouthport, MA 02675. Phone: (800) 750-7479.

National Center for Homeopathy, 801 N. Fairfax Street, Suite 306, Alexandria, VA 22314. Phone: (703) 548-7790.

National Center for Post-Traumatic Stress Disorder. V.A. Medical Center, 116D, White River Junction, VT 05001. Phone: (802) 296-5132.

National Chronic Pain Outreach Association, Inc. 7979 Old Georgetown Road, Suite 100, Bethesda, MD 20814-2429. Phone: (301) 652-4948.

National Clearinghouse on Women and Girls with Disabilities. Education Equity Concepts, Inc. 114 East 32nd Street, New York, NY 10016. Phone: (212) 725-1803.

National Family Caregivers Association. 10605 Concord Street, Suite 501, Kensington, MD 20895-2504. Phone: (800) 896-3650.

National Organization of Social Security Claims Representatives. Phone: (800) 431-2804.

National Self-Help Clearinghouse. 25 West 43rd Street, Room 620, New York, NY 10036. Phone: (212) 354-8525.

Office of Equal Employment Opportunity. Phone: (800) 669-3362. (Ask for a free booklet on the ADA.)

Pharmaceutical Research and Manufacturers of America. 1100 15th Street NW, Washington, D.C. 20005. Phone: (202) 835-3400. (They publish the *Directory of Pharmaceutical Indigent Assistance*.)

Social Security Administration. Phone: (800) 772-1213.

United States Equal Employment Opportunity Commission: Publication and Information Center. P. O. Box 12549, Cincinnati, OH 45212-0549. Phone: (800) 669-3362.

Alternative Resources

American Academy of Environmental Medicine. 10 East Randolph Street, New Hope, PA 18938. Phone: (215) 862-4544.

American Botanical Council. P.O. Box 201660, Austin TX 78720-1660. Phone: (512) 331-8868; fax: (512) 331-1924. The American Botanical Council is a nonprofit, tax-exempt research and education organization. (Their peer-reviewed scientific journal, *HerbalGram*, is not a newsletter for the casual reader. It is for readers with some degree of sophistication with herbal medicines.) They can be accessed at http://www.herbalgram.org/abcmission.html

Herbal Drugs and Phytopharmaceuticals: This is a handbook for practice on a scientific basis. Edited by Max Wichtl. Translated by Norman Grainger Bisset from the German. Published in 1994 by CRC Press, Boca Raton FL. $189 hardcover. This is the closest thing to a PDR of herbal remedies. It is very comprehensive. Ask your library to get it.

Great Smokies Diagnostic Laboratory. Great Smoky Mountain Lab. 18A Regent Park Boulevard, Asheville, NC 28806. Phone: (800) 522-4762; fax: (704) 252-9303; email cs@gsdl.com www.gsdl.com

The Great Smokies Diagnostic Laboratory is a laboratory that has the capabilities for specific testing when you are searching for perpetuating factors, or need documentation for Social Security or insurance purposes. They can test for parasitology, immunology, lactose intolerance, permeability (gut mucosal immunity) and fecal fat, candida antibodies, yeast culture, amino acid analysis, vitamin profile (requires special collection kit for serum), and elemental analysis for toxins. They also do DHEA-S, male and female hormone profiles, post-menopause profiles, detoxification profiles, adrenal stress profiles, and so forth.

Patient Products

The BackBall is an economical self-massage tool. It was designed by medical personnel, and is guaranteed to last a lifetime. It is handcrafted. Write to John Young, R.D. 2 Box 789, Bethel, VT 05032.

Decent Exposures. These are pull-on/step-in "sports" style bras, with no hardware. Write to P.O. Box 27206, Seattle, WA 98125 or call (800) 524-4949.

Devon Lake Enterprises, Inc. The Clawdia garden tool is fibro-friendly. Write to 635 Clarks Tract, Keswick VA 22947 or call (804) 293-6689.

HVGS 9000 is a personal galvanic electrical stimulator device for patient use. Contact David DeNatale, P.O. Box 97, West Pawlet, VT 05775 USA, (800) 923-0118. Rental trial available.

NMES (EMS 300) is a personal microstim device. Write to Commumed, 120 Kedron Ave., Holmes, PA 19043 or call (800) 848-5397. (Prescription required.)

Soothing Comfort, Inc. This company makes soft, microwavable, washable designer vests, comfort pads, neck wraps and warmers, mittens and "Idaho Pocket Potatoes," which may also be cooled in the freezer during summer or "FMS hot flashes." Write to 2517 Pioneer Ridge Drive, Post Falls, ID 83854 or call (888) 725-9600 or (208) 664-7931, or email morzewski@prodigy.net

(Note: The author has no connection with any of the above products or companies.)

Health Care Resources

The Gebauer Company offers a free packet of myofascial trigger point information that includes the monograph by David Simon, "Myofascial Pain Syndrome Due to Trigger Points." They also produce the Fluri-Ethyl Vapocoolant Spray for Spray and Stretch (for doctors). Write to The Gebauer Company, 9410 St. Catherine Street, Cleveland, OH 44104 or call (800) 321-9348 or (216) 271-5252.

Support

How to subscribe to the FIBROM-L Internet discussion group:

This support group is known as FIBROM-L. Anyone wishing to subscribe to the discussion group may do so by sending an e-mail message to

listserv@mitvma.mit.edu

with the following request as the body of the message:

sub FIBROM-L [your first and last name]

For example, if John Doe were a new subscriber to the Fibromyalgia Discussion Group, he would type this one-line command:

sub FIBROM-L John Doe

Warning: expect high message traffic.

Devin Starlanyl's Internet website is as follows:

http://www.sover.net/~devstar

Index

American Pain Society, 160
American Society of Addiction Medicine, 159; public policy statements from, 301–305
Americans with Disabilities Act (ADA), 216–219; definitions and requirements, 217–218; job discrimination and, 218–219, 286–287; legal rights and, 218
Anafranil, 280
Anderson, Craig, 98
anemia, 30
anesthesia, 150
anger, 201–202
angina, 106–107
ankle pain and weakness, 110
antagonists, 23
anticholinergic medications, 25
antihistamines, 24, 104
appeals process, 237–238
arthritis: as coexisting condition, 45–46; trigger points and, 12
Arthritis Foundation, 41, 170
assessment of trigger points, 57–58
asymmetry, 38–39, 118
ataxia, 108, 187
attachment trigger points, 13
August, Lynne, 30
auto accidents, 16, 206
autonomic nervous system (ANS), 22, 188
autonomic reactions, 87

B

Back Knobber, 170
back pain, 109–110
Balfour, William, 7
barometric pressure, 188, 189
Be Sick Well (Kane), 201
bed: finding the right components, 37; posture and movement in, 36
behaviors: as perpetuating factors, 37–38; in response to chronic pain, 55
"Belch button," 108, 119, 132
Belonging: A Guide to Overcoming Loneliness (Brassell), 249
Benedryl, 104, 134, 280, 289
biochemical perpetuating factors, 30
biological rhythms, 188
bite splints, 100
bladder problems: insomnia and, 152; trigger points and, 152
Blatman, Hal, 49, 171
body mechanics, 36; asymmetrical bodies and, 38–39; interconnectedness and, 188
bodywork, 85, 214
Brandis, Alan, 41
Brassell, William R., 249
breast cancer, 179

breast pain, 136
breathing: importance of, 172–173, 275; paradoxical, 34–35, 62, 107; relaxation and, 275; shortness of breath, 107, 131
bromelain, 173
bureaucracy: dealing with, 228–229; example of, 229
burning feet syndrome, 280

C

caffeine, 173, 282
calcium channels, 24
capitation, 223–225
capsaicin, 173
carbohydrates, 130–131; dietary percentage of, 33–34; effects of diets high in, 32–33; glycoproteins and, 23; insulin production and, 32–33; reactive hypoglycemia and, 30–32
cardiologists, 94–96; coexisting conditions and, 95; myofascial trigger points and, 94–95; neurotransmitter dysfunction and, 95
Carpal Tunnel Syndrome, 46, 150
CAT scan, 214
causalgia, 49
central nervous system (CNS), 54; GABA and, 26–27; multiple sclerosis and, 49; opioids and, 161; pain sensitivity and, 53, 55, 160
cervical pillows, 37, 187, 281
change: dealing with, 265; inevitability of, 287; in the weather, 188–189
checklists: for evaluating physicians, 76–77; for stressors in the workplace, 283–285
chemical sensitivities, 48, 104, 142
"chi" force, 185, 190
children: abuse and neglect of, 16; communicating with about FMS/MPS, 253–255; FMS and MPS in, 89, 289–290; parental illness and, 253
chiropractic manipulation, 168; chronic myofascial pain and, 98; trigger points and, 97
chiropractors, 97–99
chlorine sensitivity, 142
chocolate, 161, 174
cholinergic medications, 25
cholinergic receptors, 283
CHPs. *See* Community Health Plans
chromium picolinate, 31, 173, 176
Chronic Fatigue Immune Deficiency Syndrome (CFIDS), 46
"Chronic Myofascial Pain Syndrome: A Guide to the Trigger Points" (video), 82
chronic nonmalignant back pain (CNMBP), 160
chronic pain, 51–67; alternate tryptophan pathway and, 56; behaviors in response to, 55; deafferentation pain syndrome and, 55; definition of, 51–52; depression caused by, 91–92, 121, 122; diagnostic uncertainty and, 53; drug

215, 217; employment issues and, 217–219; Family and Medical Leave Act and, 219; functional difficulties list, 215–216; functional questionnaire, 311–316; Social Security benefits and, 235–238; Supplemental Security Income and, 238–239; Veterans Administration and, 220; workers' compensation benefits and, 228–230

Disability Determination Service, 235
disability insurance, 230–232
discrimination: by employers, 218–219, 286–287; by HMOs, 227
disrupted sleep, 9, 84, 121, 122, 125, 279–281; cost of, 280–281
dizziness, 11–12, 108, 186, 187
doctors. *See* physicians
documentation process: dealing with forms, 239–240; doctor's report for, 240–241; your report for, 241
dopamine, 15, 25–26
double vision, 117
dowager's hump, 62
dreams: noradrenaline and, 26; virtual, 281. *See also* sleep
driving, with FMS, 12, 117
Drug Enforcement Agency (DEA), 157, 158
drugs: addiction to, 54, 62–63, 159–160, 302–303; alcohol, 282; caffeine, 173, 282; dependence on, 62, 159–160, 302; tobacco, 184, 283; tolerance to, 302. *See also* medications
dry water massage therapy, 172
dynorphins, 27, 161
dysmenorrhea, 135
dyspnea, 95, 147

E

ear problems, 108, 115
ectopic heart rhythms, 106
educational resources, 71–72
elderly, 289
electrical stimulation, 97–98, 142, 167, 169; sample reference list on, 166–167
electromagnetic radiation (EMR), 189
electromagnetic sensitivity, 185, 188, 189–190
Electromagnetic Sensitivity Network, 188
electronic equipment problems, 190–191
Electronic Neuromuscular Stimulator (EMS), 98
emergency room visits, 106–112
emotions: expressing, 200–202; grief cycle and, 252–253
Employee Assistance Programs, 286
employment: COBRA and, 232; disability insurance and, 230–232; discrimination in, 218–219, 286; employee rights and, 250, 286; government benefits and, 236, 242–243; medical leave from, 219; retraining benefits and, 243;

workers' compensation claims and, 228–230. *See also* workplace
End to Panic, An (Zuercher–White), 77
endocrine glands, 23
endodontic therapy, 102
endorphins, 27, 63, 161
enkephalins, 27, 161
environmental factors: electromagnetic sensitivity, 185, 188, 189–190; pollution, 39, 168–169; weather changes, 188–189
epinephrine, 26, 288
Equal Employment Opportunities Commission (EEOC), 218
erectile dysfunction, 153
ERISA (Employee Retirement Income Securities Act), 232
ethics, medical, 199–200, 226
exercise: for eyes, 117; physical therapy and, 141–142; pregnancy and, 288; symptom relief through, 169; trigger points and, 58, 62, 90
exploding head syndrome, 280
expressing your feelings, 200–201
extensor hallucis brevis trigger points, 145
extensor longus trigger points, 145
extrinsic eye muscle trigger points, 65
eye doctors, 117–118
eye problems, 117–118
eyeglasses, 117
eyelid twitching, 122, 125

F

facial pain, 101–102
facial trigger points, 116, 117
failed surgical procedures, 151
fainting, 32
Fair Debt Collection Practices Act (1977), 207
Family and Medical Leave Act (FLMA), 219
family members: communicating with about FMS/MPS, 252–256; rights of, 249–251
fasiculations, 122, 125
fasting hypoglycemia, 30
fatigue, 46, 141
fats, dietary percentage of, 33–34
fear: of doctors, 197; of workplace discrimination, 286
feelings. *See* emotions
female urethral syndrome, 152
fibrofog, 14–17, 123, 126; accidents and, 16; alternate tryptophan pathway and, 56; causes of, 15–16; childhood neglect and, 16; flare and, 16–17; forgetfulness and, 15; physical therapy and, 140; reactive hypoglycemia and, 16; trigger points and, 16
Fibromyalgia & Chronic Myofascial Pain Syndrome: A Survival Guide (Starlanyl and Copeland), 3, 7, 58, 67, 71

More New Harbinger Self-Care Guides

FIBROMYAGLIA & CHRONIC MYOFASCIAL PAIN SYNDROME
A Survival Manual
This comprehensive patient guide, written by Dr. Starlanyl and coauthor Mary Ellen Copeland, shows you how to identify trigger points and helps you to cope with chronic pain, sleep problems, and the numbing effects of "fibro fog." Includes information on medications, tips for using bodywork and other treatments, and suggestions for getting help and support.   *Item FMS $19.95*

CHRONIC MYOFASCIAL PAIN SYNDROME
Guide to the Trigger Points
In this companion video, Dr. Starlanyl demonstrates the trigger points and their specific pain patterns, provides examples of self-care physical therapy techniques, and explains how to set up a treatment program. Running time: 118 minutes.   *Item 518 (VHS only) $49.95*

THE CHRONIC PAIN CONTROL WORKBOOK
Second Edition
A team of specialists in all areas of chronic pain management detail the treatment strategies for managing and recovering from specific chronic pain problems.   *Item PN2 $17.95*

THE HEADACHE AND NECK PAIN WORKBOOK
An Integrated Mind and Body Program
A step-by-step guide to managing the complex mind-body interaction underlying headaches and related neck pain.   *Item NECK $14.95*

THE DEPRESSION WORKBOOK
A Guide for Living with Depression
Mary Ellen Copeland shares insights and strategies for living with extreme mood swings. Interactive exercises teach essential coping skills, such as building a strong support system, bolstering self-esteem, fighting negative thoughts, and finding appropriate professional help.   *Item DEP $17.95*

PERIMENOPAUSE
Changes in Women's Health After 35
Beginning with subtle psychological changes in the mid-thirties and forties, perimenopause can encompass a bewildering array of symptoms. This self-care guide helps women cope with changes and assure health and vitality in the years ahead.   *Item PERI $13.95*

THOUGHTS & FEELINGS
Taking Control of Your Moods and Your Life
This workbook covers all of the most effective cognitive-behavioral techniques for treating problems ranging from depression and panic disorder to obsessional thinking and anger control.
Item TF2 $18.95

Call toll-free 1-800-748-6273 to order. Have your Visa or Mastercard number ready. Or send a check for the titles you want to New Harbinger Publications, 5674 Shattuck Avenue, Oakland, CA 94609. Include $3.80 for the first item and 75 for each additional item to cover shipping and handling. (California residents please include appropriate sales tax.) Allow four to six weeks for delivery.

Prices subject to change without notice.

Some Other New Harbinger Self-Help Titles

Dr. Carl Robinson's Basic Baby Care, $10.95
Better Boundries: Owning and Treasuring Your Life, $13.95
Goodbye Good Girl, $12.95
Being, Belonging, Doing, $10.95
Thoughts & Feelings, Second Edition, $18.95
Depression: How It Happens, How It's Healed, $14.95
Trust After Trauma, $13.95
The Chemotherapy & Radiation Survival Guide, Second Edition, $13.95
Heart Therapy, $13.95
Surviving Childhood Cancer, $12.95
The Headache & Neck Pain Workbook, $14.95
Perimenopause, $13.95
The Self-Forgiveness Handbook, $12.95
A Woman's Guide to Overcoming Sexual Fear and Pain, $14.95
Mind Over Malignancy, $12.95
Treating Panic Disorder and Agoraphobia, $44.95
Scarred Soul, $13.95
The Angry Heart, $13.95
Don't Take It Personally, $12.95
Becoming a Wise Parent For Your Grown Child, $12.95
Clear Your Past, Change Your Future, $12.95
Preparing for Surgery, $17.95
Coming Out Everyday, $13.95
Ten Things Every Parent Needs to Know, $12.95
The Power of Two, $12.95
It's Not OK Anymore, $13.95
The Daily Relaxer, $12.95
The Body Image Workbook, $17.95
Living with ADD, $17.95
Taking the Anxiety Out of Taking Tests, $12.95
The Taking Charge of Menopause Workbook, $17.95
Living with Angina, $12.95
Five Weeks to Healing Stress: The Wellness Option, $17.95
Choosing to Live: How to Defeat Suicide Through Cognitive Therapy, $12.95
Why Children Misbehave and What to Do About It, $14.95
When Anger Hurts Your Kids, $12.95
The Addiction Workbook, $17.95
The Mother's Survival Guide to Recovery, $12.95
The Chronic Pain Control Workbook, Second Edition, $17.95
Fibromyalgia & Chronic Myofascial Pain Syndrome, $19.95
Flying Without Fear, $12.95
Kid Cooperation: How to Stop Yelling, Nagging & Pleading and Get Kids to Cooperate, $12.95
The Stop Smoking Workbook: Your Guide to Healthy Quitting, $17.95
Conquering Carpal Tunnel Syndrome and Other Repetitive Strain Injuries, $17.95
Wellness at Work: Building Resilience for Job Stress, $17.95
An End to Panic: Breakthrough Techniques for Overcoming Panic Disorder, Second Edition, $17.95
Living Without Procrastination: How to Stop Postponing Your Life, $12.95
Goodbye Mother, Hello Woman: Reweaving the Daughter Mother Relationship, $14.95
Letting Go of Anger: The 10 Most Common Anger Styles and What to Do About Them, $12.95
Messages: The Communication Skills Workbook, Second Edition, $13.95
Coping With Chronic Fatigue Syndrome: Nine Things You Can Do, $12.95
The Anxiety & Phobia Workbook, Second Edition, $17.95
The Relaxation & Stress Reduction Workbook, Fourth Edition, $17.95
Living Without Depression & Manic Depression: A Workbook for Maintaining Mood Stability, $17.95
Coping With Schizophrenia: A Guide For Families, $13.95
Visualization for Change, Second Edition, $13.95
Postpartum Survival Guide, $13.95
Angry All the Time: An Emergency Guide to Anger Control, $12.95
Couple Skills: Making Your Relationship Work, $13.95
Self-Esteem, Second Edition, $13.95
I Can't Get Over It, A Handbook for Trauma Survivors, Second Edition, $15.95
Dying of Embarrassment: Help for Social Anxiety and Social Phobia, $12.95
The Depression Workbook: Living With Depression and Manic Depression, $17.95
Men & Grief: A Guide for Men Surviving the Death of a Loved One, $13.95
When the Bough Breaks: A Helping Guide for Parents of Sexually Abused Children, $11.95
When Once Is Not Enough: Help for Obsessive Compulsives, $13.95
The Three Minute Meditator, Third Edition, $12.95
Beyond Grief: A Guide for Recovering from the Death of a Loved One, $13.95
Hypnosis for Change: A Manual of Proven Techniques, Third Edition, $13.95
When Anger Hurts, $13.95

Call **toll free, 1-800-748-6273,** to order. Have your Visa or Mastercard number ready. Or send a check for the titles you want to New Harbinger Publications, Inc., 5674 Shattuck Ave., Oakland, CA 94609. Include $3.80 for the first book and 75¢ for each additional book, to cover shipping and handling. (California residents please include appropriate sales tax.) Allow two to five weeks for delivery.

Prices subject to change without notice.